Effects of Interferon on Cells, Viruses and the Immune System

Effects of Interferon on Cells, Viruses and the Immune System

Proceedings of a Meeting held at the
Gulbenkian Institute of Science, Oeiras, Portugal
on September 19 – September 21, 1973

Edited by

A. GERALDES

Laboratory of Cell Biology,
Gulbenkian Institute of Science
Oeiras, Portugal

1975

ACADEMIC PRESS

London   New York   San Francisco

A Subsidiary of Harcourt Brace Jovanovich, Publishers

ACADEMIC PRESS INC. (LONDON) LTD.
24/28 Oval Road,
London NW1 7DX

United States Edition published by
ACADEMIC PRESS INC.
111 Fifth Avenue
New York, New York 10003

Library of Congress Catalog Card Number: 75-589
ISBN: 0 12 280650 6

PRINTED IN GREAT BRITAIN BY
WHITSTABLE LITHO LTD., KENT

PREFACE

The great interest and novelty of the most recent research activity directed towards study of interferon prompted us to accept without hesitation the suggestion of Dr. C. Chany to organize a meeting on "Effects of Interferon on Cells, Viruses and the Immune System".

The intent of the program is well expressed in Dr. Chany's Introductory Remarks.

The great volume of material to be typed and illustrations to be handled, as well as some disturbance in the normal work of our Institute due to the recent events in Portugal, have slowed up the final typing of the manuscript. However, this does not diminish the interest and opportunity of these Proceedings.

Support for this meeting was given by the Gulbenkian Foundation and the Service Culturel de l'Ambassade de France in Portugal. I thank the members of the organizing committee, Dr. C. Chany, Dr. E. De Maeyer, Dr. I. Gresser, Dr. I. Kerr, and Dr. H. Pereira for their assistance.

I am especially pleased to acknowledge the assistance of Dr. C. Chany, Dr. E. De Maeyer, and Dr. J. De Maeyer-Guignard in proofreading and organizing the manuscript. I wish to thank Mrs. La Salette Costa for typing most of the final manuscript copy. I want to thank all the contributors and participants for their time and efforts expended in the preparation and presentation of their papers, which have decisively contributed to the great success of the meeting.

A. Geraldes

CONTENTS

I - CELL HYBRIDS AND UPTAKE OF INTERFERON

III - INTERFERON ACTION AT THE CELLULAR LEVEL; ANTAGONISTS

IV - INTERACTIONS WITH THE IMMUNE SYSTEM

VI - MECHANISM OF ACTION AT THE MOLECULAR LEVEL

PARTICIPANTS

Ankel, Helmut
    The Medical College of Wisconsin
    Milwaukee, Wisconsin 53233, USA
Baron, Samuel
    Department of Health, Education and Welfare
    Public Health Service, N.I.H.
    Bethesda, Maryland 20014, USA
Béládi, Ilona*
    Microbiology Institute, University Medical School
    Beloiannisz Ter 10, Szeged, Hungary
Berman, Brian
    139 East 35th Street Apt. 1 D
    New York, N.Y. 10016, USA
Besançon, F.
    INSERM, Hôpital St. Vincent de Paul
    74, avenue Denfert-Rochereau, Paris 14e, France
Boquet, P.
    INSERM, Hôpital St. Vincent de Paul
    74, avenue Denfert-Rochereau, Paris 14e, France
Bourgeade, Marie-Françoise
    Laboratoire de Virologie, Hôpital St. Vincent de Paul
    74, avenue Denfert-Rochereau, Paris 14e, France
Brouty-Boyé, Danièle
    Institut de Recherches Scientifiques sur le Cancer
    B.P. no. 8, 94800 Villejuif, France
Burke, D.C.
    Division of Biological Science
    School of Molecular and Biological Science, University

xiv   PARTICIPANTS

of Warwick

Coventry, Warwickshire CV47AL, England .

Came, Paul E.

Department of Microbiology, Schering Corporation

Bloomfield, New Jersey 07003, USA

Chany, Charles

INSERM, Hôpital St. Vincent de Paul

74, avenue Denfert-Rochereau, Paris 14e, France

Colby, Clarence

Microbiology Section, Life Sciences Building, U - 44

University of Connecticut

Storrs, Conn. 06268, USA

De Clercq, E.

Rega Institute for Medical Research

University of Leuven, Mindebroedersstraat 10

3000 Leuven, Belgium

De Maeyer, E.

Faculté des Sciences, Batiment 110

Orsay 91, France

De Maeyer-Guignard, J.

Faculté des Sciences, Batiment 110

Orsay 91, France

De Somer, P.

Rega Institute for Medical Research

University of Leuven, Mindebroedersstraat 10

3000 Leuven, Belgium

Dianzani, F.

Istituto di Microbiologia Della Via Santena, 9

Torino, Italy

Dubois, Marie-Françoise

Laboratoire de Virologie, Hôpital St. Vincent de Paul

74, avenue Denfert-Rochereau, Paris 14^{e}, France

Epstein, Lois
> University of California, School of Medicine
> Cancer Research Institute
> San Francisco, California 94122, USA

Esteban, Mariano
> National Institute for Medical Research
> Mill Hill, London NW7 1AA, England

Fauconnier, B.
> 80 Duleon - Bernard
> 35 Rennes, France

Fournier, F.
> INSERM, Hôpital St. Vincent de Paul
> 74, avenue Denfert-Rochereau, Paris 14^e, France

Friedman, R.M.
> Building 10 - 2N 116
> National Institutes of Health
> Bethesda, Maryland 20014, USA

Friedman-Kien, Alvin E.
> Department of Dermatology
> New York University, School of Medicine
> 550 First Avenue, New York, N.Y. 10016, USA

Galasso, George J.
> National Institute of Allergy and Infectious Diseases
> Building 31 - A, Room 7A - 06
> National Institutes of Health
> Bethesda, Maryland 20014, USA

Galliot, Brigitte
> Laboratoire de Virologie, Hôpital St. Vincent de Paul
> 74, avenue Denfert-Rochereau, Paris 14^e, France

Gresser, Ion*
> Institut de Recherches Scientifiques sur le Cancer
> 94 Villejuif, France

Grossberg, S.E.
    Department of Microbiology, Marquette School of Medicine
    561 North Fifteenth Street
    Milwaukee, Wisconsin 53233, USA
Huang, Kun-yen
    The George Washington University, Medical Center
    Department of Microbiology
    2300 Eye Street, N.W., Washington , D.C. 20037, USA
Kawade, Yoshimi*
    Institute for Virus Research, Kyoto University
    Yoshide-Machi, Kyoto, Japan
Kerr, Ian
    National Institute for Medical Research
    Mill Hill, London NW7, England
Léauté, Jean-Baptiste
    INSERM, Hôpital St. Vincent de Paul
    74, avenue Denfert-Rochereau, 75014 Paris, France
Lebon, Pierre
    INSERM, Hôpital St. Vincent de Paul
    74, avenue Denfert-Rochereau, 75014 Paris, France
Levy, Hilton
    National Institutes of Health
    Laboratory of Biology and Viruses
    Department of Health, Education and Welfare
    Bethesda, Maryland 20014, USA
Lindahl, Pernilla
    Institut de Recherches Scientifiques sur le Cancer
    94 Villejuif, France
Merigan, Thomas C.
    Stanford University Medical Center
    Stanford, California 94305, USA

McNeill, T.
    Department of Microbiology, University of Belfast
    Belfast, North Ireland
Mobraaten, Larry E.
    Fondation Curie - Institut du Radium
    Section de Biologie
    15, rue Georges Clemenceau, Batiment 110 - 111
    91 - Orsay, France
Morahan, Page S.
    Medical College of Virginia, Box 273
    Richmond, Virginia 23185, USA
Montagnier, Luc*
    Institut Pasteur
    25, rue du Docteur Roux, Paris 15^e, France
Mota, Miguel
    Estação Agronómica Nacional
    Oeiras, Portugal
Nagata, Ikuya
    Nagoya University, School of Medicine
    65, Tsuruma-Cho, Showa-Ku, Nagoya, Japan
Oxman, Michael
    Children's Hospital Medical Center
    300 Longwood Avenue, Boston, Massachusetts 02115, USA
Paucker, Kurt
    The Medical College of Pennsylvania
    Department of Microbiology
    3300 Henry Avenue, Philadelphia, P.A. 19129, USA
Pereira, Helio
    Animal Virus Research Institute
    Pilbright, Woking, Surrey, England

Pitha, Paula M.
        The Johns Hopkins University
        School of Medicine, Department of Medicine
        Baltimore, Maryland 21224, USA

Planterose, D.N.
        Beecham Research Laboratories
        Brockham Park, Betchworth, Surrey, England

Revel, Michel
        The Weizmann Institute of Science
        Rehovot, Israel

Rozee, K.R.
        Department of Microbiology, Faculty of Medicine
        Dalhousie University
        Halifax, Nova Scotia, Canada

Rita, Geo
        Università di Roma, Istituto di Virologia
        Viale di Porta Tiburtina 28, Roma, Italy

Stewart II, William E.
        Katholieke Universiteit de Leuven
        Minderbroedersstraat 10, Leuven 3000, Belgium

Stinebring, Warren R.
        Department of Medical Microbiology
        University of Vermont,
        105 Medical Sciences Building, Burlington
        Vermont 05401, USA

Tan, Y.H.
        Department of Biology, Kline Biological Tower
        Yale University
        New Haven, Conn. 06520, USA

Taylor-Papadimitriou, Joyce
        Cancer Institute, Theagenion Memorial
        Thessaloniki, Greece

Tovey, Michael
    Institut de Recherches Scientifiques sur le Cancer
    94 Villejuif, France
Vasconcelos-Costa, J.M.
    Gulbenkian Institute of Science
    Oeiras, Portugal
Vilček, Jan
    New York University Medical Center
    550 First Avenue
    New York, N.Y. 10016, USA
Wallen, W.C.*
    Department of Virology and Cell Biology
    Litton Bionetics, Inc.
    5510 Nicholson Lane, Kensington, Maryland 20795, USA

* Unable to participate

INTRODUCTORY REMARKS

It is now almost 20 years since the first communications describing interferon have been published. Great hopes were attached to these substances because of their inhibitory effects on the lytic and oncogenic functions of a great variety of viruses, without dramatic effects on the cell metabolism. Initial optimism rapidly declined as soon as the first difficulties appeared in the production and clinical application of interferon.

If results involving practical applications were few, international meetings in pleasant places were numerous, and there are few molecules in the organism which have procured so much pleasure to investigators interested in the field. I am sure that all of you agree that Oeiras is one of the highlights in this series of meetings, concerning the beauty of the place and the kindness of the reception.

As time progressed, much fundamental knowledge was gained in different aspects of interferon production, action, and, more recently, in regulation.

In the early sixties, workers engaged in interferon research clearly separated into two groups. This was provoked by Hilleman's calculations based on practical considerations, of which the end result was that no-one would ever be able to produce enough interferon to treat successfully a patient diseased with a virus. The difficulties are obviously related to the species specificity of interferon, to the small amount of interferon produced by the cells, possibly to its rapid degradation as a substance, and finally to the necessity of repeated inoculation of considerable amounts. It is obvious, however, that this type of calculation does not take into account our limited knowledge of interferon regulation and pharmacology.

    This observation triggered, however, a great number of in-
teresting investigations on interferon inducers with obvious
practical applications in mind. Among these inducers, poly I:C
rapidly became the most popular. Efforts to use inducers as practical therapeutic tools ran into obvious limitations. Firstly,
the regulatory mechanisms which exist in the producer and the
target cells could probably limit the maintenance of a prolonged antiviral state which is necessary for therapeutic results.
The second limitation is the toxicity of artificial polymers o-
ver a certain molecular size. Unfortunately, interferon production and toxicity are only separated by a relatively small safe-
ty margin.

    This conference will represent perhaps a new orientation
in interferon research. The relationship of interferon with cellular functions and with the immune system, and the study of
the regulatory mechanisms are new expanding fields.

    In spite of the fundamental aspects of this conference,
there is no doubt that everybody still hopes that information
gained from basic knowledge can, in one way or another, contrib-
ute to protect man and animal against the undesired consequences
of virus parasitism. The workers, however, are faced with the
problem of choosing to explore the field of inducers or to con-
centrate on interferon itself.

    This dilemma reminds me of the story of a rabbi in a Tal-
mudic School who asked his pupils to comment on these two Com-
mandments:

    Thou shalt not work on the Sabbath Day; and

    Thou shalt not covet thy neighbour's wife.

Then he found that somebody commented in the margin:

"I tried both; no comparison."

I wish to express my gratitude as well as that of my colleagues to the Gulbenkian Foundation and to the Service Culturel de l'Ambassade de France for their generous support and competent help.

C. Chany

I - CELL HYBRIDS AND UPTAKE OF INTERFERON

LINKAGE ANALYSIS OF ANIMAL CELL VIRUS INTERACTION BY SOMATIC CELL GENETICS:THE GENETICS OF HUMAN INTERFERON

Y. H. Tan

Department of Biology
Kline Biology Tower
Yale University
New Haven,Connecticut

The assignment of genes to specific loci is well established for microorganisms but only poorly substantiated in the more
complex mammalian system. For example, most of the known genetic
markers in the mammalian system have been limited to the X chromosome. It was only subsequent to the introduction of somatic
cell hybridization as a tool in gene mapping that a substantial
number of markers have been assigned to specific human autosomes
(1,2). In our present study we have applied the techniques of
somatic cell hybridization to the human interferon system. While
little is known of the genetics of the interferon system in mammalian cell, agents known to alter the primary structure of cellular DNA are also known to inhibit interferon synthesis suggesting that DNA sites contain the information for the interferon
peptides (3-8). However, it was not until recently that evidence
has been presented to support the theory that discrete genetic
sites control the production of interferon in a cell. De Maeyer
et al. (9) demonstrated that the induction of interferon in inbred mouse strains is controlled by a single codominant locus
IF-1 with two alleles IF-1^l and IF-1^h controlling low and high
production respectively, and that IF-1 is linked to the histocompatibility locus H-28. Cassingena et al.(10) utilizing mouse

monkey somatic cell hybrids provided evidence that a small subtelocentric monkey chromosome might be associated with the production of monkey interferon. Q-banding patterns identified monkey chromosome 22 as responsible for the production of monkey
interferon and perhaps monkey chromosome 29 with the expression
of the anti-viral state in monkey cells (11). Tan et al.(27)
using mouse human somatic cell hybrids showed that the human
form of indopheno-oxidase (IPO-A) and the anti-viral state (AVP)
induced in the hybrid cells by human interferon segregated concordantly in all the hybrid cells examined (12). Furthermore
both IPO-A and AVP segregated concordantly with human chromosome
21. Based on this observed association of IPO-A, AVP and chromosome 21 we postulated that the genes for IPO-A and AVP are linked to the small human G-21 chromosome. One of the questions
raised by this assignment was the biochemical nature of IPO-A
and AVP. We presumed AVP is a protein factor which initiates a
specific inhibition of viral replication but this does not eliminate the possibility that AVP is a receptor site for human interferon. IPO-A was recently shown by Beckman and by Brewer to
be a cytoplasmic form of superoxide dismutase (SOD_1) and its
presumed physiological function is to oxidise free oxygen radi-
cals (O_2-) found in aerobic organisms (13-14).

The genetics of anti-viral state in human cells

In our new series of hybrid cells (Table 1) 24 independently derived hybrid clones were selected and subjected to
treatment with human interferon and with Newcastle disease virus (NDV). Fig. 1 represents the results of this experiment.
Fifteen of the twenty-four clones were protected by human interferon but failed to produce human interferon in response to
NDV. Conversely two of the twenty-four clones tested were inducible for human interferon but were not protected by human

AVP

		+	−
Interferon	+	0	2
	−	15	7

Fig. 1 THE SEGREGATION OF ANTIVIRAL STATE AND
       INTERFERON PRODUCTION ON HYBRID CELLS

interferon against a viral challenge of Vesicular Stomatitis virus (VSV). Thus, the structural genes which control interferon
(IF) production and that which controls the expression of antiviral state are asyntenic. Following the demonstration of
asynteny of IF gene and AVP gene in our randomly selected series of hybrid clones an experiment was planned on a pre-select-
ed series of hybrid clones to characterize the localization of
AVP gene to different viral challenges. These clones were selected on the basis of their retention or loss of chromosome 21.
The hybrids were treated with human interferon and subsequently
challenged with VSV, Encephalomyocarditis virus (EMC) and Reovirus (Reo). Table 2 represents the results of this test. All the
hybrid clones which retained the human form of IPO-A and human
chromosome 21 were protected by human interferon pretreatment
against the three viral challenges used in this test. Two hybrid
clones WalX and WaV-4Rc which have simultaneously lost chromosome 21 and IPO-A were not protected by human interferon against
the viral challenge used in this study. These results in addition to confirming the assignment of AVP to chromosome 21 also
suggest that the presumed factor, AVP coded for by a gene in
chromosome 21 is effective in the inhibition of a range of viral
RNA replications. Other independent studies using somatic cell
hybrids have described the syntenic association of AVP and IPO-

A and also confirm the linkage assignment of IPO-A to human chromosome 21 (15, 16).

A natural sequel to the assignment of AVP to chromosome 21
is to compare the anti-viral response in trisomic 21 (T-21) and
diploid 21 (D-21) cells with their gene dosage. This test presents a unique opportunity of employing gene dosage relationships
to confirm a gene assignment. Skin biopsies were obtained from
fibroblast cultures established from trisomy 21 and their normal
siblings. Ten cultures of T-21 were matched with cultures established from normal siblings and processed in a double blind protocol. These were exposed for 20-24 hrs. to different concentrations of human interferon. The cells were subsequently challenged
with VSV and examined later for viral induced cytopathic effect
(CPE) or examined later for the inhibition of total viral RNA
synthesis by the method described by Skehan (17). Fig. 2 and
Table 3 represent the results of this test which show that the
threshold concentration of human interferon required to inhibit
viral replication by 50% was 3-7 times higher for the D-21 than
the T-21 cells.

To demonstrate that this was a gene dosage effect of chromosome 21 and not a generalized trisomic effect, we measured the
concentration of human interferon required to induce the antiviral state in trisomic 18 and 13 (T-18 and T-13) fibroblasts.
Table 4 shows that the threshold concentration required to induce an anti-viral state in T-18 and T-13 fibroblasts was in the
same concentration range as that required to protect normal diploid fibroblasts.

The induction of anti-viral state by human interferon was
repeated with subinducing concentrations of polyIpolyC. At these
concentrations polyIpolyC induced only an anti-viral state without detectable interferon. The anti-viral state induced by low

tion. In all the hybrid clones and the derived subclones tested
we found that human interferon production induced by NDV and by
polyIpolyC segregated concordantly, suggesting that the same genetic factors are involved in the inducibility of interferon
production by the two inducers. The assignment of HuIF to the
two human chromosomes, we believe, represents the first assignment of an inducible phenotype to more than one chromosome.

There are three primary alternatives which may account for
the assignment of HuIF to the two human chromosomes. First, one
of the two chromosomes may contain a genetic factor which codes
for a specific receptor site necessary for the processing of interferon inducers into recognizable signals to turn on the genetic factor for interferon production and the other human chromosome may contain the genetic factor for interferon production.
Secondly, both the two chromosomes may contain genetic factors
which code for interferon subunits. Third, one of the two chromosomes is involved in the processing of a precursor interferon
such as preinterferon to an active form.

The linkage assignment of the genes for interferon production reported in these experiments represents a unique opportunity to compare the homologous linkage groups in human and in monkey chromosomes. Stock and Hsu (28) utilizing the banding patterns of Q bands, heterochromatin or C bands and Giemsa or G and
R bands demonstrated that the karyotypes of two monkeys (Rhesus
and African Green monkey AGM) could be matched to a number of
human chromosomes. Human chromosome 5 was similar in banding patterns to Rhesus chromosome A_7 and Rhesus chromosome A_7 with AGM
chromosomes A_8 and A_9 (these correspond to the small subtelocentric chromosomes of the AGM karyotypes by Chany and his associates (10,11). Human chromosome 5 may thus be compared with AGM
chromosomes A_8 and A_9 by virtue of their similar banding pat-

terns with chromosome A$_7$ of the Rhesus monkey.This morphological similarity of monkey and human chromosomes can thus be correlated with the linkage groups on human chromosome 5 and on the small subtelocentric AGM chromosomes both of which have a reported association with the production of interferon.Such studies provide further insights into the evolution and conservatisms of linkage groups as suggested by similar chromosomal banding patterns observed in the primates.

Summary

Mouse human somatic cell hybrids were used to assign the gene for anti-viral expression to chromosome 21. This assignment was confirmed by gene dosage studies with human cells trisomic for chromosome 21. Similarly genetic analysis with mouse-human cell hybrid was used to dissect the genetics of human interferon. A total of 46 primary cell hybrids were tested for the production of human interferon. Ten hybrid clones produced human interferon in response to polyIpolyC and to Newcastle Disease Virus (NDV). The levels of interferon was low (1-10% of the amount produced by the parental human cell) and this could be due to the formation of a human mouse interferon heteropolymer with reduced anti-viral action on human cells. Concurrent enzymatic and chromosomal analysis of the hybrid clones indicated a concordant segregation of human interferon with human isocitrate dehydrogenase (IDH) and malate oxidoreductase (MDR) and with chromosome 5. IDH and MDR have been linked to chromosome 2. No exceptions were found in the concordant segregation of human interferon with chromosome 2 and 5. In addition hybrid clones which tested positive for the production of human interferon were shown to lose their ability to produce human interferon when they lost chromosome 5 while retaining chromosome 2. Based on these findings we postulated that there are at least 2 gene loci for the expression of interferon in human cells. This could mean that there are two interferon structural loci, alternately one of the loci is a receptor site for the uptake and processing of human interferon inducer and the other locus is the structural gene for interferon.

Acknowledgements

I wish to thank Dr. F. H. Ruddle for his encouragement and support. This work was supported by N.I.H. grant GM-19,952.

References

1. Ruddle, F.H. (1973). Nature 242:165.
2. Ruddle, F.H. (1973). Cytogenet. Cell Genet., in press.
3. De Maeyer-Guignard, J. and De Maeyer, E. (1965). Nature 205: 985.
4. Burke, D.C. (1965). Biochem. J. 94:2P.
5. Ho, M. and Breinig, M. (1965). Virology 25:231.
6. Cogniaux-LeClerc, J., Levy, A.H. and Wagner, R.R. (1966). Virology 28:497.
7. Coppey, J. and Muel, B. (1970). Int. J. Radiat. Biol. 17:431.
8. Coppey, J. (1971). Nature New Biol. 234:14.
9. De Maeyer, E., De Maeyer-Guignard, J. and Bailey, D.W. (1973). Bac. Proceed. V. 401.
10. Cassingena, R., Chany, C., Vignal, M., Suarez, H., Estrade, S. and Lazar, P. (1971). Proc. Natl. Acad. Sci. U.S.A. 68:580.
11. Chany, C. (1973), these proceedings.
12. Tan, Y.H., Tischfield, J. and Ruddle, F.H. (1973). J. Expt. Med. 137:317.

13. Beckman, G. (1973). Hereditas 73:305.

14. Brewer, G.J. (1973). Personal communication.

15. Nabholz, M. (1969). Ph.D. thesis, Stanford.

16. Westerveld, A., Pearson, P.L., Someren, H. van, Jongsma, A., Hagmeijer, A. and Bootsma, D. (1973). Genetics 74:329.

17. Skehan, P. (1972). Ph.D. thesis, Yale.

18. Chany, C., Fournier, F. and Rousset, S. (1971). Nature New Biol. 230:113.

19. Carter, W. (1971). Proc. Natl. Acad. Sci. U.S.A. 67:620.

20. Tan, Y.H., Jeng, D. and Ho, M. (1972). Virology 48:41.

21. Tan, Y.H., Ke, Y.H., Armstrong, A. and Ho, M. (1970). Proc. Natl. Acad. Sci. U.S.A. 67:464.

22. Ho, M., Tan, Y.H. and Armstrong, J. (1972). Proc. Soc. Expt. Biol. Med. 139:259.

23. Vilček, J. (1970). Ann. N.Y. Acad. Sci. 173:390.

24. Vilček, J. (1970). J. Gen. Physiol. 56:79s.

25. Havell, E.A. and Vilček, J. (1972). Biochim Biophys. Acta 2:476.

26. Vilček, J. and Ng, M.H. (1971). J. Virol. 7:588.

27. Tan, Y.H., Armstrong, J. and Ho, M. (1971). Virology 44:503.

28. Stock, D.A. and Hsu, T.C. (1973). Chromosoma 43:211.

TABLE 1

Mouse human cell hybridization by inactivated Sendai virus

Fusion between

Mouse	Human	Cell hybrid series	Selection medium
A9	skin fibroblast[*]	JFA	AA
A9	WI-38	Wa	AA
A9	leucocyte[*]	JBA	AA
RAG	leucocyte	J	HAT
RAG	spleen cell	W	HAT
RAG	skin fibroblast[†]	RK	HAT

[*] contains a 14/22 centric fusion

[†] contains a 14/X translocation

A9 = an L cell derivative lacking in adenine phosphoribosyl-
       transferase and in hypoxanthine guanine phosphoribosyl-
       transferase.

RAG = a mouse adenocarcinoma derived line lacking in hypo-
       xanthine guanine phosphoribosyltransferase.

AA = alanosine, adenine.

HAT = hypoxanthine, aminopterin, thymidine.

Y. H. TAN

TABLE 2

Concordancy of indophenol oxidase and
chromosome 21 with antiviral state

Protection Against Challenge

Cell type	Reo	VSV	EMC	IPO-A	Chr. 21
Primary clone					
WaV	+	+	+	+	+
WaIX	−	−	−	−	−
Subclones					
WaV-2Rb	+	+	+	+	+
WaV-4Rb	+	+	+	+	+
WaV-4Rc	−	−	−	−	−
WaV-5Rb	+	+	+	+	+
WaV-2Ra	+	+	+	+	+

TABLE 3

Units of human interferon required to
inhibit viral replication

Units human interferon required to inhibit

Cell Line	Virus induced CPE by 50%	Viral RNA synthesis by 50%
Trisomic 21		
Set VI	0.007	0.008
Set VII	0.007	0.011
Set VIII	0.010	0.009
Set IX	N.D.	0.009
Set X	N.D.	0.013
Diploid		
Set VI	0.042	0.044
Set VII	0.052	0.047
Set VIII	0.069	0.072
Set IX	N.D.	0.032
Set X	N.D.	0.055

TABLE 4

Induction of anti-viral state in human fibroblasts
trisomic for chromosomes 13, 18 & 21

Cell Line	Units human interferon inhibiting viral RNA synthesis by 50%
Trisomic 21	0.008, 0.009
Trisomic 21	0.007, 0.009
Trisomic 18	0.049, 0.049
Trisomic 18	0.052, 0.052
Trisomic 13	0.056, 0.045
Diploid	0.044, 0.042
Diploid	0.056, 0.047

TABLE 5

Interferon production in mouse human cell hybrids

Cell Type	Induction of Mouse Interferon by		Induction of Human Interferon by	
	PolyIpolyC + DEAE Dextran	NDV	PolyIpolyC + DEAE Dextran	NDV
Parental cells	units produced by 2×10^6 cells		units produced by 2×10^6 cells	
WI38	<2	2	4	12
Human fibroblasts*	<2	2	98	502
Human fibroblasts**	<2	2	90	256
Human leucocyte	<2	2	<2	1200
Mouse A9	<2	60	<2	<2
Mouse RAG	<2	98	<2	<2
Primary clones				
JFA 12a	N.D.	72	<2	<2
JFA 14a	<2	32	4,8,4	4,8,16
JFA 15f	<2	32	<2	<2
JFA 16a	<2	512	16,32,8	16,<4,4
JFA 19	<2	64	<2	<2
WaIa	<2	32	<2	<2
WaIIa	<2	32	<2	<2
WaIIIa	<2	48	<2	<2

TABLE 5 (continued)

Cell Type	Induction of Mouse Interferon by		Induction of Human Interferon by	
	PolyIpolyC + DEAE Dextran	NDV	PolyIpolyC + DEAE Dextran	NDV
WaIVa	<2	32	<2	<2
WaVa	<2	32	<2	<2
WaVIa	<2	48	<2	<2
WaVIIa	<2	64	<2	<2
WaVIIIa	<2	32	<2	<2
WaIXa	<2	64	<2	<2
JBA-1	<2	960	<2	<2
J3S	N.D.	256	<2	<2
J10H7	N.D.	256	<2	<2
J10H9	N.D.	256	N.D.	<2
J10H12	N.D.	256	N.D.	<2
W-1	<2	128	4,8	32,4,16
W-4	<2	120	4,8	16,16,64
W-5	<2	256	<2	<2
W-8	<2	164	<2	<2
W-10	<2	128	<2	<2

TABLE 5 (continued)

Cell Type	Induction of Mouse Interferon by		Induction of Human Interferon by	
	PolyIpolyC + DEAE Dextran	NDV	PolyIpolyC + DEAE Dextran	NDV
W-12	<2	128	<2	<2
W-13	<2	128	<2	<2
W-15	<2	164	<2	<2
W-17	<2	128	<2	<2
W-20	<2	128	<2	<2
W-21	<2	128	<2	<2
W-23	<2	128	4,8<2†	2,4,<2†
Subclones JFA-14a				
2a	<2	256	<2	<2
6b	N.D.	N.D.	<2	<2
13	N.D.	N.D.	16,4,16	4,4
23	N.D.	N.D.	<2	<2
Subclones JFA-16a				
5	<2	625	4,16	4,16
8	<2	62	64,200	4
19	<2	62	64,32	4

TABLE 5 (continued)

Cell Type	Induction of Mouse Interferon by		Induction of Human Interferon by	
	PolyIpolyC + DEAE Dextran	NDV	PolyIpolyC + DEAE Dextran	NDV
21	<2	80	<2	<2
10	<2	125	32	4

Human interferon was assayed on human foreskin fibroblasts and
Mouse interferon was assayed on mouse A9 or mouse RAG cells.

*   contain a 14/22 centric fusion

**   contain a 14/X translocation

†   subsequently lost human chromosome 5

TABLE 6

Negative correlation of human interferon
production to human chromosomes

Human Chromosome	Interferon/Chromosome				Concordant Clones (+/+ & -/-)	Discordant Clones (+/- & -/+)
	+/+	+/-	-/+	-/-		
1	2	8	12	18	20	20
2	10	0	9	21	31	9
3	2	8	6	24	26	14
4	0	10	8	22	22	18
5	10	0	2	28	38	2
6	2	8	7	23	25	15
7	1	9	9	21	22	18
8	5	5	7	23	28	12
9	0	10	0	30	30	10
10	2	8	8	22	24	16
11	7	3	7	23	30	10
12	2	8	10	20	22	18
13	2	8	5	25	27	13
14	6	4	7	23	29	11
15	-	-	-	-	-	-
16	7	3	17	13	20	20
17	7	3	11	19	26	14
18	10	0	13	17	27	13
19	2	8	6	24	26	14
20	4	6	6	24	30	10
21	2	8	10	20	22	18
22	5	5	11	19	24	16
X	0	10	14	16	16	24
Y	0	10	0	20	20	20

TABLE 7

Correlation of human interferon production
with chromosomes 2 and 5

Human chromosomes Present		NDV-induced Interferon (# clones)		Poly I/Poly C Induced Interferon (# clones)	
		+	−	+	−
2+	5+	10	0	10	0
2+	5−	0	7	0	7
2−	5+	0	2	0	2
2−	5−	0	21	0	21

TABLE 8

Correlation of human interferon production
with chromosomes 2 and 5

		Human chromosomes	
Subclones of JFA-16a	HuIF	2	5
5	+	+	+
8	+	+	+
19	+	+	+
10	+	+	+
21	−	+	−
Subclones of JFA-14a			
2a	−	+	−
6b	−	+	−
13	+	+	+
23	−	+	−

TABLE 9

Superinduction of human interferon production
in mouse human cell hybrids

	Cycloheximide (duration of exposure from hour 0 to hour)*	Actinomycin D		Human Interferon yield (units)
		Time of addition (hr.)	Duration of exposure (hr.)	
Human Skin Fibroblasts	None	None	None	112
"	5	None	None	256
"	7	None	None	256
"	7	0	7	<2
"	7	3	4	16
"	7	6	1	4912
JFA 16a	None	None	None	16
"	5	None	None	4,<4
"	7	None	None	16
"	7	0	7	<2
"	7	6	1	256
JFA-14a-13	None	None	None	16
JFA-14a-13	7	6	1	64
JFA-12a	None	None	None	<2
JFA-12a	7	6	1	<2
JFA-15f	None	None	None	<2
JFA-15f	7	6	1	<2
WaIa	None	None	None	<2
WaIa	7	6	1	<2

* Hour 0 refers to time of addition of poly I poly C

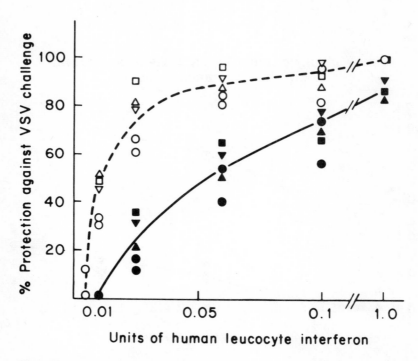

Fig. 2. The induction of anti-viral state in normal diploid fibroblasts (closed symbols) and trisomic 21 fibroblasts (open symbols) by human interferon.

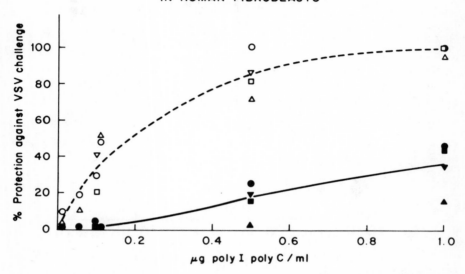

Fig. 3.   The induction of anti-viral state in normal diploid
fibroblasts (closed symbols) and trisomic 21 fibroblasts (open
symbols) by subinducing doses of polyI polyC.

DISCUSSION

Mota: I wonder if there is any line available with a translocated 21 which could help us to locate which arm of chromosome 21 carries the gene for interferon.

Tan: Yes, there are translated 21 lines that allow the regional mapping of "AVP" and "IPO-B". Currently we have used these for such a purpose.

Papadimitriou: Can I ask a technical question regarding growth of hybrids? Is there a possibility of doing biochemical work with the cells, or do you lose chromosomes in growing up a large cell population? Could one for example look at the hybrid cells that have chromosome 21 as compared to hybrid cells lacking this chromosome for content of a specific enzyme? Is this feasible?

Tan: It is possible to correlate for the presence of a human chromosome by screening for human enzymes in hybrid cells. At present more than 20 human enzyme markers are available for use as a means of scoring for the presence of about more than a dozen human chromosomes.

Burke: But I wonder if you looked at any of your hybrids for priming to see if that is separated from any of the other properties you've been looking at.

Tan: I have not yet looked at priming. I suppose it has been done.

Planterose: From your genetic analysis work, have you any comments as to whether a mutant cell exists, which produces interferon without having to be induced? Would such a cell produce vast amounts of interferon?

Tan: All our hybrid clones were tested for the presence
of a constitutive condition with reference to interferon production, but we found none. In addition from our examination of
mouse interferon production in these hybrid cells, we hope to
provide genetic evidence for the existence of a gene which regu-
lates the amount of interferon synthesized in a cell by looking
for high, intermediate and low producers of interferon. In another aspect we hope to isolate a high producer of interferon
which certainly will alleviate one major problem in the purification and isolation of interferon.

De Maeyer: It has been shown for certain lines of mouse
cells that they can make more interferon upon induction when
they have been transformed by oncorna viruses. Can you guarantee
that your different cell lines have the same background of latent virus infection, or no latent virus infection at all, or do
you think this does complicate the picture in your studies?

Tan: I think it does complicate the picture in the case
of using mouse human somatic cell hybrids to map the regulator
gene for interferon, since we do not know the effect of latent
virus activation on the production of interferon in these hybrid
cells.

De Maeyer: So you are using more than one mouse parental
cell line?

Tan: Two mouse parental cell lines and both of them produce interferon.

Chany: I would like to ask you if you have determined the
minimal number of chromosomes which are necessary to associate
them with a cellular function. Using the enzymatic marker, a
problem arises in relationship to the sensitivity of the test.

The presence of chromosomes (or fragments from them) only in 10%
of the cells is sufficient to detect activity of the corresponding enzymes. So, the enzymatic marker alone is not satisfactory
to relate chromosomes and function. I think it is absolutely
necessary to complete the assay with a classical karyotype. In
addition, it would be of interest to determine the minimal
amount of chromosomes necessary in a cell population to detect
interferon synthesis.

Tan: Perhaps the most ideal situation is to use enzyme
markers and cytogenetics jointly to identify the presence of a
specific human chromosome and more importantly that the two
approaches are complementary.

Chany: I think this is a very important point because
these hybrid cells are submitted to stress during the selection
of mutants necessary for the elimination of parental cells.
There are a great number of breaks, fragments of chromosomes,
which have apparently nothing to do morphologically with either
of the parental chromosomes. I think this is probably one of the
limitations of the somatic hybrid system as a research tool.

CONTROL OF THE INTERFERON MECHANISM IN
HAMSTER-MOUSE HETEROKARYONS[*]

S. E. Grossberg, A. J. Smith, and J. J. Sedmak

Department of Microbiology
The Medical College of Wisconsin
Milwaukee, Wisconsin 53233 U.S.A.

The golden Syrian hamster (<u>Mesocricetus auratus</u>) is highly
susceptible to many virus infections. Of all laboratory animals
it also seems to be the most susceptible host for the production
and propagation of tumors produced by tumor cells or oncogenic
viruses (1). Cultured cricetine cells are more susceptible to
productive, lytic infections with viruses, such as influenza viruses (2) and group B togaviruses (3), that replicate poorly in
most other cell cultures. The question was posed whether the unusual susceptibility of the hamster to viruses and tumors was
related to defects in its interferon mechanism.

Interferon defectiveness of the hamster

A few reports have indicated limited success in producing
low titers of interferon in the hamster or in cell cultures derived from it (4-7). Our numerous attempts to induce interferon
in this animal were largely unsuccessful using different viral
inducers as well as poly rI . poly rC. Infectious or inactivated

---

[*] Supported by United States Public Health Service Awards 70-2125
and 5 TO1-Al00239 from the National Institute of Allergy and
Infectious Disease, and by the American Cancer Society (Milwaukee division).

myxoviruses or togaviruses were only occasionally effective;
poly I . poly C consistently failed to induce interferon. The
investigation of a variety of factors that might illuminate the
basis for possible defectiveness both in vivo and in vitro were
essentially unrewarding; such factors included host age and sex,
type and dose of interferon inducer, enhancing agents, time of
bleeding or harvest of cells, cellular characteristics, and
evaluation of sensitivity of different assays to detect interferon (Table 1). The cell cultures tested were primary hamster
kidney cells, an epithelial hamster kidney (EHK) cell line obtained from Dr. Purnell Choppin at Rockefeller University, and
BHK-21 cells. The viruses used included the velogenic CG strain
of Newcastle disease virus (NDV) as well as the lentogenic Bl
strain, and poly rI . poly rC. The enhancing agents used in vitro
and in vivo included DEAE-dextran and neomycin. Although it is
possible that interferon simply deteriorated during storage, approximately a third of the interferon preparations were assayed
immediately after harvest and virus inactivation. In fact, in
all of the cases in which an interferon titer was detected, the
samples had been stored at -70° for 3 to 30 days. The fact that
some of the interferon samples (including all the plasmas) were
not treated in any way before assay, while other samples were
treated by one of two methods for partial purification, reduces
the possibility that interferon activity was destroyed by a purification process. No more than 35 units could be detected in
serum or brain of hamsters or in a variety of different hamster
cells as primary cultures or cell lines. Only four of 17 attempts
in the intact hamster and 1 out of 21 attempts in cricetine cell
cultures provided detectable interferon. The interferon used in
the studies reported here was prepared from brain of hamsters
injected with West Nile virus.

It seems curious that of the many species of animals from fishes to man that have been shown to produce interferon, the hamster appears to do so very poorly.

The formation of hamster-mouse hybrids

In order to study the apparent defectiveness of interferon production and/or action, hamster cells were hybridized with a cell line from a highly interferon-reactive animal, the mouse. Carver, Seto and Migeon (7) had reported that a hybrid cell line formed from hamster and mouse cells produced about ten times more cricetine interferon and was about eight times more sensitive to cricetine interferon than the parental hamster cells; that cell line, unfortunately, was lost (D. Carver, personal communication). Two lines of mutant cells were then obtained from Dr. John Littlefield at Harvard University: the hamster B_1 cell line lacking thymidine kinase and a mouse A_9 cell line derived from L_{929} cells but lacking hypoxanthine-guanine phosphoribosyl transferase (8). The hamster thymidine kinase-negative mutant cell can make thymidilic acid and other pyrimidines by de novo biosynthesis through a pathway that requires a folic acid derivative. The mouse hypoxanthine-guanine phosphoribosyl transferase-negative cell can make inosinic acid through de novo biosynthesis also requiring folic acid. In the presence of aminopterin which inhibits folic acid synthesis, both cells die. When the two kinds of cells are fused, they are able to complement one another even in the presence of aminopterin provided that hypoxanthine and thymidine are provided in the medium for the formation of purines and pyrimidines, respectively, through biochemical salvage reactions. Ultraviolet-irradiated Sendai virus was used to form heterokaryons from the mouse and hamster lines; the unfused parent cells were eliminated by prolonged exposure to selective medium containing aminopterin. Four of 19 clones were selected for study.

Clonal sensitivity to hamster and mouse interferons

Despite our previous efforts to use different challenge
viruses in different kinds of assays, the inability to detect
interferon in the hamster might only have reflected unresponsiveness to the action of interferon of hamster cell cultures.
In order to develop a suitable interferon assay, the mouse and
hamster cells in the hybrids were tested systematically for
their ability to produce adequate yields of several interferon-
sensitive viruses. The mouse cells produced Theiler's encephalo-
myelitis GDVII virus best, with consistently high yields of
hemagglutinin and with which the highest titers of interferon
were obtained. The hamster cells produced encephalomyocarditis
(EMC) virus best, and the highest titers of interferon were obtained with that virus. The hybrid clones, like the parental
hamster cells, produced EMC virus best. Since yield-reduction
tests are considered to be the most sensitive type of interferon
assay, we used a hemagglutinin yield-reduction test, following
the method of Oie et al. (9).

To determine if the newly derived, heterokaryotic cell
lines were interferon-sensitive, the hybrid cell clones were exposed to mouse and hamster interferons (Table 2). As expected,
mouse cells were appropriately sensitive to mouse interferon and
insensitive to hamster interferon. The hamster B_1 cell line was
consistently and completely insensitive to both hamster and
mouse interferons. Primary hamster kidney cells were insensitive
to mouse interferon but could detect 35 units of hamster brain
interferon. Clone A_9B_1 [15] did not detect activity in either
the mouse or hamster interferon preparations. However, clones 6,
10 and 12 were sensitive to mouse interferon to about the same
extent as the parent mouse line; more remarkably, these three
clones were able to measure as much as 2,300 units of hamster

interferon in the same preparation in which primary hamster
cells could detect only 35 units and in which the parental
hamster cell could detect none. Since the highest titers of
hamster interferon were obtained in clone 12, this clone was
used for subsequent assays of hamster interferons. It was not
unexpected that some of the hybrid cells would be sensitive to
interferons from species of the parents, since others (7, 12,
13) had reported similar results; rather, it is the great degree of sensitivity to interferon from one of the parents (of
hamster origin) that became apparent after hybridization.

     We thought it of interest to determine the relative re-
sponsiveness of the clone 12 hybrid to interferons from heterologous species (Table 3). Although the hamster-mouse hybrid was
about 7-fold more sensitive to human interferon than the ances-
tral L cell, and possibly more sensitive to rabbit interferon,
it was insensitive to chicken interferon. This hybrid cell
clone, unfortunately, cannot serve as a universal interferon
detector.

Clonal production of interferons

     The capacity of the hybrid cells to produce interferon
was then determined (Table 4). The hamster B_1 line failed to
produce any detectable interferon after exposure to NDV. The
mouse A_9 cells produce large amounts of mouse interferon equivalent to that detected in mouse cells, as previously noted. Clone
[15], already noted to be insensitive to exogenous interferon,
produced only small amounts of interferon, some of which was
probably of mouse origin. Clones 6 and 10 produced large amounts
of interferon detectable on clone 12 cells. More than 95% of the
interferon from clone 6 appeared to be hamster interferon since
only relatively small amounts were detectable on the mouse cells.
Clone 12 produced an interferon about 70% of which appeared to

be hamster in origin. Although it might appear fortuitously
that expressions of interferon induction and action are linked
in some clones, the finding that one clone can produce small
amounts of interferon despite persistent insensitivity to its
action argues against this, in keeping with observations in other
model systems in which interferon production and action are dissociated (13, 14).

Clonal chromosomal patterns

The A_g mouse parent cell is aneuploid, having a modal number of 56, corresponding to the number reported by Migeon (15);
there are no marker chromosomes. The B_1 hamster parent cells have
a modal number of 41, also in agreement with published data (15).
Clone 12 has a modal number of 97; this clone was most sensitive
to hamster and mouse interferons and produced both (Fig. 1).
Clone [15] has a modal number of 41, the same number as the hamster parent, but with a distinctively different chromosomal pattern (Fig. 2). This clone is resistant to mouse and hamster interferons but can produce small quantities of interferon. Further
karyologic studies of the clones, including the use of banding
techniques, are in progress. Also under study is the segregation
of enzymes, including isozymes and indophenol oxidase; the latter
has been shown to be associated with the human chromosome on
which the interferon action locus is thought to occur (16).

Studies of interferon regulation in the heterokaryons

Superinduction. In order to examine the regulatory mechanism of production of mouse or hamster interferon in the hybrid
cells, a series of experiments were begun to induce interferon,
using metabolic inhibitors in combination with priming with interferons of the two different species of the parents. The

results shown in Table 5 are from an experiment in which hybrid
cells of clone 12 were treated with hamster or mouse interferon
and then induced with NDV or poly.I.poly C. The superinduction
schedule, using cycloheximide and actinomycin D for brief periods after induction, is shown in Table 5. The culture fluids
were then assayed for interferon on clone 12 or L cells. It is
not clear that superinduction actually occurred. Certainly higher titers were obtained after pretreatment with hamster interferon than with mouse interferon. If anything, mouse interferon
may have been slightly inhibitory. Interferon induction with
poly.I.poly C in this hybrid clone was poor. These experiments
are being extended to the other clones, two of which appear to
have a disparity in the amounts produced of species specific
interferons.

Molecular interferon hybrids? Because of the possibility
that these clones would produce hybrid molecules of interferon,
the molecular weights of interferons from the two parent species
and those of the clones were measured as a function of activity
on L cells or clone 12 after Sephadex G-100 chromatography
(Table 6). Mouse interferon has a molecular weight of 26,000 and
the hamster interferon a molecular weight of 15,500. Interferons
from the clones had molecular weights that were not significantly different from the size measured for mouse interferon. The
conclusion that might be drawn from these data is at variance
with the biological activities described in Table 4. Our tentative conclusion is that it is not possible to distinguish hybrid
molecules on the basis of molecular sieve chromatography.

Hamster repressors of interferon action. Because of our
long-standing interest in repressor or inhibitory factors that
we have postulated to be present early in the development of the
chicken embryo (17) and that Chany's group has demonstrated to

exist in human amniotic membrane (18), and human sarcomas (19),
we searched for hamster factors antagonistic to interferon action (Table 7). An extract of muscle from young hamsters very
significantly reduced interferon action, whereas an extract from
older hamster had less anti-interferon activity. Significant inhibitory activity has not been demonstrated so far in unconcen-
trated preparations of hamster or mouse cells.

For comparison, the human amnion tissue antagonist provided
by Dr. C. Chany was quite potent as was an ammonium sulfate-pre-
cipitated extract obtained from very young chicken embryos
(Sedmak & Grossberg, unpublished data). It should be noted that
the method for demonstrating these activities was accomplished
by simultaneous incubation of mouse interferon and cell extract
on L cells subsequently challenged with GDVII virus, confirming
the finding of heterospecific activity of such antagonists (18).

Summary

The interferon mechanism in the golden Syrian hamster is
defective. Attempts by ordinary means with otherwise potent inducers generally failed to demonstrate interferon production as
measured in primary cell cultures or cricetine cell lines. Hybrid
cell lines were derived which appeared to carry portions of the
chromosomal complement of a mutant murine cell line, permissive
for interferon induction and action, and of a mutant cricetine
cell line, restricted in its ability to produce or respond to
interferon. Some of the hamster-mouse hybrid cell clones have
more than 200 times greater sensitivity to cricetine interferon
than the parental hamster line. The sensitivity of some of the
clones to murine interferon is roughly equivalent to that of the
parental mouse line. Certain clones can produce more than 600
times more cricetine interferon than the parental hamster line.

Thus, the interferon mechanism in hamster cells can be expressed in hamster-mouse heterokaryons, providing a valuable model for study of the controls regulating the interferon mechanism. One such control regulating interferon action may be the inhibitor of interferon action demonstrated in extracts of hamster tissue. Whether the production as well as the action of interferons in hamster cells is regulated by extractable interferon repressor substance in addition to other genetic means remains to be determined.

Acknowledgements

We thank Marcia Hilger, Mary Dixon, Joyce Fay, and Christine Kummer for excellent technical assistance.

References

1. Hoffman, R.A., Robinson, P.F., and Magalhães, H., ed.(1968). "The Golden Hamster. Its Biology and Use in Medical Research". Iowa State University Press, Ames, Iowa, 545 pp.

2. Grossberg, S.E. (1964). Human influenza A viruses: rapid plaque assay in hamster kidney cells. Science 144:1246-1247.

3. Rohitayodhin, S. and Hammon, W.M. (1962). Studies on Japanese B encephalitis virus vaccines from tissue culture. I. Virus growth and survival at 30° C. J. Immunol. 89:582-588.

4. Baron, S., Buckler, C.E., McCloskey, R.V. and Kirschstein, R.L. (1966). Role of interferon during viremia. J. Immunol. 96:12-16.

5. Talas, M., Weiszfeiler, G. and Batkai, L. (1968). Hamster interferon induced by polyoma virus.Acta Virol. 12:378-380.

6. Stewart, W.E., Scott, W.D. and Sulkin, S.E. (1969). Relative sensitivity of viruses to different species of interferon. J. Virol. 4:147-153.

7. Carver, D.H., Seto, D.Y. and Migeon, B.R. (1968). Interferon production and action in mouse, hamster, and somatic hybrid mouse-hamster cells. Science 160:558-559.

8. Littlefield, J.W. (1966). The use of drug-resistant markers to study the hybridization of mouse fibroblasts. Exptl. Cell Res. 41:190-

9. Oie, H., Buckler, C.,Uhlendorf, C.P., Hill, D.A., and Baron, S. (1972). Improved assays for a variety of interferons. Proc. Soc. Exp. Biol. Med. 140:1178-1181.

10. Grossberg, S.E., Jameson, P., and Sedmak, J.J. (1974). Interferon bioassay methods and the development of standard procedures: a critique and analysis of current observations. In Vitro (in press).

11. Sedmak, J.J. and Grossberg, S.E. (1973). Interferon bioassay: reduction in yield of myxoviral neuarminidases. J. Gen. Virol. 21:1-7, 1973.

12. Guggenheim, M.A., Friedman, R.M., and Rabson, A.S. (1969). Interferon action in heterokaryons. Proc. Soc. Exp. Biol. Med. 130:1242-1245.

13. Cassingena, R., Chany, C., Vignal, M., Suarez, H., Estrade, S. and Lazar, P. (1971). Use of monkey-mouse hybrid cells for the study of the cellular regulation of interferon production and action. Proc. Natl. Acad. Sci. U.S.A. 68:580-584.

14. Desmyter, J., Melnick, J.L. and Rawls, W.E. (1968). Defectiveness of interferon production and of rubella virus interference in a line of African green monkey cells (Vero). J. Virol. 2:955-961.

15. Migeon, B.R. (1968). Hybridization of somatic cells derived from mouse and Syrian hamster: evolution of karyotype and enzyme studies. Biochem. Genetics $\underline{1}$:305-322.

16. Tan, Y.H., Tischfield, J. and Ruddle, F.H. (1973). The linkage of genes for the human interferon-induced antiviral protein and indophenol oxidase-B traits to chromosome G-21. J. Exptl. Med. $\underline{137}$:317-339.

17. Grossberg, S.E. and Morahan, P.S. (1971). Repression of interferon action: induced dedifferentiation of embryonic cells. Science $\underline{171}$:77-79.

18. Fournier, F., Rousset, S., and Chany, C. (1969). Investigations on a tissue antagonist of interferon. Proc. Soc. Exp. Biol. Med. $\underline{132}$:943-950.

19. Chany, C., Lemaitre, J., and Galliot, B. Use of interferon antagonists for the study of animal and human sarcomas (1971). Perspectives in Virology, Vol. 7, M. Pollard, ed., Academic Press, New York, pp. 111-126.

TABLE 1

Attempts to induce serum interferon in hamsters

Inducer[1]	Age & Sex of Hamster[2]	Dose of Inducer[3]	Bleeding Time	Type of Assay[4]	Assay Cell[5]	Challenge Virus[6]	Interferon Titer[7]
WS-UV	4 mos – M	HA-1024	5 hrs	PR	HK	SFV	20
"	15 mos – M	HA-1024	5 hrs	PR	EHK	VSV	20
			24 hrs	PR	EHK	VSV	<4
NDV-B1	21 mos – M	3.6×10^8 PFU	7 hrs	PR	HK	VSV	<8
NDV-CG	4 wks – M	3.9×10^8 PFU	5 hrs	PR	HK	SFV	<4
				YR	BHK-21	Sindbis	<5
"	7 mos – M	3.9×10^8 PFU	5 hrs	PR	HK	SFV	<4
				YR	BHK-21	Sindbis	<5
"	21 mos – M	1.3×10^9 PFU	5 hrs	PR	HK	VSV	10
"	24 mos – M	3.9×10^8 PFU	7 hrs	PR	HK	SFV	<4
				YR	BHK-21	Sindbis	<5
pI.pC	4 mos – M	200 µg(with and without DEAE-dx)[8]	2, 7, 12,24 hrs	PR	HK	SFV	<4
"	4 mos – M	500 µg	"	PR	HK	SFV	<4

pI.pC	4 mos - M	1 mg	2, 7, 12,24 hrs	PR	HK	SFV	<4
"	8 mos - F	200 µg	3 hrs	PR	HK	VSV	<4
"	17 mos - F	500 µg(with DEAE-dx)8/	3 hrs	PR	HK	VSV	<4

1/ WS-UV = Influenza A_0/WS/33 HONI, inactivated by ultraviolet light.
  NDV = Newcastle disease virus, strain B1 or CG.
  pI.pC = polyriboinosinic - polycytodilic acid homopolymer pair.
2/ M = male; F = female.
3/ HA = Hemagglutinin titer; PFU = Plaque forming units.
4/ PR = Plaque reduction assay; YR = Hemagglutinin Yield-reduction assay.
5/ HK = primary hamster kidney cell cultures; EHK = epithelial hamster kidney cell line;
  BHK-21 = baby hamster kidney cell line.
6/ SFV = Semliki forest virus; VSV = vesicular stomatitis virus.
7/ Reciprocal of dilution; available sample size determined lowest dilution used.
8/ DEAE-dx = diethyaminoethyl - dextran combined with inducer in ratio 10:1.

TABLE 2

The sensitivity to hamster and mouse interferons of
hamster-mouse heterokaryons

Cell of assay	Titer[1] of interferon [2] from indicated source		
	A_9 cells	B_1 cells	Hamster brain
Mouse A_9	6000	<10	<10
Hamster B_1	<10	<10	<10
A_9B_1 [15]	<10	<10	<10
A_9B_1 [6]	3000	<10	1200
A_9B_1 [10]	7000	<10	450
A_9B_1 [12]	10,000	<10	2300

1/ Titers are expressed as 0.5 $\log_{10}$ hemagglutinin yield-
reduction units/ml. The challenge virus used in hamster
cells was encephalomyocarditis virus and in mouse cells
GD-VII virus.

2/ Interferons in B_1, A_9, and L_{929} were prepared by infection with Newcastle disease virus (strain OG). B_1 and A_9
preparations were dialyzed against pH 2 buffer for 5
days. Hamster interferon was prepared from brains of
hamsters injected intracranially with West Nile virus;
residual virus was inactivated by dialysis against pH 2
buffer for 24 hours.

TABLE 3

Relative reactivity of the $A_9 B_1 [12]$
clone to heterologous interferons

Species of interferon	Homologous interferon		Heterologous titer in:	
	Cells of assay	Titer	Mouse L_{929}	Hamster-mouse $A_9B_1 [12]$
Human	BUD-8	300,000	340	2100
Rabbit	RK-13	14,000	<10	16
Chicken	CEC	1,300	<10	<10

1/ Human leukocyte interferon (CIF) from Dr. K. Cantell was
titrated in BUD-8, a diploid cell strain from Dr. S. Baron,
by the EMC viral hemagglutinin (HA) yield-reduction test
(10, and Jameson et al, unpublished). Rabbit serum reference
standard interferon from the NIH was assayed in the RK-13
cell line by the EMC yield-reduction test. Partially purified chicken embryo interferon was titrated in primary
chicken embryo cultures (CEC) by the neuraminidase yield-
reduction assay (11).

TABLE 4

The production of hamster and mouse interferons
in hamster-mouse heterokaryons

Cells producing interferon	Titer[1] of interferon assayed in indicated cells		
	$\underline{A}_9$	$\underline{B}_1$	$\underline{A_9B_1}$ [12]
A_9B_1 [15]	61	<10	240
A_9B_1 [6]	180	<10	6300
A_9B_1 [12]	680	<10	2400

1/ Titers are expressed as 0.5 $\log_{10}$ hemagglutinin yield-reduction units/ml. The challenge used in the B_1 line and A_9B_1 12
clone was encephalomyocarditis virus and A_9 cells GD VII
virus.

TABLE 5

Results of superinduction with priming[1] on interferon
production by hybrid clone A_9B_1 12

Species	Dose (units)	Inducer	Interferon titer assayed in L_{929}	Interferon titer assayed in $A_9B_1[12]$
None	0	NDV	1,000	2,400
Hamster	10	"	1,500	4,000
"	100	"	2,100	6,400
"	10	pI.pC (50µg)	11	<5
"	100	"	56	27
Mouse	14	NDV	2,500	850
"	140	"	1,250	270

[1]   Schedule of superinduction:

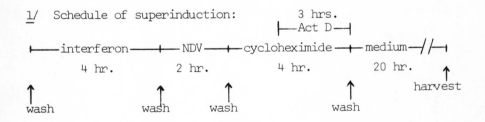

TABLE 6

Molecular weight determinations of interferons from
hamster-mouse heterokaryons using Sephadex G-100 chromatography

Source of interferon	Approximate molecular weight as assayed on:	
	L_{929}	A_9B_1 [12]
A_9 cells	26,000	26,000
Hamster	no activity	15,500
A_9B_1 [6]	28,000	28,000
A_9B_1 [10]	28,000	28,000
A_9B_1 [12]	22,000	22,000
A_9B_1 [15]	28,000	28,000

TABLE 7

Interferon antagonistic activity of cellular
extracts in L_{929} cells[1]

Source	Reduction in interferon activity vs. indicated interferon dose	
	Interferon units	Fold-reduction
Hamster muscle(4-wk-old)-2.5%dw	7	8-16
Hamster muscle(4-wk-old)-1% dw	7	8
Hamster muscle(12-wk-old)-2.5%dw	7	8
Hamster muscle(12-wk-old)-1% dw	7	0
Hamster BHK-21 cells -5% ww	16	1-2
Human amnion TAI (Chany) -1% dw	16	16

dw = dry weight; ww = wet weight

[1] L_{929} cells were exposed to mouse interferon and cellular
extracts simultaneously for 18 hr., washed, and challenged
with GD VII virus. Extracts were either prepared from freeze-
dried tissues, which were broken up in a Waring blender followed by Dounce homogenization or from cultured cells which
were Dounce homogenized. The final extract consisted of
supernatant fluid from 30,000 x g centrifugation. Tissue
antagonist of interferon (TAI) was obtained from Dr. Charles
Chany.

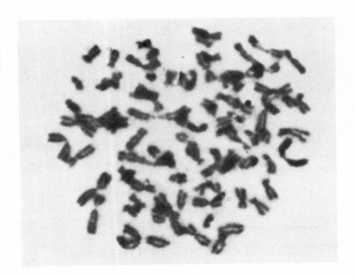

Fig. 1. Metaphase of clone A_9B_1 12 .

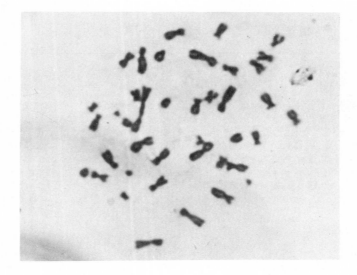

Fig. 2. Metaphase of clone A_9B_1 15 .

DISCUSSION

Tan: We have also generated mouse hamster hybrid but there is no electrophoretic difference between the mouse and hamster form of indophenol oxidase B. This creates difficulty for the time being when one attempts to establish a syntenny between AVP and IPO-B in the mouse.

Grossberg: That is too bad.

Stinebring: This is not directed at what you said, but I would just like to know if you or anyone else in the audience has worked with guinea-pigs. You know there are reports in the literature that guinea-pigs produce interferon, but I've never been able to find this to be true, and I just wondered whether or not guinea-pigs are an animal that is deficient in this type of system.

Grossberg: No, I have no personal information about guinea-pig interferon production.

Planterose: Some years ago we looked to see if we could detect guinea-pig interferon. If you give guinea pigs Sendai virus, you can detect interferon in their serum.

Grossberg: Administered in what fashion?

Planterose: Sendai virus given intravenously.

Chany: What was the virus titer?

Planterose: I forget, but I think something like 200 units, but then what's a unit? It was detected on guinea-pig kidney cells, challenged with EMC virus.

INTERFERON CELL RECEPTOR INTERACTIONS IN
SOMATIC MONKEY-MOUSE HYBRID CELLS

C. Chany and M.-F. Bourgeade

Institut National de la Santé et de la Recherche Médicale
U. 43 de Recherches sur les Infections Virales
Hôpital St. Vincent de Paul
74, Avenue Denfert-Rochereau, 75014 Paris, France

It is well established that interferon production and
action are dissociated phenomena (1,2). Genetic information for
monkey interferon synthesis can be located in a small subtelocentric chromosome. This chromosome was recently identified by mod-
ern band staining methods (3).

Events involved in interferon action are, however, related
to cellular products of which no genetic information is carried
in the same monkey chromosome. Thus, interferon is a diffusible
substance which appears after induction in the tissue culture
medium or in the bloodstream of animals.

In some of its aspects, interferon recalls hormones. Unlike hormones, this protein is not produced by a specialized
cell (however, the reticulo-endothelial cell system is especially competent for its production); but like hormones, it acts at
distance on cells carrying available and appropriate recognition
sites. When mouse sarcoma virus-transformed cells are grown in
the presence of interferon for long periods, genetic and somatic
changes might appear. The transformed cells recover characteristics (ie. recovery of contact inhibition, incapacity to produce

colonies in a gelified medium, etc.), usually attributed to normal cells (4).

The problem we wish to investigate is how the interferon
protein induces in the cells the series of events which finally
result in the above mentioned changes.

In the present publication, the mechanism of interferon-cell
interaction is analyzed by studying the response of somatic monkey-mouse hybrid cells to both of the parental interferons. Because of their well-known cell species specificity, they protect
only homologous and not heterologous cell types in the parental
cells.

We demonstrate for the first time the existence of a proteinaceous interferon receptor located on monkey cell membranes
and postulate that: 1) solely the cell receptor system is responsible for the cell species specificity of interferon; and 2)
the receptor interacts with the active site of the interferon
molecule and an activator site responsible for switching on the
series of events induced by interferon in the cell. The effect of
interferon is thus of a cooperative type.

It is of interest that as reported in another presentation
at this meeting, interferon might activate the receptor-activator
system, probably by contact or perhaps by detachment from the
molecule of an active component (5).

Material and Methods

Hybrid cell lines. The establishment, development, and
karyotype analysis of the somatic monkey-mouse hybrid cell clone
(MKCV-III) used here were described (1). In Figure 1 a brief summary is presented showing the different clonal populations

studied, which all originated from the parental hybrid MKCV-III
clone. All clones were isolated by the soft agar method. Clone 2
(25th passage) and clone 4 (27th passage) were subsequently re-
cloned. Two subclones derived from clone 2 were designated clones
M and W, and four clones isolated from clone 4 were called clones
3, 33, 34 and 35.

Other cell lines. Mouse L cells and monkey BSC-1 cells
used were routinely propagated in this laboratory. The MSV-inter-
feron[+] cells were BALB/c embryonic fibroblasts transformed by the
Mouse Sarcoma Virus (MSV-M strain) and grown in vitro for over
200 passages in the presence of mouse interferon (4).

Medium. All cells were propagated in Eagle's medium with
10% calf serum. For maintenance, serum concentration was reduced
to 2%. Somatic hybrid cells were grown in the presence of HATG
(100 μM hypoxanthine-10 μM aminopterin-40 μM thymidine-10 μM
glycine) medium (1).

Viruses. Newcastle Disease Virus (NDV), Hertsfordshire
strain, was used to induce interferon (m.o.i.= 100 plaque-forming
units (PFU). The Indiana strain of Vesicular Stomatitis Virus
(VSV) and the Encephalomyocarditis (EMC) Virus were routinely
passaged in the laboratory with L cells.

Interferon preparation. Interferon from primate (human)
white blood cells and mice was obtained as described (6). Interferon from human amniotic membrane (HAM) was prepared according
to Fournier et al. (7). Mouse and human interferon were purified
by a single passage through a Sephadex gel G-100 chromatographic
column.

Interferon assay. In all experiments, interferon preparations were assayed by serial 2-fold dilutions of interferon and
incubated with sensitive cells for 18-20 h at $37^{\circ}C$. The preparations were washed and challenged with VSV at a m.o.i. = 0.1 PFU,
and incubated for an additional 16 h at $37^{\circ}C$. For each dilution,
total virus yield was established by plaque titration in L cells.
The results were expressed as log inhibition of the control/
treated cells for each dilution. The interferon titer was the
dilution that inhibited 90% of the yield of the challenge virus
and is expressed in NIH reference units for mouse interferon and
INSERM reference units for human interferon.

Results

A. Demonstration of separate monkey and mouse receptors
on the hybrid cells.

Subclone M, CV-1, MKS-BU-100, and L cells were trypsinized
(150 μg/ml) (Choay twice cristallized), and 2×10^{6} cells were suspended in serum-free Eagle's medium. Parallel series of cells were
suspended in the same medium plus 2% calf serum. After incubation
with 100 units of interferon for 4 h at $37^{\circ}C$, VSV was diluted in
Eagle's medium plus 5% calf serum (m.o.i. = 0.1), and the cells
were further incubated for 16 h at $37^{\circ}C$. Then the cultures were
frozen and kept at $-80^{\circ}C$ until titration.

As summarized in Table 1, primate interferon had no antiviral activity in CV-1 cells and was significantly impaired in the
hybrid cells when the freshly trypsinized cells were kept in
serum-free medium during the 4-h incubation period with interferon. The presence of 2% calf serum in the medium restored full
interferon sensitivity in the same cells. In contrast, after tryp-
sination, mouse interferon was fully active in the parental MKS-

BU-100 cells, in reference L cells, and in hybrid clone M, with
or without serum in the medium.

When EDTA (200 µg/ml) was used instead of trypsin in similar
experiments, the antiviral effect of primate interferon was, in
both cases, fully expressed.

The best interpretation of these results is that trypsin
destroys monkey interferon receptors, while mouse interferon receptors are resistant to its action. Receptors are missing in
cells fed with medium containing no serum, but rapidly restored
in the presence of 2% calf serum. In the same cells, mouse receptors are completely insensitive to trypsin.

B. Cooperative dose-response curves in normal and hybrid
cells for mouse interferon. Lack of cooperative effect in hybrid
cells for monkey interferon.

The shape of the dose-response curves of mouse and human
interferon tested in various mouse and monkey (or human) cells
was regularly found to be sigmoidal (2), provided that the cells
were free of latent infectious agents and the experimental conditions were carefully controlled. This result was found even when
the same pool of mouse interferon preparation was repeatedly assayed in different batches of L cells (between 25 April 1970 and
10 February 1971), although up to 10-fold variations of the 90%
inhibition end-point were observed (unpublished experiments).

When mouse interferon was assayed in different somatic
monkey-mouse hybrid cell clones or in the parental cells, the
curves were sigmoidal and parallel. When primate interferon was
assayed in parental monkey CV-1 cells, the dose-response curves
obtained were parallel to those of mouse interferon assayed in
hybrid clone 4. On the contrary, the slope of the dose-response

curves for primate interferon simultaneously assayed in hybrid
clone 4 (92nd passage) was completely different. At high concentrations of interferon, the antiviral state was 10- to 20-times
lower in hybrid clone 4 than in parental CV-1 cells. At low concentrations, the opposite was observed: the antiviral protection
was 10- to 20-times greater in the hybrid clone. Thus, the slope
of the dose-response curves was decreased and crossed the sigmoidal curve observed in parental CV-1 cells.

It is of interest that, in spite of different slopes, the
90% inhibition end-point for primate interferon was higher in
hybrid clone 4 than in parental CV-1 cells (Figure 2).

The results reported here were regularly reproducible in
different subclones of clone 2 (M and W) and clone 4 (3, 33 and
35). As in the previous experiments, in all of these hybrid subclones the dose-response effect for mouse interferon was clearly
sigmoidal and parallel to the curves obtained in mouse L cells.
The shape of the dose-response curves for primate interferon in
all the hybrid clones was comparable to that obtained in hybrid
clone 4 (Figure 3). The slopes of the curves varied from one clone
to the other, but were not parallel to that obtained in monkey
CV-1 cells (representative examples are given in Figure 4).

The use of a different challenge virus did not affect the
shape of the dose-response curves in monkey-mouse hybrids. In all
experiments, when EMC virus was used instead of VSV as challenge
virus, the results were similar to those obtained with VSV (unpublished experiments).

The distribution of biarmed chromosomes in the different
hybrid clones suggested that none of the monkey chromosomes are
responsible for the antiviral protein induced by either of the two
interferons. A very very small subtelocentric chromosome (VVSST)

could, however, carry information necessary for the interferon-receptor system.

C. Cooperative response of the monkey and mouse interferon
added simultaneously to hybrid cells.

Cells, MKCV-III clone 2, were treated simultaneously with
increasing concentrations of mouse interferon and a constant
amount of primate interferon (50 reference units) for 24 h. The
amount of primate interferon, when employed alone, induced only a
2-4-fold increase in the hybrids. As shown in Figure 5, 15 or 30
reference units of mouse interferon, for example, had practically
no antiviral effect. Combined with the above mentioned amount of
human interferon, the antiviral state increased 50-100-fold. Similar results were obtained in the presence of a small amount of
murine interferon and increasing concentrations of primate interferon (8).

Discussion

The data here presented clearly show that the receptors for
primate interferon are different from the receptors for murine
interferon. In the parental and hybrid cells, primate receptors
are trypsin-sensitive, while mouse receptors are not. This could
either be related to differences in the chemical nature of the
receptors or to the positioning of the receptors in the cell membrane, making them accessible or not to the proteolytic enzymes.
The analysis of the dose-response curves in the hybrid and parental cells seem to suggest that the antiviral effect is cooperative, involving probably a receptor site which interacts with the
active site of the interferon molecule and an activator site
which triggers the events leading to the antiviral state. The
switch on of the activator site might require interferon mole-

cules, thus explaining the low efficiency of hybrid cells in the
presence of a high concentration of primate interferon and, on the
contrary, their high efficiency when the concentration of interferon molecules is low in the preparation. This could be due to
the decreased number of receptor sites for primate interferon in
the cell membrane or to an inactivation of the activator site related to interactions between monkey and mouse antigens. It is
also feasible that different receptor-activator systems spread
over the cell membrane are interacting with each other and are
successively activated with increasing concentrations of interferon molecules.

Another argument in favor of the cooperative effect of interferon is the result obtained with the combined application of the
two interferons. These two interferons act obviously on different
receptor sites, but since the antiviral effects are potentiated,
it is very likely that only the cell receptors are responsible for
cell species specificity, while all the events following membrane
receptor-activator interactions are not cell species specific. Thus,
none of the chromosomes present in hybrids contain any genetic information involving special primate antiviral protein (see model
represented in Figure 6). The very very small subtelocentric chromosome, previously mentioned as participating at least partially
in the establishment of the antiviral state, is probably involved
in the genetic information responsible for the receptor sites.
Other yet unidentified chromosomes could equally contain genetic
information necessary for the establishment of the antiviral state.

Another implication of this observation is that interferon
probably does not participate as such in the antiviral state it
induces. This is in agreement with the findings presented by Dr.
Ankel on the antiviral effect of insoluble interferon. All these
data do not exclude, nevertheless, the possibility that fragments

from interferon or a modified molecule play a role in the induction of the antiviral state.

As stated in the introductory remarks, it is of interest to compare interferon to hormones. The interferon molecule could thus be a part of a regulatory system including tissue antagonists (9), involved in a yet unidentified manner in the regulation of cell growth.

References

1. Cassingena, R., Chany, C., Vignal, M., Suarez, H., Estrade, S., and Lazar, P. (1971). Proc. Nat. Acad. Sci. USA 68, 580-584.

2. Chany, C., Grégoire, A., Vignal, M., Lemaitre-Moncuit, J., Brown, P., Besançon, F., Suarez, H., and Cassingena, R. (1973). Proc. Nat. Acad. Sci. USA 70, 557-561.

3. Bobrow, M., Madan, K., and Pearson, P.L. (1972). Nature New Biol. 238, 122-124.

4. Chany, C. and Vignal, M. (1968). C.R.H. Acad. Sci. 267, 1798-1800.

5. Ankel, H., Chany, C., Galliot, B., Chevalier, M.J., and Robert, M. (1973). Proc. Nat. Acad. Sci. USA 70, 2360-2363.

6. Gresser, I. (1961). Proc. Soc. Exp. Biol. Med. 108,799.

7. Fournier, F., Falcoff, E., and Chany, C. (1967). J. Immunol. 99, 302-309.

8. Bourgeade, M.F. (1974). C.R.H. Acad. Sci. 278, 165-168.

9. Fournier, F., Rousset, S., and Chany, C. (1969). Proc. Soc. Exp. Biol. Med. 132, 943-950.

TABLE 1

Antiviral effect of primate and of mouse interferon

| | | Interferon | | | |
| | | Human white blood cell | | Mouse | |
Cell type	Dispersing agent	No Serum	2% Calf Serum	No Serum	2% Calf Serum
CV-1	Trypsin	0.07	3.42	N.D.	N.D.
Clone M	Trypsin	0.49	2.06	2.76	2.86
MKS-BU-100	Trypsin	N.D.	N.D.	1.13	1.75
L	Trypsin	N.D.	N.D.	2.80	2.97
CV-1	EDTA	2.86	3.07	N.D.	N.D.
Clone M	EDTA	2.23	2.25	N.D.	N.D.

Antiviral effect of primate and mouse interferon in trypsinized or EDTA-dispersed parental and clone cells. Numbers represent $\log_{10}$ inhibition of VSV yield in interferon-treated cells as compared to contact cells subjected to the same experimental conditions but incubated with media containing no interferon. N.D. means Not Done.

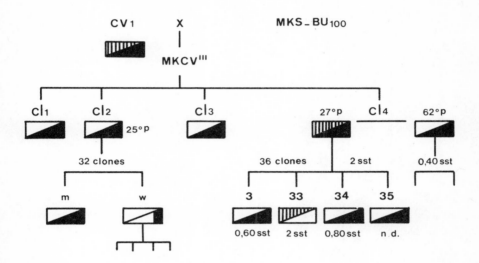

Fig. 1. Selection of clonal populations from MKCV III (monkey-mouse hybrid) clone:

Clones that produce primate interferon and are sensitive to it.

Clones that do not produce primate interferon but are sensitive to it.

Clone (33) producing primate interferon but not sensitive to it.

Clone (W) not producing interferon and only weakly sensitive to it.

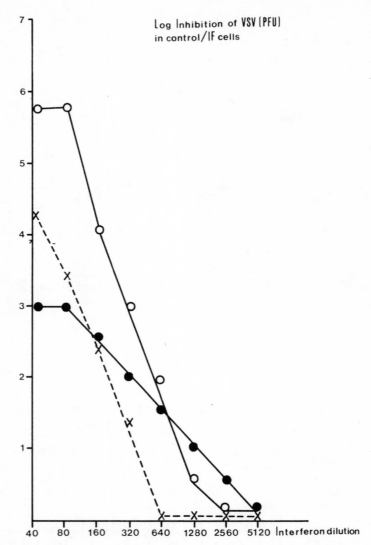

Fig. 2. Dose-response curves (log 10 inhibition) in hybrid clone 4 (92nd passage). O——O, hybrid cl. 4 (mouse interferon); ✗---✗, parental monkey cells (primate interferon); ●——●, hybrid cl. 4 (primate interferon).

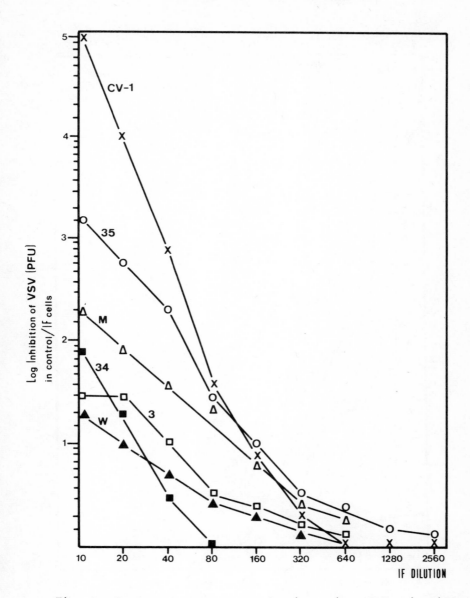

Fig. 3. Dose-response curves of primate interferon in different subclones of hybrid clones 2 and 4: Clone 2 = M and W; Clone 4 = 3, 34 and 35; CV-1 = parental monkey cell lines (See Figure 1 for reference). The slopes of the curves are not parallel and lose their sigmoidicity.

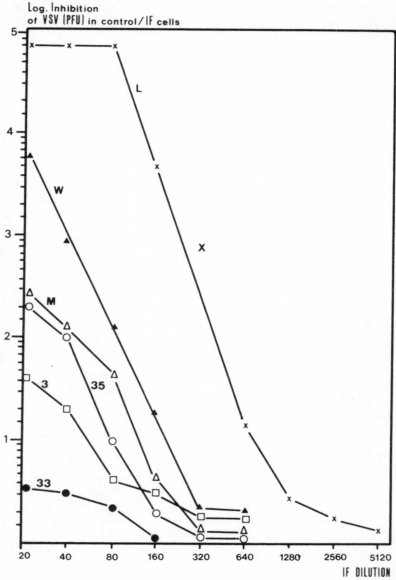

Fig. 4. See legend for Figure 3. Dose-response curves for mouse interferon in the same hybrid cells and in reference L cells. Although significantly different in their sensitivity, the slopes run roughly in parallel.

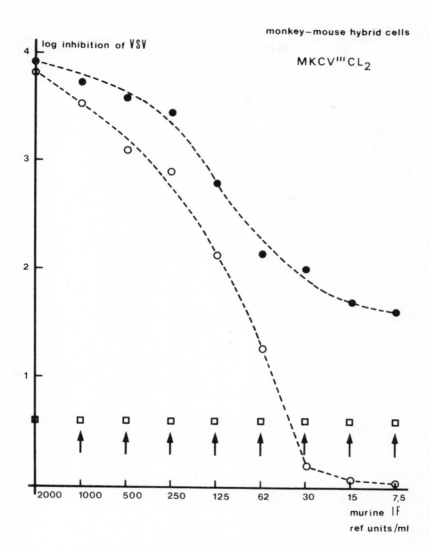

Fig. 5. Dose-response relationship between the amount of interferon is expressed in reference units as the log of the viral yield in control/the log of the viral yield in interferon-treated cells. ●----● Cells treated with murine and primate interferons; O----O Cells treated with murine interferon; □   □ Cells treated with a constant amount of primate interferon.

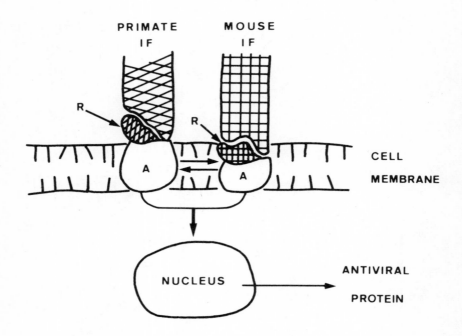

IF- INTERFERON ; A-ACTIVATOR SITE ; R- RECEPTOR SITE

Fig. 6. Model of the receptor-activator system in somatic mon-key-mouse hybrid cells. Both receptors are closely connected to activator sites. The receptor site for primate interferon could become extruded from the cell membrane, thus accessible to trypsin. Both primate and mouse interferon are able to interact only with their own receptor sites and trigger activator sites. Each indi-vidual receptor-activator system could affect neighboring sites, thus cooperating with each other, spreading their effect all over the cell membrane. The subsequent events follow a common pathway, explaining the potentiation of mouse by primate interferon and vice versa. This can only be obtained in hybrid cells and stipu-late the integrity of the two receptor systems.

DISCUSSION

Pereira: Have you analyzed your dose-response curves to see how they fit with Poisson distribution?

Chany: We haven't performed any detailed mathematical analysis of the curves. The shape of the curve is sigmoidal whatever scale (arithmetical or logarithmic) is used.

Pereira: What about the slope?

Chany: The slope itself is variable. For instance, in some cells the slope might change after the use of mutagens. The slope is probably in relationship with the number of receptor sites available on cell membranes.

Pereira: I can visualize that irrespective of the number of receptor sites available, the number of interferon molecules required to produce an effect might lead to either a single hit or a multiple hit curve.

Chany: Well, a single hit curve should give a linear dose-response, which is never observed.

Pereira: This is what I wanted to know, because I suppose you can decide according to Poisson distribution whether one of these curves fits with a single hit or a multiple hit, and I wondered whether such an analysis was possible or not.

Levy: This single hit versus multiple hit may be totally confusing in this situation. If the interferon molecule reacts momentarily with the cell, then comes off and comes back and keeps biting at the cell, nibbling at it frequently, I think that type of analysis is not going to be applicable.

Chany: But then we get back to the multiple hit system. If the same molecule hits only once or several times I think the end results on the cell are the same.

Tan: I understand that one of your hybrid clones produces monkey interferon but is insensitive to monkey interferon.

Chany: Yes indeed.

Tan: How do you establish the independence of the interferon receptor site and the antiviral protein?

Chany: Well, the antiviral protein is certainly synthesized, since the cell is highly sensitive to mouse interferon. However, in the clone you mentioned, the antiviral state cannot be induced with human interferon. The most satisfactory explanation is that the receptor site is probably missing. We have subcloned these cells and have clearly segregated, about 50%-50%, cell clones with or without monkey receptors. The study of chromosomal segregation seems to indicate that chromosome 29, which resembles the human G 21, is perhaps involved. In answer to Dr. Levy's question about the cooperative effect, Dr. Bourgeade has found that small amounts of interferon of both types, added simultaneously to the cells, were 10-100-fold more active, as expected when comparing the results to the antiviral state obtained with each interferon alone. In addition, we have shown in this study that receptor sites for monkey-mouse interferon are separate. Thus, no competition occurs, in this hybrid, between the two interferons for the receptors.

Burke: I was thinking of the Sheaff and Stewart paper (Can. J. Microbiol. 14, 965) where they showed that the interferon pretreatment with a very small dose affected the subsequent action of interferon. I wondered if you had looked at the dose-response curves after pre-treatment with very small doses, because they might get an alteration of the slope.

Chany: Exactly. We have published this with Dr. Besançon and found the pre-treatment with small doses of interferon changes the slopes of the dose-response curves of interferon added 4 hours later. The slope is more and more horizontal, depending on the amount of interferon used for pre-treatment.

Tovey: I was wondering if in the interpretation of your dose-response curves, it might not help to plot probits instead of your sigmoidal curve; then you would get a linear relationship over a wider range.

Chany: This is true, but this would only be a mathematical transformation of the curve.

Tovey: Yes, but with probits you can then take into consideration the two ends of the curve. You get a linear relationship over a wider range.

Chany: Yes.

UPTAKE OF INTERFERON :
THE FATE OF CELL-BOUND INTERFERON DURING INDUCTION
OF ANTIVIRAL AND NON-ANTIVIRAL ACTIVITIES

(Dedicated to the Memory of Professor S.Edward SULKIN,1908-1972)

William E. Stewart II[*]

Rega Institute for Medical Research
University of Leuven
Leuven, Belgium

The interaction of interferon with cells leads to alterations that are both antiviral and non-antiviral (1), but it has
not yet been resolved whether interferon itself takes a direct
part in the expression of any of the alterations it induces.

On the one hand, de novo protein synthesis is required in
interferon-treated cells for them to become resistant to viruses
(2, 3, 4, 5), and it has, therefore, been widely accepted that
interferon is not itself antiviral but rather induces cells to
produce a purported antiviral protein.

On the other hand, it has been proferred that interferon is
itself antiviral but that cells require an induced product (possibly a permease) to get interferon into its antiviral location
within the cell (6, 7). However, Stewart and Lockart (8) have
argued that if such were the case, the relative antiviral resist-

[*] Aided by Grant DRG-1219 from the Damon Runyon Memorial Fund for
     Cancer Research, and Grant 310 from the Jane Coffin Childs
     Memorial Fund for Medical Research.

ance induced by cross-reactive interferons should be specified by
the interferon, not by the treated cell; these authors, however,
found the contrary: the relative antiviral resistance induced by
heterologous interferon is characteristic of the resistance induced in the treated cells by homologous interferon (9). This led
the author to agree with the prevalent presumption that interferon
was not itself involved in the antiviral activity it induces. However, as Colby and Morgan (10) and, more recently, Weber and
Stewart (7), have correctly pointed out, the data to date have not
excluded the possibility that interferon might itself be involved
as a co-antiviral substance with the induced cell component(s)
which would determine the characteristics of the resistance. Thus,
though an induced cell product is needed (as further evidenced by
the requirement of a nucleus in the cell (11)) it still remains a
possibility that interferon is itself involved in the antiviral
activity it induces in cells.

With regard to the non-antiviral activities induced by interferon, Stewart et al. (12, 13), and, more recently Barmak and
Vilcek (14), have reported that de novo protein synthesis is not
required for cells to become primed by interferon, and it appears
also that protein synthesis is not required for interferon-treated
cells to develop enhanced susceptibility to the toxicity of ds-RNA
(W.E. Stewart II, unpublished data). These findings increase the
likelihood that interferon might itself directly take part in at
least some of the alterations it induces.

To resolve the possible role played by interferon in the activities it induces, I have attempted to determine the nature of
the interaction of interferon with cells and to determine its
presence in, or on, cells under conditions allowing development
of antiviral and/or non-antiviral activities.

The initial interaction of interferon with cells has previously been studied in several ways (reviewed by Stewart et al.,
15). Attempts to determine adsorption of interferon by measuring
its disappearance from the medium applied to cells have been particularly fruitless. Some workers have shown that interferon is
taken up in appreciable amounts; others have shown it was not de-
tectably taken up; some have found it was inactivated by cells,
and some found that it adsorbed non-specifically to various sur-
faces.

Several studies have provided indirect evidence that interferon binds to cells. Cells exposed to interferon in the cold and
washed prior to incubation at 37 C develop antiviral activity and
become primed; however, cells exposed to interferon in the cold
and treated with trypsin prior to transfer to 37 C fail to develop
antiviral activity (16, 17) or priming (W.E. Stewart II, unpublished data). These indirect data suggested that interferon binds
to cells, but it was also possible that interferon had acted as a
catalyst to initiate a superficial alteration that was itself trypsin sensitive.

Attempts to directly measure the presence of interferon in
cells have been few. Levine (18) and Friedman (16) have both reported recovering antiviral activity (presumably the applied interferon) from interferon-treated cells, provided sufficiently high
concentrations of interferon were applied to the cells. However,
it remained uncertain what amount, if any, of the recovered activity represented interferon that was involved in a meaningful relationship with the cells.

I have previously reported (Stewart et al., 40) that the
amounts of interferon that can be recovered from interferon-treated cells is in good correlation with the relative sensitivities of

the cells to the antiviral activity of the interferon (Table I).
However, due to the conditions used in such experiments (that is,
monolayer cultures of cells exposed to relatively large volumes
of interferon), these data did not allow correlations of the ability to recover interferon from cells with a corresponding reduction of activity of the applied interferon, most probably owing
to imprecisions in assaying interferons. The calculated recovery
of applied interferon represents total applied units minus recovered cell-bound units; obviously it would require a more precise interferon assay to confidently distinguish between initial
titers of 100 units/ml and residual titers of 99, 97 or even 85
units/ml. Therefore, the possibility remained that the failure to
recover interferon from heterologous cells and the recovery of
different amounts of interferon from cells with different interferon sensitivities could merely have reflected differences in
the abilities of the cells to inactivate interferon after it was
bound, though identical amounts could have bound to each cell
type. This inactivation of bound interferon by insensitive cells
would also explain its inactivity or lesser activity in such
cells.

Preliminary studies using the type of interferon-binding
system employed in Table I (that is, monolayer cultures exposed
to large volumes of interferon) showed that binding was complete
within a short time and that the amount of interferon bound was
dependent on both numbers of cells and interferon concentration,
but was independent of the total amount of interferon applied
(Stewart et al., 15). This suggested that by applying interferon
to large numbers of cells in small volumes, it might be possible
to correlate the amount of interferon recovered from cells with
losses of the activity from the applied interferon. Such a relationship would be dependent on interferon-cell interactions following the law of mass action and would imply that the increased

sensitivity of some cells to interferon results from the presence of excess numbers of receptors on such cells. Such a situation has been reported for interactions of polypeptide hormones with their target cells (19, 20, 21, 22, 23).

To determine whether this relationship also exists between interferon and cells, experiments were directed toward better defining the nature of the initial interaction of interferons and cells.

For these experiments, suspension culture cells were employed, as these were better suited for studies involving high concentrations of cells. Lpa-cells, harvested during logarithmic growth, were resuspended at 10^8 cells in 1 ml of medium containing 10^4 units of interferon. At 37°C binding was maximal by about 10 minutes (Fig. 1); the binding rate was slower at 4°C, but by 30 minutes the amounts of interferon recoverable were the same at 4°C and 37°C. In other experiments, binding kinetics were similar for L-929 cells, but the plateau of recoverable interferon was approximately 3 times higher, in agreement with the greater sensitivity of L-929 cells to interferon. The reported kinetics of binding of insulin to target cells are very similar to the interaction shown here, and the rate of hormone-receptor interaction is also temperature dependent (19, 21, 22, 23, 24).

When a constant number of cells was incubated for 1 hour with 1 ml containing increasing concentrations of interferon, binding was seen to be a function of interferon concentration (Fig. 2), and increasing amounts of interferon could be recovered from cells. In these experiments, about 10^4 units/ml appeared to be the saturating concentration of interferon for 10^8 cells of either Lpa or L-929. In the presence or absence of saturating concentrations, L-929 cells consistently bound more interferon than did Lpa cells. Since L-929 cells are more sensitive to both the

antiviral and non-antiviral effects of interferon, these data are
consistent with the interpretation that cells equipped with a
larger number of interferon receptors are more sensitive to interferon; since, according to the law of mass action, such cells
would be able to bind the amount of interferon necessary to induce
its effects even when the interferon concentration is low. Of
course, this interpretation would, again, be contingent upon relative recoveries of interferon from these cells not merely reflecting relative abilities of the cells to inactivate interferon while
they bound similar amounts.

When a constant concentration of interferon in 1 ml was incubated with increasing numbers of cells, binding was seen as a
function of cell concentration (Fig. 3). With each concentration
of interferon (except the apparent saturating concentration) it
is possible to plot the amount of interferon recoverable from any
given number of cells. The linear relationships of binding to
these cells (in the absence of saturating concentration), which
occurred irrespective of the purity of the interferon preparation
used, appears to be a relationship reflecting the specificity of
interferon binding. In view of these data, and by extrapolating
the plots, it is not surprising that several workers, using relatively low concentrations of interferon or low numbers of cells,
or both, have been unable to demonstrate either reduction of activity of applied interferon or recovery of measurable cell-bound
interferon.

In view of these findings, the initial studies comparing
relative amounts of interferon recoverable from different cells
with different interferon sensitivities were repeated, this time
using optimal conditions for determining whether the differences
in amounts of interferon recovered merely reflected differences
in abilities of different cells to inactivate bound interferon.

Pellets containing approximately 10^8 Lpa cells or L-929 cells were
incubated for 1 hour with increasing concentrations of interferon
in 1 ml of medium (Table 2). Applied interferon was recovered and
assayed for residual activity, and cell-associated activity was
determined. Even with the imprecisions of interferon assays, it
can be seen that, in the absence of saturating concentrations of
interferon, there is a good correlation between the amount of
interferon recoverable from cells and the amount lost from the applied interferon. If the different amounts recovered from cells
merely reflected differences in abilities of cells to inactivate
interferon, residual supernatant titers would not be additive with
cell-bound interferon, as is the case. These data, therefore, substantiate the interpretation that the interferon binding is specific and relates quantitatively to the cellular alterations induced by interferon.

Experiments were, therefore, designed to determine the location of interferon during the development of the activities it
induces. Previous studies have demonstrated that interferon binds
to cells at both 4°C and 37°C; however, if interferon is bound to
cells in the cold and removed by trypsin before they are incubated at 37°C, cells do not become primed or virus resistant.This
suggests there are two stages in effective binding: the first,
occurring in the cold, cannot be washed off but is reversed by
trypsin. The second stage proceeds from the first very rapidly as
cells are transferred to 37°C, and its effects are not reversible
by trypsin. I, therefore, determined the effects of trypsin on the
recovery of bound interferon from cells in the two stages of binding. Cells were incubated at 4°C with interferon and at intervals
were washed and assayed for cell-bound interferon, or they were
treated with trypsin at 4°C, washed and assayed for cell-bound
interferon. At all times, interferon bound to cells at 4°C was accessible to removal by trypsin (Fig. 4). However, when interferon

was bound to cells at 37°C, it was largely protected from removal
by trypsin. Thus it appears that at 37°C, other reactions in addition to superficial binding take place, and since interferon's
presence is required during these events for induction of antiviral or non-antiviral activities, it is tempting to speculate
that the uptake observed to occur here is also a requirement. However, these data, showing uptake of soluble interferon, do not exclude that uptake could be prevented by binding interferon to an
insoluble matrix and still have effective binding at 37°C. Indeed,
the interpretation of Ankel et al. (25) is that no uptake is required, though 37°C-binding is required; it should be pointed out,
however, that their interpretation was based on the assumption
that no 'leakage' of matrix-bound interferon had occurred, a possibility not excluded by their data.

Since our experiments seemed to suggest a requirement for
uptake, experiments were performed to follow interferon into
cells, to determine its localization under conditions allowing development of the alterations it induces. Interferon was bound to
cells for various times at 4°C and at 37°C; washed cells were
broken up and separated into 'nuclear' fractions, 'membrane' fraction and 'sap' fractions, which were assayed for interferon content (Fig. 5). At 4°C all the cell-bound interferon was recovered
in the membrane fraction at $2\frac{1}{2}$ and 5 minutes. Thus, like the
receptor for polypeptide hormones (19, 20, 21, 26, 27, 28), interferon receptors are apparently located on the plasma membrane.This
is not surprising in view of the trypsin sensitivity of interferon
bound to cells at 4°C (Fig. 4). By 10 minutes enough interferon
was bound that interferon also appeared in the nuclear pellets;it
seems likely that this resulted from contamination of the nuclear
pellets with membrane. At 4°C, no soluble or 'sap' interferon was
found at any time during binding. At 37°C, interferon was recovered in the nuclear pellet and this could not be attributed to con-

taminating membrane: nuclear and membrane interferon levels were
about the same at 2 $\frac{1}{2}$ and 5 minutes, but by 10 minutes, nuclear
interferon levels were much higher than the membrane interferon
titers. Also, 'sap' interferon levels were about the same as membrane interferon levels. These experiments suggest, therefore,
that at 37°C, under conditions allowing induction and development
of antiviral and non-antiviral activities, interferon that initially bound to membrane receptors quickly became associated with
the nuclear fraction, perhaps after first being released from the
membranes into the cytoplasmic sap. Such release from membrane
receptors apparently does not occur at 4°C.

Since, in the experiments shown in Fig. 5, the applied
interferon was constantly present in the medium, continued binding perhaps maintained the levels recovered in the fractions and
masked the eclipse, loss, or movement of interferon. Therefore,it
seemed that by binding interferon to cells and chasing it with
interferon-free medium, it would be possible to determine its location at intervals after binding and during development and expression of antiviral and non-antiviral activity. Therefore,cells
incubated for 1 hour with interferon were washed, re-incubated
with interferon-free medium and assayed at intervals thereafter
for cell-associated interferon. Cultures similarly treated with
interferon were washed and at intervals were appropriately challenged to determine the development of antiviral activity, priming, or enhanced susceptibility to the toxicity of ds-RNA. Virus
challenge was VSV containing actinomycin D to prevent subsequent
development of antiviral activity after adding the challenge;
priming challenge was poly I.poly C which does not induce interferon in L-cells in the absence of DEAE-dextran unless they are
first treated with interferon (29, 30, 31). It was not possible
to arrest cell syntheses along with the priming challenge since
these processes are required for the interferon production; tox-

icity challenge was poly I.poly C containing actinomycin D and
cycloheximide to prevent further development of this activity
after adding the toxic challenge (this is possible since cell
synthetic processes are not required for development of ds-RNA
toxicity in interferon-treated cells) (32). Both priming and toxicity enhancement were fully developed by the time the applied
interferon was removed and the interferon-free medium was added
to the cultures (Fig. 6). However, no detectable antiviral activity had developed at this time, and virus resistance did not
begin to develop for another hour. Virus resistance was completely developed by 3 hours after addition of the interferon-free
medium. All the induced activities (antiviral resistance, priming,
and toxicity-enhancement) remained at maximum levels as long as 8
hours after addition of the interferon-free medium. However, cell-
associated interferon levels began falling almost as soon as the
interferon was removed from the environment, and by 3 hours interferon was no longer detectable in cell pellets.

Thus, while the non-antiviral activities induced by the
interferon remained at maximal levels, the cell-associated interferon levels declined rapidly, and while the cell-bound interferon
level was rapidly decreasing, the antiviral activity induced by
interferon was rapidly increasing. These data, showing an inverse
relationship between the development of the effects induced by
interferon and the presence of cell-associated interferon suggested that either the cells rapidly inactivated the bound interferon
or that interferon became bound in cell components in such a way
that activity was not recoverable.

However, when the interferon-free chase media were recovered and assayed for interferon, it became apparent that the cells
did not inactivate the bound interferon or bind it in some unre-
coverable manner (Fig. 7). Rather, virtually all of the cell-bound

interferon disappearing from the cells at each interval after
binding was recovered in the chase medium. Therefore, the interferon-cell interaction (again, like those involving polypeptide
hormones and their target cells) (19, 23) is a dissociable process with an interferon-receptor half-life of about 30 minutes.
These data, showing that interferon is dissociating from cells as
the levels of its induced activities are increasing, strongly
suggest that interferon is not itself involved in any of the alterations it induces in cells.

In conclusion, the following statements appear to apply to
the interaction of interferon with homologous cells and to the
interactions of polypeptide hormones with their target cells. The
first step in action appears to be interaction with specific receptors that are located in the plasma membranes (19, 20, 21, 27,
26, 28). The binding is a time and temperature dependent process
that follows the law of mass action and is saturable (19, 21, 22,
23, 24). The binding does not involve formation of stable covalent
bonds but is a dissociable process which does not result in degradation of the effector molecule (19, 28, 22, 23).

Several analogies can also be found in hormone and interferon systems regarding the quantitative aspects of binding and
activation of the cellular effects induced. In the systems reported here, the amounts of interferon binding correlated with the
sensitivity of the cells to interferon; apparently this relationship also exists in certain other interferon-cell systems (33, 34,
35). Similarly, several studies have shown a correlation between
hormone receptor numbers and hormone responsiveness. Independent
studies have shown a striking decrease in insulin binding sites
in liver and adipose cells from genetically obese mice (27, 24)
and in lymphocytes of insulin-resistant patients with acromegaly
(23). However, it should be evident from the scheme shown in Fig.8

(which could relate to hormone-cell interactions as well) (36)
that differences in the numbers of receptors is only one of the
ways in which responsiveness can be altered. Biological potency
would be a measure of binding and the efficacy of the effector-
receptor complex in activating cellular processes. Therefore, alterations in receptor affinity or in the coupling of receptors to
each of the more distal cellular processes could also explain
differences in responsiveness of cells. For example, while differences in binding appear to explain some differences in inter-
feron-sensitivities, it does not appear to explain all cases (34;
Stewart II, unpublished data). Also, insulin-resistant cells from
starved rats showed no reduction in either quantity or affinity
of insulin-binding (37); therefore, this difference likely
results from changes in processes which occur after the initial
interaction. Such cells could, for example, possess receptors
that are not coupled to an effector system, such as the adenyl
cyclase system found in many of the hormone-sensitive tissues
(38, 39). To induce any cellular alterations, antiviral or non-
antiviral, interferon (IF; Fig. 8) must bind to receptors (R) in
the plasma membrane; and the interferon-receptor complex (IF.R)
must be activated (Fig. 8,a) at 37 C to induce any of the alterations. However, once the activation has occurred the sequences of
events leading to the various alterations may become diversified.
For example, while development of antiviral activity requires me-
diation through the nucleus (11), with subsequent m-RNA and protein synthesis, development of certain of the other alterations
induced by interferon (for instance priming and toxicity-enhancement), which do not appear to depend on such processes (12, 30,
14), may proceed directly from activation or perhaps from any of
the more distal processes.

While the data do show that interferon goes into cells under
conditions allowing it to exert cellular alterations, they do not

show that it is necessary for interferon to do so to exert these effects. The data suggest that interferon could itself participate in some of the events leading to the expression of the alterations, since interferon appears to become associated with internal components subsequent to interferon-receptor activation. However, the complete dissociation of interferon from cells, while the effects it induces are maintained at maximal levels or are still increasing, strongly suggest that interferon is not itself participating in the alterations it induces.

References

1. Stewart, W.E. II, and De Clercq, E. (1973). Medikon 2, 279.
2. Levine, S. (1964). Virology 24, 586.
3. Lockart, R.Z. Jr. (1964). Biochem. Biophys. Res. Commun. 15, 513.
4. Taylor, J. (1964). Biochem. Biophys. Res. Commun. 14, 447.
5. Friedman, R.M., and Sonnabend, J.A. (1965). J. Immunol. 95, 696.
6. Sheaff, E.T., and Stewart, R.B. (1969). Can. J. Microbiol. 15, 941.
7. Weber, J.M., and Stewart, R.B. (1973). J. Gen. Virol. 19, 165.
8. Stewart, W.E. II, and Lockart, R.Z. Jr. (1970). J.Virol. 6, 795.
9. Stewart, W.E. II, Scott, W.D., and Sulkin, S.E. (1969). J. Virol. 4, 147.
10. Colby, C., and Morgan, M.J. (1971). Ann. Rev. Microbiol. 25, 333.

11. Kates, J.R., Radke, K.L., and Colby, C. (1973). Abstr. Ann. Meeting Amer. Soc. Microbiol. V. 267.

12. Stewart, W.E. II, Gosser, L.B., and Lockart, R.Z. Jr. (1971). J. Virol. 7, 792.

13. Stewart, W.E. II, Gosser, L.B., and Lockart, R.Z. Jr. (1972). J. Gen. Virol. 15, 85.

14. Barmak, S.L., and Vilcek, J. (1973). Arch. Ges. Virusforsch., in press.

15. Stewart, W.E. II, De Clercq, E., and De Somer, P. (1972). J. Virol. 10, 707.

16. Friedman, R.M. (1967). Science 156, 1760.

17. Goldsby, R.A. (1967). Experientia 23, 1073.

18. Levine, S. (1966). Proc. Soc. Exp. Biol. Med. 121, 1041.

19. Cuatrecasas, P. (1971). Proc. Nat. Acad. Sci. USA 68, 1264.

20. Cuatrecasas, P., Desbuquois, B., and Krug, F. (1971). Biochem. Biophys. Res. Commun. 44, 333.

21. Freychet, P., Roth, J., and Neville, D.M. Jr. (1971). Proc. Nat. Acad. Sci. USA 68, 1833.

22. Kono, T., and Barham, F.W. (1971). J. Biol. Chem. 246, 6210.

23. Gavin, J.R. III, Roth, J., Jen, P., and Freychet, P. (1972). Proc. Nat. Acad. Sci. USA 69, 747.

24. Kahn, C.R., Neville, D.M. Jr., Gorden, P., Freychet, P., and Roth, J. (1972). Biochem. Biophys. Res. Commun. 48, 135.

25. Ankel, H., Chany, C., Galliot, B., Chevalier, M.J., and Robert, M. (1973). Proc. Nat. Acad. Sci. USA 70, 2360.

26. Hall, Z.W. (1972). Ann. Rev. Biochem. 41, 925.

27. Freychet, P., Laudat, M.H., and Laudat, P. (1972). FEBS Letters 25, 339.

28. Cuatrecasas, P. (1972). J. Biol. Chem. 24, 1980.

29. Rosztoczy, I. (1971). Acta Virol. <u>15</u>, 431.

30. Stewart, W.E. II, De Clercq, E., Billiau, A., Desmyter, J., and De Somer, P. (1972). Proc. Nat. Acad. Sci. USA <u>69</u>, 1851.

31. Stewart, W.E. II, De Clercq, E., and De Somer, P. (1972). J. Virol. <u>10</u>, 896.

32. Stewart, W.E. II, De Clercq, E., and De Somer, P.(1973). J. Gen. Virol. <u>18</u>, 237.

33. Berman, B., and Vilcek, J. (1973). Personal communication.

34. Gresser, I. (1973). Personal communication.

35. Weil, R. (1973). Personal communication.

36. Lefkowitz, R.J. (1973). New Engl. J. Med. <u>288</u>, 1061.

37. Bennett, G.V., and Cuatrecasas, P. (1972). Science <u>176</u>, 805.

38. Sutherland, E.W., Robison, G.A., and Butcher, R.W. (1968). Circulation <u>37</u>, 279.

39. Illiano, G., and Cuatrecasas, P. (1972). Science <u>175</u>, 906.

40. Stewart, W.E. II, Gosser, L.B., and Lockart, R.Z. Jr. (1971). J. Gen. Virol. <u>13</u>, 35.

WILLIAM E. STEWART II

TABLE 1

CORRELATION OF SENSITIVITIES OF CELLS TO MOUSE INTERFERON AND AMOUNT
OF INTERFERON RECOVERABLE FROM CELLS

| CELLS | ANTIVIRAL TITER ON INDICATED CELLS | UNITS APPLIED * | | UNITS RECOVERED | | |
| | | UNITS/ml | TOTAL (units/ml×50) | CELL BOUND | SUPERNATANT | |
					CALCULATED (TOTAL-CELL BOUND)	EXPERIMENTAL
MOUSE Lpa	$10^{1.5}$	100	5000	50	4950 (99 UNITS/ml)	~5000
MOUSE L929	10^{2}	100	5000	150	4850 (97 UNITS/ml)	~5000
PRIMARY MOUSE EMBRYO FIBROBLASTS	$10^{2.5}$	100	5000	750	4250 (85 UNITS/ml)	~5000
PRIMARY RABBIT KIDNEY	$<10^{0.5}$	100	5000	<15	~5000	~5000
HUMAN DIPLOID	$<10^{0.5}$	100	5000	<15	~5000	~5000

* UNITS ASSAYED ON L929 CELLS

TABLE 2

COMPARISONS OF ABILITY TO RECOVER INTERFERON FROM CELLS AND
ABILITIES OF CELLS TO REDUCE ACTIVITY OF APPLIED INTERFERON

INTERFERON APPLIED (UNITS IN 1 ml) *	CELLS	INTERFERON CELL-BOUND	RECOVERED SUPERNATANT
10^{1}	Lpa	<10	<10
	L929	15	<10
10^{2}	Lpa	30	50
	L929	100	<10
10^{3}	Lpa	300	1000
	L929	1000	100
10^{4}	Lpa	300	10,000
	L929	2000	10,000
10^{5}	Lpa	500	100,000
	L929	2000	100,000

* PDD$_{50}$ - VSV ON L929 CELLS.

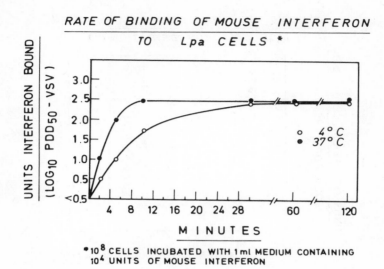

Fig. 1.   Kinetics of binding of mouse interferon to mouse Lpa
cells.

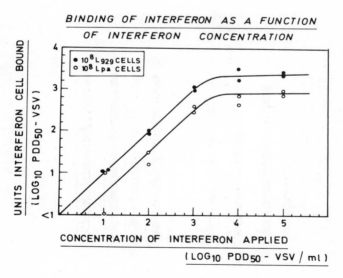

Fig. 2.   Binding of mouse interferon to mouse cells as a function of the concentration of interferon in the medium.

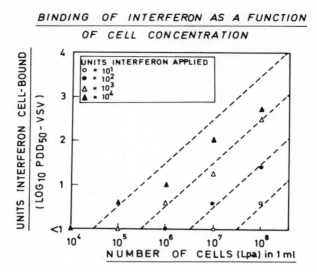

Fig. 3. Binding of mouse interferon to mouse Lpa cells as a function of the concentration of cells in the medium.

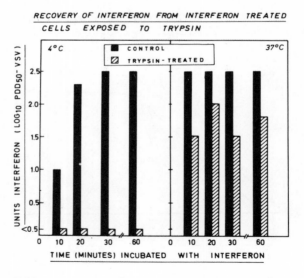

Fig. 4. Effect of trypsin on the recovery of interferon from cells exposed to interferon at 4° C and 37° C.

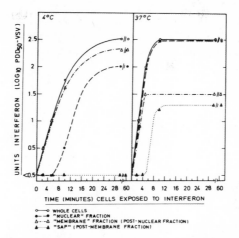

Fig. 5.   Localization of cell-bound interferon under conditions preventing or allowing development of the alterations it induces in cells.

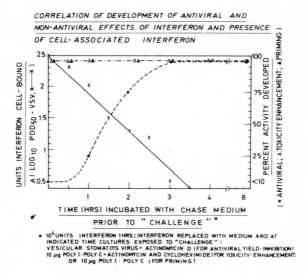

Fig. 6.   Fate of cell-bound interferon during induction and expression of antiviral and non-antiviral activities: inverse relationship between cellular alterations induced by interferon and the ability to recover cell-associated interferon.

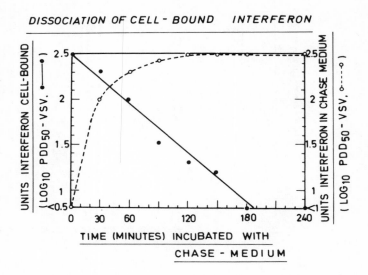

Fig. 7. Fate of cell-bound interferon during induction and expression of antiviral and non-antiviral activities: dissociation of interferon from cells.

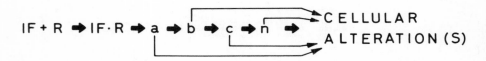

Fig. 8. Sequencies of reactions leading to cellular alterations induced by interferon.

DISCUSSION

Ankel: Is the material that you recover from the cells the
same interferon that you added originally, or could it be possible
that it is generated after the cells have been in contact with
interferon? In other words, have you checked whether it has the
same properties as the added interferon, like for example, the
same molecular weight?

Stewart: We haven't done molecular weight determinations,
but we've fully characterized this recoverable antiviral activity
as interferon, and the inhibitor is also recoverable from metabolically inactive cells, indicating that it is not an induced
product, and it has the physical and chemical characteristics of
interferon.

Burke: Maybe I have missed this, but when you talked about
the events which are not dependent upon cycloheximide-toxicity
enhancement, for example, you said that a nuclear event is not
involved. Did you show that there was no binding to the nucleus
at 37° C in the presence of cycloheximide?

Stewart: I've done these experiments, but I didn't show
them here. Binding is identical in interferon-treated cells with
cycloheximide; nuclear association appears the same also.

Burke: So if that binds...

Stewart: It doesn't appear to be inhibitory to the uptake.

Vilcek: Don't you find it is somewhat strange that you get
the recovery of interferon in your interferon-free medium from

cells after the binding and yet you find that interferon is taken
up and reaches the nucleus? This would mean that interferon goes
in, goes through the nucleus, and then again comes out unaltered.

Stewart: I made several analogies to the polypeptide hormone situation, and this does not appear to be one of the con-
formities to that hypothesis. This appears more like the steroid
hormones which apparently have cytoplasmic receptors and migrate
to the nucleus after complexing with this cytoplasmic receptor;
but they also elute from the nucleus after the external environment has been freed of the effector.

Grossberg: It seems that you are recovering relatively low
quantities of interferon. Technical details of how you recover
your interferon can make a difference in how you draw your conclusions. How do you recover your membranes? Do you sonicate in
order to recover interferon from the membranes?

Stewart: Let me answer your last question first. The sonication is a convenient procedure that I use to assure a homogeneous distribution of the sampling; sonication has no effect on
the amount of recovery. This appears to be because the interferon
in the assay system elutes from the particles to which it is
bound. The first question was regarding the quantitative aspect: In some of our experiments, the recovery is as much as two
or three thousand units from the cells and these are sufficient
quantities to assure that I'm not dealing with obscure numbers.

Grossberg: The question is whether this amount of recovery is related to treatment of the membranes in order to dis-
lodge the interferon.

Stewart: The amount recoverable from the precipitable membranes is of course dependent on the speed of the experimentation,

for example. These procedures involving rapid recovery of interferon have to be done under hurried conditions. You have to precipitate before the material elutes and the half life of elution
is approximately half an hour; so this is possible because I only
swell the cells in RSB (reticulocyte standard buffer) for five
minutes; I dounce these and pellet membranes after the nucleus.
The nuclear pellet is a hundred gs for two minutes. The membrane
pellet is then approximately two thousand gs for half an hour at
4° C.

Pitha: I was wondering, when you tested the nuclei bound
interferon, whether you treated the nuclei in some special way?
If we look at the steroid hormones, the receptors have high affinity for the steroid, and if you have the interferon bound to
the nuclei, you can assume that it would bind to some part very
strongly. It rather surprises me that the interferon could be
bound to nucleochromatine and still be biologically active unless
you redissociated it in some way.

Stewart: I haven't checked this possibility. The only thing
is that it appears to me that the elution from nuclei or dissociation is identical to that from intact cells or from cytoplasmic
membranes.

Friedman: How far have you pursued the specificity of the
binding? In most cases I think people who have looked for this
have not found as great a specificity as you found. It is really
rather central to the issue that you are raising.

Stewart: Yes, I mentioned that briefly, that there are
situations where this binding does not appear to relate to the
effects induced. I have no ready explanation. I have also systems
where I get some binding, where there is no induction of these activities. The systems that I picked here to demonstrate the point

show this specificity of binding, and I believe Dr. Berman has some results that are consistent with this interpretation, too.

ANTIVIRAL EFFECT OF INTERFERON COVALENTLY BOUND TO SEPHAROSE

H. Ankel[*], C. Chany, B. Galliot,
M.J. Chevalier, and M. Robert

Institut National de la Santé et de la Recherche Médicale,
U.43, Hôpital St. Vincent de Paul,
74, avenue Denfert Rochereau, 75014 Paris, France

We should like to report some experiments which strongly
suggest that Interferon does not enter the cell in order to induce the antiviral state. Cuatrecasas has shown that insulin covalently attached to Sepharose-beads several times bigger than
cells retains its hormonal effect (1). These experiments demonstrate that insulin does not penetrate into the cell to exert its
activity. We have used the same approach in our attempts to investigate whether Interferon reacts after penetration or not.

Crude mouse Interferon obtained by induction of L-cells
with NDV (Hertfordshire) or polyIC was concentrated by pressure
dialysis and incubated with cyanogen bromide-activated Sepharose
4-B, as described for other proteins by Porath et al. (2). After
incubation at room temperature for two hours, unreacted immino
ester groups were reacted with ethanolamine and the beads were
exhaustively washed with buffer at pH 2 and 8 in alternating se-
quence to remove any noncovalently linked protein. Control preparations were prepared identically, only that in this case in-

---

[*] On leave from the Medical College of Wisconsin, Milwaukee,
Wisconsin USA.

cubation was first with ethanolamine, than with Interferon. The
Interferon titers in the supernate before and after incubation
with cyanogen bromide-activated Sepharose are shown in the first
table (Table 1), also the amounts of protein that remained after
treatment. As seen in the table, practically all of the Interferon originally present and approximately 50% of the protein had
disappeared from the supernate. Washed Interferon beads or control beads were then layered on top of monolayers of sensitive
L-cells and incubated for 18 hrs at 37° as shown in Fig. 1. When
observed with an optical microscope in phase contrast, one bead
covered an average area of about 14 cells; however, because of
its spherical shape, one bead probably touched one or a very small
number of cells at any given time. It is of importance to note
that control as well as Interferon-beads did not attach strongly
to the cell surface, but were rolling on the tissue culture sheet
with the movements of currents in the culture medium.

    Interferon activity was only associated with washed Inter-
feron-Sepharose particles. Cyanogen bromide-activated Sepharose
that was inactivated with ethanolamine before incubation with
Interferon had no antiviral effect. These data indicate that
Interferon binds covalently through the immino ester sites on the
Sepharose, since the binding of Interferon was abolished by saturating these sites with ethanolamine. When the dose response relationship between the number of Interferon-Sepharose beads employed
and the antiviral state was studied, the surprising observation
was made that one bead per 40 cells was sufficient to induce maximal inhibition of the replication of Encephalomyocarditis virus.
Even one bead per 400 cells resulted in 99% inhibition of viral
yield. When VSV instead of EMC was employed as challenge virus, the
number of beads that caused maximal inhibition was even smaller
(Figure 2).

In order to demonstrate that indeed Interferon was covalently attached to Sepharose, several experiments were carried out. As
shown in Table 2, the antiviral effect of Sepharose-bound Interferon, like that of free Interferon, was completely neutralized
by Interferon-specific antiserum. Subsequent treatment of the
Sepharose-bound antigen-antibody complex at pH 2.25 for 40 minutes
at 20° with 1 molar propionic acid almost completely restored the
antiviral effect of the particles. The slight decrease of the
antiviral activity is due to loss of some beads during these manipulations.

Friedman has shown that cells treated with Interferon at 4°
for 4 hours will develop the antiviral state after removal of
Interferon and subsequent incubation of the cells at 37° (3). No
antiviral effect is observed when the cells are challenged with
virus immediately after removal of Interferon. These data suggest
that cellular metabolism at 37° is required to establish the antiviral state. When similarly tested, Sepharose-bound Interferon, in
contrast to free Interferon, could be completely removed from the
cells. The data in Table 3 indicate, that under conditions similar
to those of Friedman (3), free Interferon protects the cells
against Mengo virus, whereas Sepharose-bound Interferon is inactive.

We attempted to demonstrate the necessity of contact between
the cells and Sepharose-bound Interferon for antiviral activity.
In such experiments porous membranes were placed between cells and
beads. In control sets Interferon was inoculated on top of these
filters in such a manner that soluble material had to pass through
to interact with the cells. The presence of filters abolished the
antiviral effect of insoluble Interferon, but the effect of free
Interferon, although reduced, was still measurable (Table 4). The
loss of activity of free Interferon was probably due to adsorption

to the filters.

The results so far presented can be interpreted in two different ways. Firstly, a small amount of Interferon is detached from the beads in contact with the cells and the solubilized antiviral material diffuses to neighboring cells. This antiviral material could be Interferon itself, an active fragment therefrom, or the substance induced in the cells by Interferon. Secondly, only contact with the Interferon-beads themselves, which are able to move freely over the cell monolayer, could induce one or a series of modifications in the cells, which lead to a fully expressed antiviral state.

In order to explore these possibilities, free movement of the Interferon-Sepharose beads was prevented by restricting the beads in the center of a plastic ring, which was placed on top of a cell monolayer. As shown in Fig. 3, when soluble Interferon was applied inside the plastic ring, all cells, inside as well as outside, were completely protected from viral infection. When however, Sepharose-bound Interferon was applied inside the plastic ring, only the cells inside the ring were protected. 310 plaques compared to 390 plaques in the control were counted on the outside of the imprint of the ring. A significant number of plaques was found in close contact with the border line. These results demonstrate that, in contrast to the situation with free Interferon, in the case of Sepharose-bound Interferon no material, Interferon or antiviral protein, diffused outside of the ring in detectable amounts.

These experiments do not exclude the possibility, however, that small amounts of Interferon, or fragments of the molecule, could have been detached during contact with the cells. If this were the case, it would be expected that after serial passages,

the antiviral effect of the beads should progressively decrease
and eventually disappear.

Therefore, Interferon-Sepharose beads were incubated for 24
hrs with sensitive L-cells at a concentration of about 1 bead per
20 cells. The beads were then washed, resuspended in medium and
transferred to fresh cells for another 24 hours of incubation.
This transfer was repeated 2 more times and after each passage,
the antiviral state was measured, comparing the effect to fresh
Interferon-Sepharose beads. The results are shown in Table 5. They
indicate, that after 4 cell-to-cell transfers over a period of 96
hours, the antiviral properties of the Interferon-Sepharose beads
remained unchanged. A small loss of activity occurred, when the
Interferon-Sepharose beads alone were kept in suspension at 37°
during the same period probably due to some terminal inactivation
at higher pH. No detectable amount of Interferon was found in the
supernate of control Interferon-Sepharose beads after five days
at 37°. It therefore appears likely that Sepharose-bound Interferon induces the antiviral state by simple cell contact and that
full protection of the cells can only be obtained, when the beads
are freely moving on the cell surface.

In comparing the physicochemical properties of free and
Sepharose-bound Interferon it was observed that in contrast to
free Interferon, Sepharose-bound Interferon retained full activity
after heating at 56° for one hour. Free Interferon was completely
destroyed under these conditions. Using more drastic conditions,
free Interferon and Interferon bound to Sepharose were autoclaved
for 30 min at 110° with 1 kilogram per square centimeter pressure
at different pH values between 2 and 7 or 4 and 8. The results are
shown in Table 6. Sepharose-bound Interferon lost very little of
its antiviral potency at pH 3. However, its biological activity
gradually diminished at increasing pH values. Surprisingly soluble

mouse Interferon was also quite resistant to heat at low pH values, but at pH values from 5-7, the antiviral activity was completely destroyed.

The effect of crystalline pepsin and of crystalline trypsin was also assayed. Pepsin almost completely inactivated Interferon-Sepharose, while the amount of trypsin which completely destroyed soluble Interferon, was less effective in the case of Sepharose-bound Interferon as shown in Table 7.

Discussion

Our experiments show that the biological properties of Interferon covalently bound to Sepharose are fully expressed. The fact that a relatively small number of Interferon-Sepharose beads is sufficient to block almost completely the replication of the virus, could be due to small amounts of Interferon that become separated from the beads during contact with the cells. It also might be possible that only active fragments of the Interferon molecule could be detached. A cell-to-cell spread of an Interferon-induced antiviral protein is also among the possibilities. Apparently a more attractive hypothesis is, that Interferon induces the antiviral state solely after contact with cell receptors. This second hypothesis is substantiated by the lack of detectable antiviral activity diffusing out of a plastic ring used to restrict the Sepharose-bound Interferon. This interpretation is also supported by the maintenance of unchanged antiviral properties of Sepharose-bound Interferon after four 24 hrs cell-to-cell transfers. Since the dose-response relationship of soluble Interferon is sigmoidal, it is unlikely that small amounts of Interferon, which could become detached from the beads at each 24 hr period, could induce such a strong antiviral state. Thus our data are in agreement with the hypothesis that Interferon acts merely by contact with cell membrane receptors without penetration into the cell.

It is interesting to compare some of the properties of Interferon and insulin. Both are proteins of low molecular weight diffusing in the tissue and the circulation and the biological effects of both are inhibited by ouabain (4,5). In addition both are active when bound to Sepharose, suggesting that for their biological effect no penetration is required (1,6).

Future work on the mechanism of Interferon action should address itself to three fundamental questions: A, What are the cell membrane receptors that interact with Interferon; B, What is the message generated after contact of Interferon with the cell surface; and C, How is this message translated into a biochemical event that renders the cell antiviral.

References

1. Cuatrecasas, P. (1969). Proc. Nat. Acad. Sci. USA 63, 450-451.

2. Porath, J., Axen, R. and Ernbank, S. (1967). Nature 215, 1491-1492.

3. Friedman, R. (1967). Science 156, 1760-1761.

4. Blatt, L.M., McVerry, P.H. and Kim, K.H. (1972). J. Biol. Chem. 247, 6551-6554.

5. Lebon, R. and Moreau, M.-C. (1973). C.R.H. Acad. Sci. 276, 3061-3064.

6. Ankel, H., Chany, C., Galliot, B., Chevalier, M.J. and
    Robert, M. (1973). Proc. Nat. Acad. Sci. USA 70, 2360-
    2363.

TABLE 1

Antiviral activity of mouse interferon before
and after incubation with CN Br-Sepharose

Interferon preparation	Antiviral titer (reference units per 0.1 ml)	Protein (mg/0.1 ml)
Starting material	2×10^4	0.6
Supernatant after incubation with CNBr-Sepharose	2×10^2	0.33
Supernatant after Sepharose inactivated by ethanolamine	2×10^4	0.57

The antiviral effect of interferon was expressed in units
adjusted to N.I.H. mouse reference interferon.

TABLE 2

Neutralization of antiviral effect of interferon-
Sepharose by antiserum to interferon and its
recovery at pH 2.25

	Soluble interferon		Interferon-Sepharose	
	HA	PFU/0.5ml	HA	PFU/0.5ml
Control	<2	2.8×10^5	≤2	4.9×10^5
+ Antiserum	2048	2.1×10^8	2048	2.2×10^8
+ Antiserum Treated at pH 2.25	ND	ND	4[*]	2.1×10^6
Treated at pH 2.25	ND	ND	4[*]	3.5×10^6
Control EMC	4096	2.8×10^8		
+ Interferon antiserum	2048	1.7×10^8		

The amount of antibody used is equivalent to that required to neutralize 800 units of soluble interferon.EMC
virus titers are expressed in hemagglutinating (HA) and
plaque-forming (PFU) units.
*The slight decrease of the antiviral activity is most
likely due to a 20% loss of the number of beads during
the manipulations.
ND = not done.

TABLE 3

Lack of establishment of the antiviral
state by interferon-Sepharose previously
incubated with the cells at 4°

	Preincubated 5 hr at 4°		Preincubated 5 hr at 37°	
	HA	PFU/0.5ml	HA	PFU/0.5ml
Interferon-Sepharose	>2048	6.8×10^8	512	1.6×10^8
Interferon	256	7.7×10^7	256	6.2×10^7
	512			
Control EMC	>4096	5×10^8	>4096	6.5×10^8

L cells were incubated at 4° or 37° for 4 hr. Then they were
washed three times, replenished with fresh medium, and incubated
for a further 18 hr at 37°. Then they were challenged with EMC,
multiplicity of infection = 1.

TABLE 4

Separation of Sepharose-bound interferon
from the cells by filters

	EMC (PFU/0.5 ml)	
	With filter	Without filter
Interferon-Sepharose	3.9×10^8	4.8×10^5
Soluble interferon	5.2×10^7	1.7×10^5
Control EMC	3.5×10^8	3×10^8

Antiviral effect of insoluble and soluble
interferon separated from the cells by a filter. The small loss of soluble interferon activity is probably due to unspecific adsorption to the filter.

TABLE 5

Antiviral activity of interferon-Sepharose
before and after four cell-to-cell transfers

	EMC (PFU/0.5ml)	VSV (PFU/0.5ml)
Interferon-Sepharose control 4°	1.5×10^7	7.4×10^3
Interferon-Sepharose control 37°	3.7×10^7	1.2×10^4
Interferon-Sepharose at the fourth cell-to-cell transfer	4×10^7	2×10^4
Control virus	5.6×10^8	1.2×10^7

TABLE 6

Effect of autoclaving at different pH levels at
110° C (1 kg/mm pressure) on the antiviral
properties of Sepharose-bound Interferon

Interferon	pH								Control
	2	3	4	5 ·	6	7	8	9	
Soluble	3.2^x	3	2	0	0	0	–	–	5
Sepharose-Bound	–	5.8	4.6	3.8	3.5	1.7	–	–	6.5
	–	–	–	3.7	–	2.3	2	0	4.1

x
  Log Single Cycle VSV Yield Control/Treated Cells

TABLE 7

Effect of pepsin and trypsin on Sepharose-
bound and soluble Interferon

	Interferon Sepharose-Bound			Interferon Soluble	
Pepsin	0.4^x	–	–	–	–
Trypsin	–	1	0.5	0	0
Control	3.2	2.9	3.2	3.2	4.2

x
  Log Single Cycle VSV Yield Control/
Treated Cells

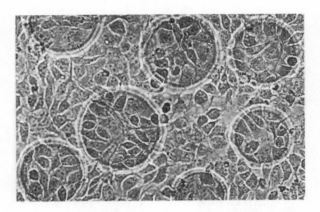

Fig. 1.   Interferon-Sepharose beads partially covering mouse L cells in culture. Cell to bead ratio approximately 50:1 (phase contrast, magnification 160x).

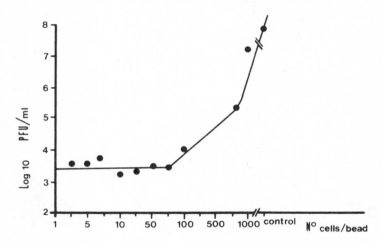

Fig. 2.   Dose-response relationship between the number of interferon-Sepharose beads per cell and the antiviral state induced. Decreasing numbers of Interferon-bound Sepharose beads were incubated with sensitive L cells grown in Eagle's medium in 35 mm plastic petri dishes. After 22 hrs of contact, the beads were removed; the cells were washed twice with medium and infected with VSV at a m.o.i. = 0.1. After incubation for 16 h at 37°C, the viral yield was measured in each preparation, using a routine plaque technique in L cells.

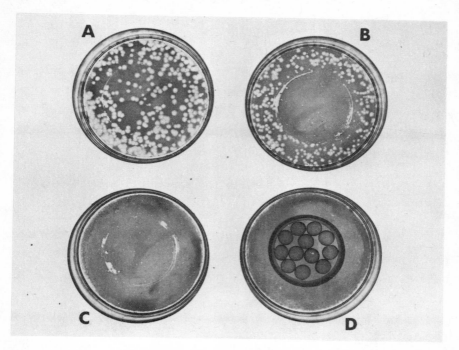

Fig. 3.   A polythylene ring was placed in the center of a 60
mm plastic petri dish containing a monolayer of mouse L cells. In
one set of experiments, Interferon-Sepharose beads (1 bead/10
cells) were placed in the center of the ring, which kept them
from escaping into the surrounding area (B). In another set, free
Interferon (8×10^4 reference units/ml) was added to the center of
the ring (C). After 22 h, the beads or free Interferon were removed and about 400 infectious units of VSV were added. In the
control not treated with Interferon(A), about 390 plaques were
counted, of which about 70 were found in the area corresponding
to the interior of the ring used in B and C. In B, about 310
plaques were counted outside of the ring and only small, hardly
visible microplaques inside of the ring. In B and C, the imprint
of the ring is easily detectable. Thus, no antiviral material diffused outside of the ring when free Interferon was used (C), but
remained restricted to the interior of the ring when Sepharose-
bound Interferon was applied (B). For the purpose of illustration
of the experiment, glass beads of distinguishable size, enclosed
by the same type of plastic ring as used in B and C, are shown
in D.

DISCUSSION

Stewart: Obviously we had the same problem that people have
had trying to show the disappearance of interferon from the supernatant of cells: we had to have a lot of cells to bind a little
bit of interferon. The thing is, you used a small number of cells
in these experiments, about 10^4, I believe, 10^6 maybe.

Ankel: The number of cells for the actual assay was about
one million cells.

Stewart: Is there any possibility that you could, for example, use a large number of cells passed through exposure to these
beads and attempt to recover any interferon activity from the
cells? 10^8 cells, for example?

Ankel: Yes. It seems to me there is no technical problem
in incubating any number of cells with the beads. What you want
to recover then is free interferon released from the cells?

Stewart: Yes, if you could recover, or not recover, interferon from an appreciable number of cells, it would aid the interpretation of these data. I mean, is there a possibility, the same
with Dr. Cuatrecasas' work with insulin, for a small release of
insulin or interferon from the beads? And this small amount which
would be released in any of the experiments, I believe it's not
reaching cells could be explained by absorption to either the
plastic rings or the membranes that prevent this small amount from
reaching the cells.

Ankel: If you are talking in terms of very small amounts,
they probably would not be detected under these conditions. However, it could also be possible that the sepharose-bound interferon would induce the production of interferon. It depends on how

to differentiate between these two possibilities.

Stewart: Well, mainly metabolically inert cells that wouldn't produce interferon. You would be able to distinguish this because you would still have binding.

Ankel: I do not exclude the possibility that the interferon may penetrate into the cell.

Stewart: I am not excluding the possibility that it does not, but I would like to be able to resolve it because if you could bind for example to the same number of beads and just use enough cells to be able to either recover or not recover interferon from the cells, I think it would resolve the question.

Chany: I should like to stress the following point: In the cell-to-cell transfer experiments, the number of beads used was about ten thousand and the total volume of ten thousand beads is about 1/100 of ml. After 4 cell-to-cell transfers with such a small volume, if something is detached from the beads, a loss in antiviral activity should appear. I realize, however, that at the present stage, it is impossible to answer definitely this question of penetration.

Tan: Do you get interferon diffusing out of those rings?

Ankel: If I've put free interferon on the inside of those rings? I showed that when free interferon was placed inside of the ring, the cells both inside and outside of the ring were protected.

De Clercq: I don't think you excluded the possibility of a direct transfer of interferon from the sepharose beads to the cells. Interferon may have been transferred directly from the sepharose to the cell without entering into the supernatant fluid.

Ankel: You mean it doesn't have to be detached to be transferred?

De Clercq: It doesn't have to be released into the supernatant to be transferred. This means that, if you wish to evaluate
whether sepharose-bound interferon is active per se from the outside of the cell, you should rather focus on what portion of interferon is eventually taken up by the cells and not on the amounts
released into the supernatant fluid. I have a second question. Can
you recover interferon from the sepharose after it has been bound
to the sepharose?

Ankel: In order to measure the bound interferon, you can
measure its titer. When you do it after several cell-to-cell transfers, you find that it is unchanged. But, we have not treated the
sepharose-interferon with a proteolytic enzyme and then recovered
soluble interferon.

De Clercq: Can you recover it again?

Ankel: That we have not attempted. It's a little difficult
to do it.

De Clercq: That's just what I wanted to know, because if
you cannot do it, how do you know how much interferon is actually
bound to the sepharose?

Ankel: I measure it by the antiviral titer. I count the
beads, I put the beads in contact with cells, and I measure the
viral yield after infection with virus. Then, I use the same
beads, put them on another set of cells, and again measure the
antiviral state, and so on. I can compare the antiviral activity
of the beads which, as you saw, doesn't change after several cell-
to-cell transfers. But, I cannot detach the interferon from the

beads and measure the stuff which is soluble. That I cannot do.

De Clercq: How far did you go with your transfers? 4 times? or did you go further?

Ankel: I did it up to four 24-hour transfers, a total of something like 96 hours.

De Clercq: This means 4 times.

Ankel: We haven't done more than 4 times. 5 times?

Chany: 5 times.

De Clercq: I don't think it is sufficient.

Ankel: I see. How many times would you think would be necessary?

De Clercq: Maybe 100 times.

Chany: You have to take into consideration, as I just mentioned, that we used ten thousand beads, which is 1/100 ml of insoluble interferon of which 90% is inactive material. If you would do 100 passages with the same amount of soluble interferon, I wonder what would be left?

Ankel: It can be done. You just have to start with a large batch of beads and then work the way down. If not, then you'll lose them all.

Stewart: But there is always the possibility that you can have a polymer of interferon that bound onto a bead can be functional as one unit of interferon.

Ankel: Yes.

Stewart: And so a partial elution, or hydrolysis of this at 37° C (it wouldn't occur at 4° C) could still account for your not detecting loss from the beads, but still losing it. You have to have binding at 37° C; so you have to have specific hydrolysis after contact.

Merigan: I think that these are a set of very interesting experiments, but I think it is very important to recognize that you really don't know whether a certain small amount is cleaved off or not, and that it might be active. I think it has been very clear in the hormone systems and in other areas where insoluble materials have been studied that it is often a very efficient way of delivering anything to cells. You're the first one in the interferon area trying to evaluate what could be a much more efficient system. Whether it is delivery with cision of a small amount off the carrier or just better delivery to the cell's surface you really can't tell. It would be nice obviously to have radioactive markers and do very careful stoichiometry experiments to back up your claim that the biological activity is not lost from the sephadex. But obviously that's for the future.

Ankel: In the case of Cuatrecasas, of course, he has been attacked on the same grounds.

Merigan: Yes.

Ankel: But the action of insulin occurs without any measurable penetration of insulin into the cells. So, the conclusion from these experiments is that insulin might enter the cell for the purpose of degradation and not necessarily for the purpose of action.

Merigan: There is one other set of experiments that you can
also do that are unique now, and that is to shake the plates, because you're working with a new diffusion constant, obviously not
insoluble interferon, and so the physical measurement of the apparent diffusion constant of your material and how it is influenced by shaking and heating, I think it would be all unique and
interesting.

Chany: We have done this experiment.

Ankel: We took a small number of beads, let's say one thousand beads per one million of cells, and we agitated them slowly.
We found inhibition of viral yield of about one log when the beads
were agitated. When we didn't shake them, we didn't find any protection.

Merigan: Have you tried it in suspension culture?

Ankel: No.

Pitha: I only wanted to say that interferon bound to solid
support is a much more clearer system than that of poly IC. If you
would postulate that you have detachment, it would have to be in
the place of an attachment because any hydrolytic cleavage would
inactivate interferon. It is similar to the peptide hormones. They
can be cleaved by hydrolytic enzymes present in the membrane, but
would lose the biological activity. Poly IC, on the other hand,
can be cleaved in any place and the remaining piece of poly IC may
still be active.

Colby: A word of caution in addition to what Dr. Merigan
said. We do not really need to concern ourselves exclusively with
the problem of potential cleavage. The model that Dr. Carter and
Dr. Pitha (Carter, W.A., Pitha, P.M., in "Biological Effects of

Polynucleotides", Ed. R.F. Beers, W. Braun 1971, Springer Verlag,
New York) postulated a few years ago is that interferon is a mono
subunit molecule which can form dimers, tetramers, octimers and
dodecamers. The chemical binding of one such subunit to sepharose
could then be followed by this type of oligomeric association,
such that you could have one subunit covalently bound to the
sepharose beads and a number of other subunits then attached noncovalently to it. If, in fact, monomeric or dimeric molecules are
active, one could have the dissociation of the oligomeric form on
interaction with the cell surface, and one would not even need an
hydrolytic cleavage. I think it directly relates to Dr. Stawart's
question of: can you look at the molecule that is attached to the
bead? Can you put it on and then get it back? Is there any way
that you can do experiments to ask whether it is in a dimeric or
polemeric form?

Ankel: Many proteins that consist of subunits are dissociated at low pH. We have treated sepharose-bound interferon at
pH 3 and 110°, for instance, without loss of activity. I mean any
similar protein composed of several subunits is probably dissociated under these conditions. The other possibility that exists,
if you have such a situation, is that you will constantly lose
interferon so you should conceivably find decrease in the antiviral titer of the beads after sufficient cell-to-cell transfers.
It is still the same argument.

Revel: My question is quite similar to that of Dr. Colby's.
Have you taken into account the role of the other proteins which
are contaminating your interferon preparation? What I have in mind
is that if the interferon is too close to the beads, it should not
work very efficiently. It is probable that you have some distance
between the interferon molecule and the bead itself, and you might

have some other proteins intercalated between the two.

Ankel: That would not be possible. If you have 99% of inert proteins and a very small amount of interferon, you would bind all the other proteins also to the sepharose. But you could not bind covalently another protein molecule to a protein molecule which is already bound to the sepharose. That is not possible.

Stewart: It just seems that the only way to resolve whether interferon is actually bound to the cells and is lost from the beads is to recover it from cells, but with 10^6 cells or less, you can't detect recoverable interferon; it is not bound enough to be a unit. But if you use 10^8 cells, you should be able to recover interferon from them.

Ankel: Yes, I should do this.

STUDIES OF THE ROLE OF CELL-BOUND INTERFERON
IN THE INDUCTION OF ANTIVIRAL ACTIVITY

Seiya Kohno[1], Charles E. Buckler,
Hilton B. Levy and Samuel Baron

National Institute of Allergy and Infectious Diseases
Laboratory of Viral Diseases
National Institutes of Health
Bethesda,Maryland 20014

ABSTRACT

The role of the fraction of applied mouse interferon which
becomes cell-bound in the development of the antiviral state in
cultured mouse L cells was studied. The findings confirmed previous observations that only about 1% of applied interferon is
bound to cells, the bound interferon is probably at the cell surface since it is digestable by trypsin, and antiviral activity
continues to develop after removal of unbound interferon. The
development of resistance after removal of unbound interferon was
probably not a direct function of the level of initially bound
interferon since most of the cell-associated interferon eluted
within 15 to 30 minutes after washing but resistance developed
much later; the concentration of eluted interferon was quantitatively sufficient to account for the lower level of resistance
which was induced eventually in washed cultures; repeated washings or continuous replacement of medium to remove dissociated

---

1) Present address: Department of Measles Virus, National Institute of Health, 3260 Nakato, Musashi-murayama-shi, Tokyo 190-
12 Japan.

interferon during the elution period blocked further development
of resistance; and increasing the elution volume, to dilute the
dissociated interferon, decreased the development of antiviral activity. This supports the interpretation that the previously reported development of resistance after removal of unbound interferon was probably a function of a new equilibrium in which 99% of
the originally bound interferon is in the culture medium. Most of
the 1% of cell bound interferon may be bound nonspecifically since
human albumin, with no known specific interaction with cells,bound
to and eluted from cells in a manner quantitatively similar to
interferon and there was no correlation between the levels of
interferon bound to a variety of cell types and the level of antiviral activity. The hypothesized smaller fraction of cell-bound
interferon which may be effective in inducing resistance probably
exists either as a fairly rapidly dissociating or rapidly decaying
complex to account for the inhibition of continued development of
resistance after removal of interferon from the culture medium.

Introduction

It is known that part of the added interferon becomes cell-
bound after exposure to sensitive cells (4, 6, 9, 11). Cell cultures which had been exposed to interferon and washed extensively
to remove unbound interferon were found to increase their antiviral resistance during subsequent incubation. In another study
there was a positive correlation between the relative sensitivity
to interferon of 5 cell types and the amount of cell-bound interferon. It therefore was postulated that firm binding of interferon
with cells was a prerequisite to the development of the antiviral
state. A study was undertaken to further define the role of cell-
bound interferon in the development of antiviral activity.

Materials and Methods

Cells. Mouse L cells (obtained from Dr. J. Youngner, University of Pittsburgh), primary and secondary mouse embryo cells, human U cells (obtained from Dr. K. Cantell, State Serum Institute, Helsinki, Finland), HeLa cells, human foreskin fibroblasts, monkey CCL-MK2 cells, monkey MA-104 cells (Microbiological Associates), monkey Vero cells and guinea pig (strain 2) embryo heart fibroblasts were cultured in Eagle's minimal essential medium containing 10% fetal bovine serum and antibiotics. During experiments the concentration of fetal bovine serum was reduced to 5% unless otherwise specified.

Interferon. A stock mouse interferon, titering approximately 100,000 units per ml, was used without purification. This interferon had been prepared by infecting mouse C-243-3 cells with Newcastle disease virus (7). Interferon potency was determined by hemagglutinin yield reduction of GD-7 virus as reported elsewhere (8). Although a calculated concentration of interferon was applied during experiments, the actual potency was determined in each experiment. The level of antiviral activity was measured similarly by determining the inhibition of hemagglutinin yield of GD-7 virus in a single step growth cycle. I-131-labeled human albumin (molecular weight: 67,000), of which the specific activity was 100 microcuries per mg, was obtained from Abbott Laboratories, and dialyzed against Eagle's MEM overnight to remove unbound iodine.

The actinomycin D used in this study was shown to be active by (a) inhibiting the action of interferon at 1 through 20 µg/ml and (b) inhibiting RNA synthesis by 95% within 45 minutes at 1 µg/ml.

Results

Time course of binding of mouse interferon to mouse L cells.
Tube cultures of mouse L cells were each inoculated with 1 ml of
medium containing 3,500 units of mouse interferon. After varying
periods of time at 37C or 4C, 4 replicate cultures were washed 6
times with 3 ml per wash of Earle's balanced salt solution (EBSS).
This removed unbound interferon since the last washing fluid contained no detectable interferon. 1 ml of medium was added to the
washed monolayers and at varying times they were frozen and thawed 6 times to disrupt the cells. The pooled homogenate of 4 tubes
was assayed for interferon titer. This basic procedure was used
throughout the study unless otherwise specified.

As previously reported (4, 6) binding to cells was rapid and
reached a maximum of 0.6% of the input interferon after 30 minutes
at 37C. In comparison, at ice bath temperatures the maximum binding was of similar magnitude but delayed until 3 hours (Fig. 1).
Only 20 units of the 3500 units of interferon applied were found
in the homogenate. However the volume of the cells from which the
interferon was extracted represented only a small fraction of the
volume of the homogenate. Calculating from the volume of cells
(0.002 ml per tube) the concentration of cell bound interferon ap-
proximates the concentration originally applied to the cells (3500
units/ml). This is in agreement with the previous findings of
others using mouse L cells (9). It would therefore appear that applied interferon is not concentrated in or on the cells.

The maximum amounts of interferon bound were similar in the
presence or absence of 5 μg/ml of actinomycin D. Also no more
interferon could be recovered from cells when the homogenates were
sonicated. Finally we were able to confirm that treatment of cells
with bound interferon for 10 minutes at room temperature with 0.3%

trypsin, decreased bound interferon from 30 units to 6 units. The
latter finding indicates that most of the bound interferon is at
the surface of the cell as previously suggested (4).

Binding of interferon as a function of concentration of
suspended cells. To determine whether interferon binding was a
function of cell concentration, 1300 units of interferon in 1 ml
was mixed with varying concentrations of suspended mouse L cells
in 1 ml and held at 37°C for 1 hour. The cells were then collected
and washed 3 times by centrifugation, with 10 ml per wash of EBSS,
suspended in 1 ml of culture medium and disrupted by 3 cycles of
freezing and thawing prior to assay for interferon. As shown in
Figure 2 there is a linear relationship between the cell number
and the total amount of interferon bound. Assuming that this relationship holds true for other cell types, it may be possible to
normalize data on cell-bound interferon to compensate for variation in cell number between different cell cultures (see below).

Binding of mouse interferon to a variety of cell types. As
a preliminary to testing the possibility that the concentration
of cell-associated interferon influenced the degree of induced
antiviral activity, the amount of interferon bound to a variety
of cells was determined. Cells in 32 oz bottles were washed once
with EBSS and treated with 10 ml per bottle of mouse interferon
for 1 hour on a horizontal rocking device at 37°C. Treated cultures
were then washed twice with 100 ml per wash of EBSS, scraped off
with a rubber policeman, collected and washed twice by centrifugation (1,500 rpm 5 minutes at 4°C) with 50 ml of culture medium.
They were subsequently suspended in 10 ml of culture medium, counted and disrupted by one cycle of freezing and thawing and sonicated
before assaying for interferon. Table 1 shows the total amount of
interferon bound and the ratio of bound interferon to cell number.

It may be seen that mouse L cells consistently bound more total interferon than did the other cell types. However this may be misleading because the L cell density was greater than the other cell densities and therefore amounts of interferon bound per cell (ratio column in table) was only moderately different among the cell types.

With this information it was possible to compare interferon bound per cell with antiviral activity. In our laboratory mouse interferon induces equal antiviral activity in mouse L cells and in mouse embryo cells (8). However, mouse embryo cells bind one-sixth as much interferon per cell as do mouse L cells. Similarly there is little (less than 10%) or no induction of the antiviral state by mouse interferon in the heterologous cell types in table 1 (2, 10) but a substantial amount of interferon is bound to many of these cell types. Thus the interferon bound per heterologous cell is generally about one-fourth the amount bound to homologous cells but the antiviral activity on heterologous cells is one-tenth to less than one-ten thousandth the activity on homologous cells. There appears to be little correlation between concentration of cell-bound interferon and induction of antiviral activity in the present study.

Binding of a less specific protein, human albumin, to mouse L cells. Experiments were performed to compare the amount of interferon bound to cells with that of another protein with no known specific interaction with cells--human albumin. Tube cultures of mouse L cells were incubated with 1 ml per tube of various concentrations of labeled human albumin in Eagle's MEM for 1 hr at $37^{\circ}C$ or at $4^{\circ}C$. The cells were then washed 6 times with 3 ml of EBSS per wash. For each experimental point cells from 6 replicate cultures were scraped from the glass with a rubber policeman,

pooled, suspended in 9 ml of Dulbecco's phosphate buffered saline
(pH7.2), and centrifuged. The pellet was dissolved in 0.2 ml of
1N NaOH by gentle warming and diluted immediately with 0.8 ml of
distilled water. Recoveries of cellular protein were monitored by
measuring optical densities (280 nm), which were employed for
comparisons of radioactivity measurements. Seven tenths ml aliquots were assayed for radioactivity in a Packard Tricarb liquid
scintillation counter.

    The results are summarized in Figure 3. The percent binding
of albumin increased as its applied concentration was increased.
To compare the uptake of the interferon protein with that of albumin, the following calculations were made. Assuming that the
specific activity of pure mouse interferon is ca 10^9 units/mg, then
5000 interferon units applied would correspond to ca 0.05 µg/ml
of interferon protein. When the experimental lines in Figure 3 are
extrapolated (linearity is assumed) to 0.05 µg/ml of applied concentration of protein (vertical line) (to simulate the calculated
concentration of interferon protein) an uptake of ca 1% is projec-
ted at 37°C and ca 0.1% at 4C. These estimated values at 37°C are
comparable to the observed binding of interferon to mouse cells
calculated from column 1 of table 1 to be 0.7 to 2%. The decreased
binding of albumin at 4°C as compared with 37°C for 1 hour is similar to the delayed binding of interferon in the cold (Figure 1).
These findings indicate that the degree of binding of interferon
to mouse L cells is comparable in magnitude to that of human serum
albumin, a protein with no known specific interaction with cells.

    Effect of removal of unbound interferon on the development
of antiviral activity. Experiments were performed which confirmed
the previous observation that the antiviral state developed approximately 6 hours after removal of unbound interferon (4). Tube

cultures of mouse L cells were treated with interferon for 1 hour
at 37°C, washed six times to remove unbound interferon, refed 1 ml
of medium and incubated at 37°C. At the times shown in Figure 4,
groups of 4 cultures were infected with GD-7 virus, washed after
1 hour and reincubated. Viral HA yields were determined at 20
hours after infection. Figure 4 confirms rising curves of moderate
resistance which peak at 6-8 hours after removal of unbound interferon. The addition of 5 µg/ml of actinomycin D at 1 hour after
addition of interferon blocked further development of resistance.
This indicates that the mRNA for the hypothetical antiviral protein is being transcribed after removal of unbound interferon.
These findings are consistent with the interpretation that the
eventual development of resistance was related to the action of
the interferon remaining in the cultures after washing. It is
noteworthy that the level of maximal resistance is much less after
removal of the unbound interferon as compared with its continuous
presence. This will be considered later.

     Elution of cell-bound interferon. To help determine whether
the interferon originally bound to cells remains so during development of antiviral activity, the amounts of cell-bound and eluted
interferon were determined. Tube cultures of mouse L cells were
treated with 5,000 units of interferon, washed and refed as in
earlier experiments, and incubated at 37°C. At each time indicated
in Figure 5, media from 4 tubes were pooled and assayed for interferon. The remaining cells were immediately washed once with 3 ml
of EBSS, frozen and thawed 6 times with 1 ml of medium per tube.
Homogenates of 4 tubes were pooled and titrated for interferon.

     A typical result is shown in Figure 5. Most of the cell-
bound interferon was released after 15 minutes incubation at 37°C.
Elution was virtually complete between 1 and 2 hours. A large

portion but perhaps not all the cell-associated interferon could eventually be recovered in the culture medium at the time that the cells had lost most of their interferon. The inability to recover all the eluted interferon in the medium in some experiments may be due to the limitation of accuracy of the assay or inactivation. The dissociated interferon was characterized as interferon by the inability of washing to reverse its induced resistance and by the inhibition of its action by actinomycin D. The level of resistance which develops can be accounted for by the concentration of eluted interferon in the medium. For example in Figure 4 the maximum level of resistance which developed by 6 hours after washing (1) averaged 2^{10} decrease of yield of viral HA. An average of twenty units/ml of interferon was eluted from these cells into the medium (Figure 5). This concentration of interferon when reacted with previously untreated cells for 6 or more hours induced the same 2^{10} decrease in HA yield.

Examination of elution of cell-bound, radio-labelled albumin by the same method used to study the elution of interferon, demonstrated that 30% of bound albumin was disassociated from cells held at 37°C for 1 hour after binding.

The observation that the cell-associated interferon eluted before development of maximal resistance (c.f. Figures 4 and 5) suggests that the initially bound interferon was not directly responsible for the development of the subsequent resistance. It seems more likely that the eluted interferon establishes a new equilibrium with approximately 1% of the remaining interferon being cell-bound at any one time. Resistance would develop during this proposed second equilibrium. This hypothesis can be partially tested by determining the effect on development of resistance of removal of eluted interferon (see below).

Kinetics of development of antiviral activity after removal
of eluted interferon. To test the hypothesis that the original
cell-bound interferon might not induce resistance from the site
where it is bound but rather functioned after most of it eluted
into the culture medium, 3 experimental approaches were used. In
general cultures were incubated with interferon to allow binding
and then they were washed 6 times to remove unbound interferon.
Since (a) most of the cell-bound interferon elutes within the
next 30 minutes (Figure 5) and (b) it requires 6 hours of interferon-cell reaction for cells to develop maximal resistance
(Figure 4), the rapid removal or dilution of the eluting interferon should decrease the degree of resistance attained if the
eluted interferon continues to react with the cells to induce the
resistance. Alternatively if the interferon acts from the initial
binding site to trigger the production of antiviral protein the
subsequent removal of the eluting interferon should not decrease
the final level of resistance. The 3 procedures used to remove or
dilute the eluting interferon were repeated washings, continuous
replacement of medium and increasing the volume of eluting medium.

The first experiments examined the effect of repeated washings during the dissociation period. Four thousand units of interferon were incubated with tube cultures of L cells for 30 minutes.
The cultures were then washed 6 times and fed with 0.75ml of medium containing 10% fetal bovine serum. Half of the cultures were
washed for 3 minutes with 2 ml of warmed culture medium every 5
minutes to remove eluted interferon. To block further development
of resistance 3 replicate cultures in each group were treated at
$37^{\circ}C$ with 10 µg/ml of actinomycin D at the times indicated in Figure 6. One hour after addition of actinomycin D, cultures were
challenged with GD-7 virus for 1 hour, washed and the viral HA
yield determined after 20 hours. As shown in Figure 6 antiviral

activity of the experimental groups increased until shortly after completion of the additional washings and then resistance stopped developing. In comparison the cultures which did not have the eluted interferon washed away continued to develop significantly more resistance. Similar results were obtained in a number of repeated experiments. This finding is consistent with the hypothesis that the initially cell-bound interferon induced most of its antiviral activity after most of the interferon eluted into the medium.

The second experiments examined the effect of continuous replacement of culture medium during the dissociation period. Two hundred and fifty units of interferon were added to cultures of L cells and held at $4°C$ for 1 hour. The cultures were then washed 6 times and the experimental group received replacement with medium (2 ml per minute per tube) at $37°C$ to continuously remove eluted interferon. Control cultures were not washed continuously but were fed 1 ml of medium and held at $37°C$. At the times indicated in Figure 7, duplicate cultures were challenged with GD-7 virus containing 3 µg/ml actinomycin D, incubated for 1 hour, washed, refed with culture medium containing 10% fetal bovine serum and harvested after 20 hours for assay of viral HA. It was determined that the continuous replacement of medium prior to infection did not alter virus HA yield in control cultures.

As demonstrated in Figure 7, the level of resistance did not increase after initiation of continuous replacement of medium. In comparison the controls developed significantly greater antiviral activity.

The last experiments examined the effect of varying the volume of culture medium during the period of dissociation of interferon. It is known that the degree of induced resistance is proportional to the concentration of applied interferon (1, 5).

Therefore the level of resistance which develops should decrease
with increasing volume if the cell-bound interferon elutes into
the medium before it induces resistance. The results of 3 experiments in which the eluting volume was varied from 0.1 to 10.0 ml,
are presented in Figure 8. Appropriate controls demonstrated that
the different volumes of medium with constant interferon concentration did not influence virus HA yield or sensitivity of the
cells to interferon. The decreased development of the antiviral
state with increased volumes of eluting medium is also consistent
with the hypothesis that the observed resistance was not due to
the action of the original cell-bound interferon as its original
site.

Thus all 3 types of experimental results from experiments
designed to decrease the concentration of eluted interferon, support the hypothesis that cell-bound interferon did not induce the
ongoing development of resistance from the site where it was initially bound. Instead the interferon probably acts after establishing a new equilibrium with 99% of the originally bound interferon in the culture medium.

Discussion

This study was to further define the role in the development of the antiviral state, of that fraction of applied interferon which becomes cell-bound (4, 6). Results confirm that only
about 1% of applied interferon is bound to cells (4, 6). The
binding site is probably at the cell surface since others (4) and
we have found that bound interferon is digestable by trypsin. The
present findings also substantiate that antiviral activity continues to develop after removal of unbound interferon (4). However
it does so at a reduced rate. In addition binding of interferon to

actinomycin D treated cells indicates that binding does not require transcription.

The present findings indicate that the development of resistance after removal of unbound interferon is not a direct function of the level of initially bound interferon. Studies of dissociation of cell-bound interferon demonstrated that most of the interferon eluted from mouse L cells within 15 to 30 minutes after washing. This was long before the maximal development of antiviral activity which reached a peak at 6 to 8 hours as also reported previously (1, 3). The concentration of the eluted interferon was sufficient to account for the lower level of resistance which was eventually induced. These findings supported but did not establish the hypothesis that the interferon which initially bound to cells did not induce subsequent cellular resistance from the bound site but subsequently eluted and induced resistance as a function of a new equilibrium in which approximately 1% of the originally bound interferon is cell-associated.

To further test the hypothesis that the bound interferon induced resistance after most of it eluted into the medium, 3 experimental approaches were used to reduce the concentration of eluted interferon. Firstly repeated washings to remove dissociated interferon during the elution period blocked the further development of resistance. Secondly, continuous replacement of culture medium during the elution period also blocked further development of resistance. Finally, increasing the elution volume, to dilute the disassociated interferon, decreased the development of antiviral activity. These findings tend to substantiate the hypothesis that the observed, cell-associated interferon did not induce resistance from the bound site but instead acted sometime after most of it eluted into the culture medium.

Some of the present findings suggest that most of the observed 1% binding of interferon to cells during any of equilibri-
ums may not be specific for induction of the antiviral state.Most
of the observed binding might actually represent nonspecific binding of protein with cells. Specifically, a comparison of the
levels of interferon bound with the degree of induction of antiviral activity in a variety of homologous and heterologous cells,
failed to establish a correlation. Another protein with no known
specific interaction with cells, radioisotopically labelled human
albumin, was observed to bind to and elute from cells in a manner
quantitatively similar to interferon. This lack of specificity of
the bound interferon suggests, but does not establish, that most
of the 1% that is bound may not serve as the driving force which
causes the cells to develop the virus resistant state. Instead, a
smaller but specifically acting fraction may be inducing resistance.

The present interpretations do not imply that interferon
acts from the culture medium without making specific contact with
the cell. Neither does it exclude the existance of specific cellular binding sites for interferon. The present findings do indicate that (a) the previously reported development of resistance
after removal of unbound interferon was probably a function of a
new equilibrium in which 99% of the initially bound interferon is
in the culture medium and (b) most of the 1% of cell-bound interferon may be bound nonspecifically. Further, since resistance
stops developing shortly after removal of interferon from the
culture medium (3), the specific reaction of interferon with cells
is probably short lived. The hypothesized short life of this reaction could be due to rapid dissociation of a specific cell-
interferon complex or to rapid inactivation of the specifically
bound interferon. Since no loss of interferon can be detected in

this system then if the rapid inactivation hypothesis is true, the number of specific interaction sites must be small. Finally the dependence of the level of resistance on the concentration of extracellular interferon (1) and the interruption of continued development of resistance by removal of extracellular interferon are compatible with the interpretation that the ongoing frequency of collision of interferon molecules with cells determines the level to which the antiviral state will develop.

Further understanding of the specific interaction of interferon with cells probably will require more sensitive and precise assay methods.

Acknowledgement

The authors wish to acknowledge the excellent suggestions made by Dr. C.F.T. Mattern.

References

1. Baron, S., C.E. Buckler, H.B. Levy and R.M. Friedman (1967). Some factors affecting the interferon induced antiviral state. Proc. Soc. Exp. Biol. Med. 125:1320-1326.

2. Buckler, C.E. and S. Baron (1966). Antiviral action of mouse interferon in heterologous cells. J. Bact. 91:231-235.

3. Dianzani, F., C.E. Buckler and S. Baron (1968). Kinetics of the development of factors responsible for inter-

feron-induced resistance. Proc. Soc. Exp. Biol. Med. 129:535-538.

4. Friedman, R.M. (1967). Interferon binding: The first step in establishment of antiviral activity. Science 156:1760-1761.

5. Hallum, J.V. and J.S. Youngner (1971). Personal communication.

6. Levine, S. (1966). Persistence of active interferon in cells washed after treatment with interferon. Proc. Soc. Exp. Biol. Med. 121:1041-1045.

7. Oie, H.K., A.F. Gazdar, C.E. Buckler and S. Baron (1972). High interferon producing line of transformed murine cells. J. Gen. Virol. 17:107-109.

8. Oie, H.K., C.E. Buckler, C.P. Uhlendorf, D.A. Hill and S. Baron (1972). Improved assays for a variety of interferons. Proc. Soc. Exp. Biol. Med. 140:1178-1181.

9. Stewart II, W.E., E. De Clercq and P. De Somer (1972). Recovery of cell-bound interferon. J. Virol. 10:707-712.

10. Sutton, R.N.P. and D.A.J. Tyrell (1961). Some observations on interferon prepared in tissue cultures. Brit. J. Exp. Pathol. 42:99-105.

11. Vilcek, J. and B. Rada (1962). Studies on an interferon from tick-borne encephalitis virus-infected cells. III. Antiviral action of interferon. Acta. Virol. 6:9-16.

TABLE 1

Amount of Mouse Interferon Bound to Cells
After Reaction for 1 Hour at 37°C

Experiment Number	Cell Types	Bound Interferon	Cell Number $\times 10^5$	Ratio: Bound Interferon Cell number $\times 10^5$
1	HeLa	0	12	0
	Human Foreskin	3	4.6	0.6
	Monkey CCL-MK2	4	8	0.5
	Monkey MA-104	4	5.4	0.8
	Guinea Pig Heart	8	5.8	1.4
	Mouse L	80	56	1.4
2	Human Foreskin	3	6	0.5
	Mouse Embryo	13	40	0.3
	Mouse L	90	50	1.8
3	Mouse L	25	60	0.42
	Monkey Vero	3	18	0.17
	Human U	1	24	0.04

Input interferon: experiment 1 = 40,000 units
experiment 2 = 5,000 units
experiment 3 = 1,600 units

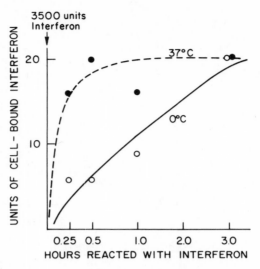

Fig. 1. Kinetics of binding of mouse interferon to mouse L
cells at 37°C or 4°C.

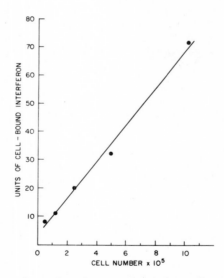

Fig. 2. Relationship of concentration of suspended mouse L
cells with amount of interferon bound.

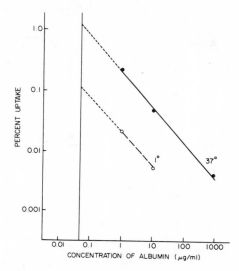

Fig. 3. Binding of human albumin to mouse L and human U cells.

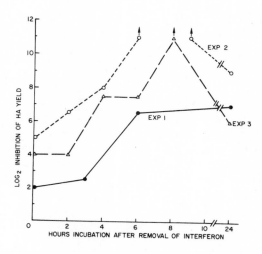

Fig. 4. Development of antiviral activity in mouse L cells after exposure to large amounts of interferon for 1 hour and subsequent removal of unbound interferon. In experiment 1 the initial interferon concentration was 1,300 units and in experiment 2 and 3 the interferon concentration was 5,000 units.

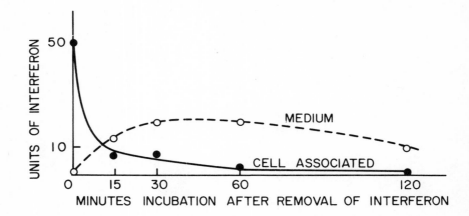

Fig. 5. Kinetics of dissociation of cell-bound interferon from mouse L cells. Cells were exposed to 5,000 units/ml of interferon for 1 hour at 37°C and then washed 6 times and refed. Subsequently interferon levels in cells and fluid were determined at intervals.

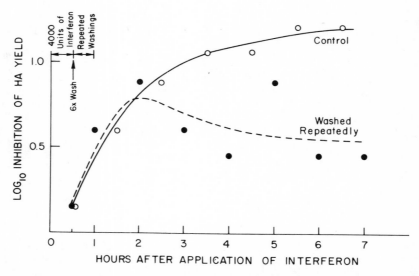

Fig. 6. Effect of repeated washings during the disassociation period on the development of antiviral activity in mouse L cells.

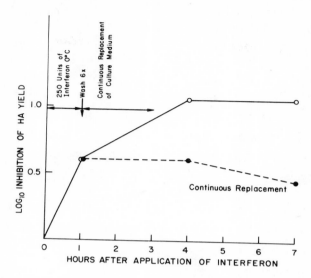

Fig. 7. Effect of continuous replacement of culture medium during the dissociation period on the development of antiviral activity.

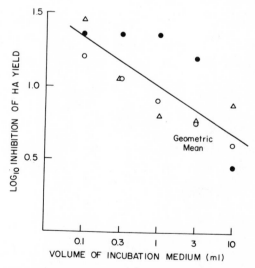

Fig. 8. Effect of volume of culture medium during and after the disassociation period on the development of antiviral activity.

DISCUSSION

Chany: I think that most people would agree with saying
that what really counts for the establishment of the antiviral
state is the concentration of the active molecules at the receptor sites. The volume would interfere only if interferon is con-
sumed by the cell. I think these data are very much in agreement
with this concept.

Stinebring: I just wonder how you control pinocytosis in
this. Assuming that there is a specific binding site, what you've
described, Dr. Baron, looks as though this all could be reverse
pinocytosis followed by pinocytosis again.

Baron: Yes. Although I didn't use that term, that's very
much in our thinking. There are a number of ways of binding of
proteins like interferon to cells which would be non-specific and
pinocytosis is one of them. It's an important differential because pinocytotic vacuoles, although within the cytoplasm, contain
materials which are still outside the cell membrane.

Stinebring: In other words, this could be in separate com-
partments and not necessarily inside?

Baron: Right, and it would tend to confuse the issue, because it might falsely appear to be intracellular interferon when
it was actually nonspecifically pinocytosed.

II - INTERFERON INDUCTION, MECHANISM AND ITS REGULATION

INDUCTION OF INTERFERON BY SEPHAROSE-BOUND POLY I:C

Joyce Taylor-Papadimitriou and John Kallos

Theagenion Cancer Institute
Thessaloniki,Greece

The double stranded polyribonucleotide poly I:C can induce viral resistance in chick embryo fibroblasts (CEF) (1), although detectable amounts of interferon are produced only be cells induced in the presence of DEAE-dextran (2, 3). An attempt has been made to determine whether the ability of poly I:C to induce interferon in this system depends on its entry into the cell. Poly I:C was coupled to "Sepharose" beads, which are too large to enter the cell, and the induction of interferon by the solid inducer was followed.

Under the conditions used to couple poly I:C to cyanogen-bromide activated "Sepharose" 4B (4, 5), between 10 and 20% of the soluble polynucleotide remained attached to the beads after extensive washing. The stability of "Sepharose"-bound tritium-labelled poly I:C was studied by following the liberation of radioactivity after treating the beads in various ways. Table 1 shows that very little radioactivity was released after treatment with alkali or RNAse; after incubation with cultures of CEF 3% was solubilized of which one third was associated with the cells. The actual number of counts on the gel was determined accurately after solubilizing the gel with 6N HCl. It seems therefore that poly I:C is strongly bound to "Sepharose" beads by multipoint attachment.

Table 2 shows the results of an experiment done to test the interferon-stimulating ability of poly I:C-"Sepharose" in the presence and absence of DEAE-dextran. Clearly, the solid inducer is an effective inducer of interferon in CEF, and, unlike soluble poly I:C, its effectiveness is inhibited, and not enhanced by the presence of DEAE-dextran. The inhibitory effect of DEAE-dextran on the interferon-inducing capacity of poly I:C suggests that it is the bound nucleotide and not released soluble material which is responsible for the induction.

The "Sepharose" beads can be visualized in the microscope interacting with the cells, and after incubation for 3-5 hours, very little binding was observed under the conditions of the experiment reported in Table 2. The transient contact resulting from the colision between beads and cells appears to be enough to result in interferon induction.

The above results suggest that poly I:C is able to induce interferon in chick embryo fibroblasts, merely by interaction with the cell membrane. However, to deduce from these observations that poly I:C does not need to enter the cell in order to induce interferon, we must assume that there is no direct transfer of poly I:C from the beads across the cell membrane. The material associated with the cells after induction corresponds to approximately 0.5 µg of poly I:C per cell culture. Although this is only 1% of the total bound poly I:C added to the culture, it is a finite amount of inducer which could conceivably be responsible for the interferon induction.

References

1. Field, A.K., Tytell, A.A., Lampson, G.P. and Hilleman,
    M.R. (1967). Proc. Nat. Acad. Sci. USA, 58:1004.
2. Colby, C., and Chamberlin, M.J. (1969). Proc. Nat. Acad.
    Sci. Washington, 63:160.
3. Long, W.F. and Burke, D.C. (1971). J. Gen. Virology, 12:
    1.
4. Axen, R., Porath, J., and Ernback, S. (1967). Nature,
    214:1302.
5. Porath, J., Axen, R., and Ernback, S. (1967). Nature,
    215:1491.
6. Poonian, M.S., Schlabach, A.J., Weissbach, A. (1971).
    Biochemistry, 10:424.

TABLE 1

Stability of ^{3}H poly I:C-Sepharose

Treatment procedure	Radioactivity liberated (c.p.m.)	% total counts
1 hr 37°C with 40 µg/ml of pancreatic RNAase	15	1
0.3 NaOH 16 hrs 37°C	50	3
5 hrs 37°C in MEM with Monolayer CEF	56	3
6N HCl overnight	1,600	100

0.1 ml samples of ^{3}H-poly I:C Sepharose were incubated with RNAase, NaOH or cells as indicated and the number of counts released into the supernatant estimated. The Sepharose sample which was incubated with HCl was dried and total counts estimated.

TABLE 2

Induction of interferon in chick embryo fibroblasts
by poly I:C coupled to Sepharose

Concentration of poly I:C[a]	Units of interferon produced after incubation with:					
	Soluble poly I:C		Sepharose-poly I:C		Sepharose	
	alone	+DEAE-dextran	alone	+DEAE-dextran	alone	+DEAE-dextran
50µg/ml	8	18	192	40		
20µg/ml	8	25	192	33		
10µg/ml	5	31	80	25		
					<5	<5

Sepharose 4B was activated with cyanogen bromide (5) and coupled to poly I:C in 0.1 M phosphate buffer pH 8.0 containing 0.03 M NaCl Equal volumes of poly I:C (1 mg/ml) and packed beads were mixed overnight at 4°C. After extensive washing, the beads were suspended in PBS A. The amount of coupling was determined by following the disappearance of UV-absorbing material (260 mµ) or isotope and efficiency of coupling was usually 10-20%. Five day old cultures of CEF grown in Dulbecco's MEM + 5% calf serum were incubated for 5 hours at 37°C with soluble or Sepharose bound poly I:C, in MEM with or without DEAE-dextran (10 µg/ml) in the absence of serum. After removal of inducer, cultures were washed extensively, and incubated with fresh MEM (3 ml) without serum for 16 hrs at 37°C. The supernatants were harvested, incubated with RNAase (40 µg/ml) for 1 hour at 37°C, UV irradiated for 15 mins after the addition of 0.1% albumen, and titrated for interferon against Vaccinia virus.

[a] made by mixing homopolymers in equal amounts and incubating 10 mins at 37°C.

DISCUSSION

From the audience: I am surprised by the resistance to ribonuclease of the Sepharose-bound poly I:C. Do you have an explanation for this?

Papadimitriou: Well, there is not one point of attachment.
Presumably bonds can still be broken, and the small molecular
weight products could still be attached to the "Sepharose" if
there are many sites of attachment. Poonian, who coupled nucleic
acids to Sepharose also observed a multipoint-attachment and very
strong binding. Also we must remember that we are dealing with a
bead which is full of holes. The molecules interacting with cells
are presumably on the surface, whereas those bound inside the
bead may be very well protected from any kind of enzyme action.

MECHANISM OF INTERFERON INDUCTION BY POLY IC: DEPENDENCE ON CELL MEMBRANE INTEGRITY

Paula M. Pitha[*], Harry D. Harper[*], and Josef Pitha[†]

[*]Department of Medicine and Microbiology,
The Johns Hopkins University, School of Medicine,
Baltimore, Maryland 21205
[†]National Institute of Child Health and Human Development,
Gerontology Research Center, Baltimore, Maryland 21224

Cells exposed to the complex of poly IC develop resistance to direct challenge and simultaneously release interferon in the medium (1, 2). The mechanism by which polynucleotides trigger interferon induction is still not very clear. It was shown recently that poly IC induces synthesis of specific mRNAs for interferon which can be translated with fidelity in heterologous cell systems (3). However, nothing much is known about the pretranscriptional steps which lead to the formation of interferon mRNA.

There are numerous mechanisms by which foreign molecules control the activity and rate of synthesis of specific proteins in the host cell. Nearly all of these could be theoretically applied to interferon systems as well. A few examples are in Fig. 1. There are primarily two ways in which foreign macromolecules can get into the cytoplasm. One is through the damaged places in cellular membrane; and it is interesting to note that dead or even slightly damaged cells can take up even 100x more RNA than the living ones (4). The second entry is through pinocytotic vesicles and secondary lysosomes (5). It was shown on double-stranded reovirus RNA complexed with poly lysine that all endocytosed RNA was conserved in vacuolar systems (5). By the same route, soluble proteins are taken up by the cell (6). The orthodox view is that endocytes macromolecules remain within this system until they are degraded to nucleotides or small peptides (7). However, the fact that both single- and double-stranded viral RNAs can form infectious centers indicates that penetration of intact RNA into animal cells can happen (8).

While the entry of nucleic acid into cytoplasm seems to be rather non-specific, the way hormones regulate the expression of cellular genome shows high specificity from the very beginning. Each of the peptide hormones seem to have a specific binding site on cellular membrane of the target cell. The bound hormones then activate the adenylcyclase, which is a membrane associated enzyme regulating the levels of cyclic AMP in the cytoplasm. This either directly activates the cytoplasmic enzymes, or interacts with the nucleohistones (9). On the other hand, the steroid hormones work through a different mechanism. The transport through the membrane is non-specific, but they bind to specific high m.w. protein in the cytoplasm, which transports them to the nucleus where they interact with acidic proteins of the chromatin (10).

In most described effects, the cellular membrane plays a crucial role. The basis of membrane forms a lipid monolayer with choline phospholipids in the external half and amino phospholipids in the cytoplasmic part. The majority of the proteins are located in the cytoplasmic part, but some extend across the monolayer. These generally have carbohydrates on their surface remote from the cytoplasm (11). The membrane lipids are in fluid state, which brings a large degree of mobility to the whole membrane (12). The structural and functional integrity of the membrane not only af-

fects membrane receptors mediated processes, but also a general
one as pinocytosis (13).

If we come back to the interferon system, we can see that
here much less knowledge is available.

Studies of the interaction between the inducer molecule and
the inducible cells indicated that the critical absorption of
$rI_n \cdot rC_n$ molecules to the cells is a very rapid event (14), but
a rather nonspecific one since biologically inactive single-
stranded polyribonucleotides and polydeoxyribonucleotides became
cell-associated at rates comparable to that of $rI_n \cdot rC_n$ (15).
Furthermore, no quantitative differences in the binding of the
inducer to the sensitive and insensitive cells have been demonstrated (16). Autoradiographic analysis has revealed that
$rI_n \cdot rC_n$ is taken up by the cells, but no critical information
concerning the triggering site was obtained (17).

The attempts to isolate biologically active poly IC from
the cytoplasm has been also unsuccessful and, therefore, a number
of indirect approaches have been designed. Polycations have been
reported to enhance the antiviral activity of poly IC (18, 19).
Whether this is due to the enhancement of binding, uptake, or due
to the specific effect on cellular membrane has not been completely clear. We assumed that the particular nature of complexes formed between poly IC and DEAE-dextran may be pinocytosied more extensively than poly IC (19). To see if any substantial increase
in the molecular weight of poly IC would have the same effect, we
linked covalently to poly IC neutral macromolecules, such as BSA
or high m.w. dextran. However, these modifications completely
abolished the antiviral effect of poly IC. Thus, the stimulation
of polycations is probably due to the effect on cell rather than
on the poly IC complex only.

Poly IC retained its antiviral activity when coupled to large particles, which apparently cannot enter the cell (20,21). The antiviral activity did not depend in a critical way on the stability of attachment. Separation of poly IC from mica was nearly complete during the experiments, but the biological ability was low. On the other hand, the release of polynucleotide from cellulose, Sephadex or Sepharose, was not substantial, yet the complex had the same or higher activity than when induction was carried out by poly IC in solution only.

This may indicate that the interferon induction site is located on the outer part of the cellular membrane and suggest that for the interferon induction, poly IC does not have to enter the cell. However, since minute quantities of double-stranded RNA are capable of interferon induction, we felt that our results did not conclusively prove that mere contact of inducer with the external membrane is sufficient for interferon induction.

From this reason we approach the problem from a different direction and studied how the antiviral effect of poly IC and its binding depend on structural integrity of cellular membrane.

Since Con A is one of the lectins which interact with surface receptors of a number of cells, we analyzed the effects of such interaction on the binding and antiviral effect of poly IC (22). We used mouse 3T3 cells since Con A interaction with these cells has been well characterized, and compared results obtained with this system to results using human fibroblasts. The results in Figure 2 show that pretreatment of mouse 3T3 cells with 10-100 µg/ml Con A caused a profound decrease in interferon production. If Con A was added to the cells after poly IC, the effect was less profound. To see whether the inhibition was due specifically to Con A, we tested the capacity of hapten inhibitors to block its

effect. When methyl-D glucose was incubated simultaneously with
Con A, no inhibition was observed.

Under the same conditions, the binding of poly IC alone or
in the presence of DEAE-dextran was not greatly affected by the
low concentrations of Con A that have a significant effect on
interferon production. Only when high concentrations of Con A
were used, the binding of poly IC decreased. Also, the binding of
radioactive Con A was not affected by pretreatment with poly IC.
These results indicate that Con A and poly IC do not bind to the
same site on the membrane of 3T3 cells. However, the effect was
not specific for mouse 3T3 cells; a similar pattern of inhibition
was observed in human fibroblast cells as well.

Figure 3 shows the dose response analysis studied in human
fibroblasts. These are the typical dose response curves for poly
IC in the absence and the presence of Con A as measured by the
resistance of the cells against virus infection and virus yield.
The curves are similar in shape and reach the same maximum which
is typical for a competitive inhibition. This indicates that poly
IC and Con A compete for a common cellular target, which probably
is not as the earlier experiments have shown the binding site on
cellular membrane. It is too early to say at this point where
this common receptor is located, but it might be a component of
cell membrane involved with the specific recognition of poly IC
or its subsequent entry into cytoplasm.

To examine further the nature of the recognition site for
interferon induction, the possible role of cell surface glycoproteins and phospholipids was studied (23). Although the mild
digestion with trypsin was shown at first to stimulate and later
abolish the antiviral effect of poly IC, the lack of specificity
of trypsin digestion made the result difficult to interpret. How-

ever, neuraminidase, often called the receptor destroying enzyme,
has a specificity for sialic acid residues which are part of many
glycoproteins forming cell membrane receptors.

Pretreatment of the cells with low concentrations of neuraminidase inhibited the antiviral effect of poly IC (Fig. 4). Concentrations of neuraminidase sufficient for inhibition of poly IC
stimulated antiviral response did not cause cell toxicity and
were without effect on the binding of inducer. When cells were
treated with neuraminidase after being exposed to poly IC, no inhibition was observed. This may indicate that sialic acid residues
of cell surface glycoproteins are somehow critical in the series
of events which trigger interferon induction, but are not part of
receptor structure; or that sialic acid residues are necessary for
receptor activity, but not for poly IC binding. The same results
were observed when cells were treated with subtoxic concentrations
of phospholipase C. Once again, the interferon induction, but not
the binding of inducer, was affected.

There is a possibility that enzymatic treatments destroy the
specific sites of polynucleotide binding that are required for
biological effect, thus implying that a very small amount of inducer is bound to active receptors; the rest being nonspecifically bound and inactive. However, the fact that a wide variety of
agents inhibit poly IC activity makes it unlikely that there is a
specific site destruction.

The question then arises whether the binding of inducer to
the cellular membrane is through specific binding with a limited
number of binding sites, or whether all the binding we measured
is due to the nonspecific adsorbtion only. The effects of polynucleotide pretreatment on the subsequent binding of poly IC is
shown in Table 1. Both double- and single-stranded RNAs at re-

latively high concentrations caused only partial inhibition of
poly IC binding. This indicates that both specific and nonspecific binding occurs.

In conclusion, we would like to point out that although the
present studies did not locate the triggering site for interferon
induction unambiguously, they demonstrate clearly that it is possible to completely interrupt the antiviral effect of $rI_n \cdot rC_n$
either by specific membrane treatments or by pretreatment with Con
A without modifying the binding function of the membrane receptors.

The approach used in these studies - modification of cell
surface receptors and measurement of resulting biological effect
-- may be of some value in further elucidation of the mechanism
and site of interferon induction.

References

1. Field, A.K., Tyttel, A.A., Lampson, G.P., and Hilleman,
    M.R. (1967). Proc. Natl. Acad. Sci. 58:1004.

2. Younger, J.S. and Hallum, T.V. (1968). Virology 35:177.

3. De Maeyer-Guignard, J., De Maeyer, E. and Montagnier,
    L. (1972). Proc. Natl. Acad. Sci. 69:1203.

4. Juliano, R. and Mayhew, E. (1972). Experimental Cell
    Res. 73:3.

5. Seljelid, R., Silverstein, S.C., and Cohen, Z.A. (1973).
    J. Cell. Biol. 57:484.

6. Steinman, R. and Cohen, Z.A. (1972). J. Cell. Biol. 55:
    616.

7. Cohen, Z.A. and Ehrenreich, B.A. (1969). J. Expt. Med.
    129:201.

8. Bishop, J.M. and Koch, G. (1971). J. Biol. Chem. 242: 1736.

9. Pastan, I. and Rerlman, R.L. (1971). Nature New Biology 229:15.

10. Jensen, E.V. and De Sombre, E.R. (1973). Science 182:126.

11. Bretcher, M.S. (1973). Science 181:622.

12. Singer, S.J. and Nicolson, G.L. (1973). Science 175:720.

13. Edelman, G.M., Yahara, I., and Wang, J.L. (1973). Proc. Natl. Acad. Sci. 70:1442.

14. Pitha, P.M., Marshall, L.W., and Carter, W.A. (1972). J. Gen. Virol. 15:89.

15. Colby, C. and Chamberlin, M.J. (1969). Proc. Natl. Acad. Sci. 63:160.

16. De Clercq, C.E. and De Sommer, P. (1973). J. Gen. Virol. 19:113.

17. Prose, P.H., Friedman-Kien, A., and Vilček, J. (1970). J. Gen. Physiol. 56:995.

18. Dianzani, F., Contagalli, P., Gagironi, S., and Rita, G. (1968). Proc. Soc. Exp. Biol., N.Y. 128:708.

19. Pitha, P.M. and Carter, W.A. (1971). Virology 45:777.

20. Pitha, P.M. and Pitha, J. (1973). J. Gen. Virol., In Press.

21. Taylor-Papadimitriou, J. and Kallos, J. (1973). Nature, In Press.

22. Harper, H.D. and Pitha, P.M. (1973). Biochem. Biophys. Res. Commun. 53:1220.

23. Pitha, P.M., Harper, H.D., and Pitha, J. (1973). Virology, Submitted.

TABLE 1

The effect of polynucleotide pretreatment
on subsequent binding of $rI_n \cdot rC_n$ to human fibroblasts cells

Pretreatment (µg of poly-nucleotide/ml)		cpm/ 10^6 Cells	ng $rI_n \cdot rC_n$ Bound/10^6 Cells	Inhibition (%)
-	-	945	20.3	0
$r(IG)_n \cdot rC_n$	300	438	9.4	50
	30	945	20.3	0
$rA_n \cdot rU_n$	300	366	7.8	60
	30	459	9.8	50
rI_n	300	480	10.1	50
	30	906	19.4	4
rC_n	300	213	4.5	80
	30	645	13.8	30

Human fibroblast cells grown in Packard scintillation vials
(3×10^5 cells/vial) were pretreated with given concentration of
unlabeled polynucleotide for 1 hr, 37°C. The cells were washed
with PBS and incubated with 1 ml of $rI_n \cdot (^3H)rC_n$ (30 µg/ml,
1.4×10^6 cpm/ml) for 1 hr, 37°C and radioactivity counted as described in Methods.

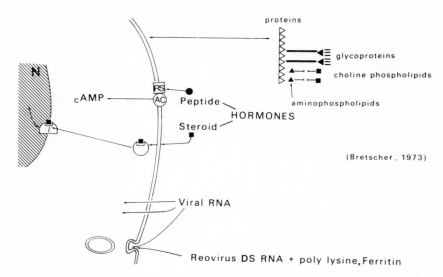

Fig. 1. Various modes of interaction of macromolecules with cells.

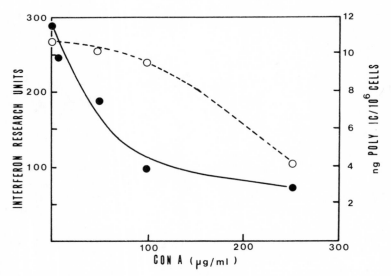

Fig. 2. The effect of Con A pretreatment on interferon induction by poly IC in mouse 3T3 cells (22).

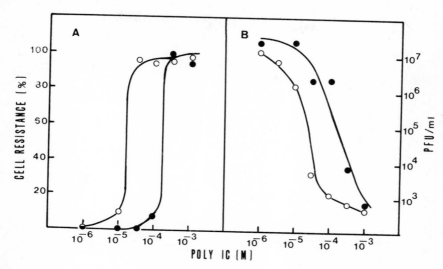

Fig. 3. The dose-response curve for poly IC in human fibroblasts in the absence and presence of Con A (22) o——o controls; ●——● 50 µg/ml of Con A.

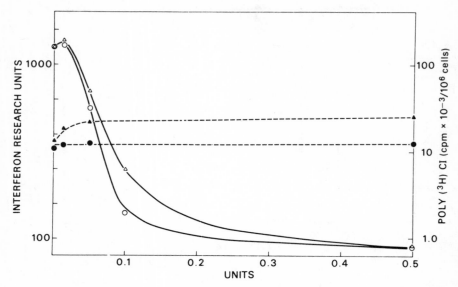

Fig. 4. The effect of neuraminidase and phospholipase C pretreatment on interferon induction by poly IC in mouse 3T3 cells
(23). Full lines represent interferon units; dotted lines represent binding of poly (^{3}H)IC; o represent neuraminidase treatment;
Δ represent phospholipase treatment.

DISCUSSION

Levy: Dr. Kelly, working in my laboratory on a PHD thesis, did some experiments to study the nature of the bound poly I:C. What he looked for was the presence of biologically active poly I:C as Dr. Pitha just alluded to. We, in agreement with Dr. Pitha, were not able to find any biologically active poly I:C in RNA from cells that were exposed to large quantities of poly I:C. If we used radioactive poly I:C, we were indeed able to find radio-activity, but if you looked at the radioactivity in poly acrila-mide gels, it was not radioactive poly I:C anymore, it was broken down poly I:C, largely re-incorporated into cellular RNA. So, in these various experiments, where one attempts to study the effect of modifying agents on poly I:C uptake, I think it is a little risky to say that, when you measure radioactivity uptake, this is uptake of poly I:C. I think such correlations are really not totally justified.

Pitha: I agree, but in our experiment, we treated the cells with poly I:C in phosphate buffer for a very short period of time and we know that under these conditions, there is no substantial degradation. However, if you open the cells, you may not be able to find the poly IC free for several reasons. As soon as you open the cells, you may release and activate all the nu-cleases; also, if you assume that if only a few molecules of poly IC get inside the cell, you would not expect to find them free. Poly IC may interact with some proteins, and then it depends on the methods used, if you defect them or not.

Levy: Yes, this is certainly correct. What we did though was: we exposed cells to poly I:C for periods of time ranging

from 5 minutes to 3 hours and in quantities ranging from 1 microgram to a couple of hundred micrograms, and then we immediately
exposed the washed cells to hot phenol. I think this would protect
it from ribonuclease action.

Pitha: That's right, but even in the 5 minutes you did not
find any high molecular weight of poly I:C.

Levy: No biologically active poly I:C down to .03μg, the
limit of sensitivity of the test.

De Clercq: I would like to make a remark in regard to Dr.
Levy's comment about the uptake of radioactive poly I:C by the
cells. I have looked at the radioactivity associated with the
cells after incubation of rabbit kidney cells with radioactive
poly I:C for 1 hour. The cells were homogenized by ultrasonic disintegration and the radioactivity was analysed by velocity ultracentrifugation in a sucrose gradient. The radioactive material in
the cell homogenates showed the same peak as control preparations
of poly I:C, suggesting that it was actually poly I:C that was recovered from the cells in this particular case.

May I add some comments on Dr. Pitha's presentation? She
found that the several treatments of the cells with trypsin, with
neuraminidase, with phospholipase and even with concanavalin A inhibited the interferon response to poly I:C, and interpreted these
findings in terms of an inactivation of the receptor site for
interferon induction by poly I:C. This would suggest that the receptor site for poly I:C is a very aspecific one because it can
be affected by so many different enzymes and even by concanavalin
A. I would not expect such a lack of specificity for this receptor site, because it has been postulated repeatedly that it should
be a very specific one (cfr. Colby and Chamberlin, 1969, Proc.

INTERFERON PRODUCTION AS A MODEL OF INDUCED
PROTEIN SYNTHESIS IN EUKARYOTIC CELLS

Jan Vilček and Edward A. Havell

Department of Microbiology, New York University
School of Medicine, New York, New York 10016

Introduction

In studying the mechanism of interferon induction, poly I.
poly C offers some advantages over viral inducers. While the actual trigger molecule responsible for interferon induction by
viruses is not known, synthetic polynucleotide inducers are chemically and structurally defined entities. Furthermore, for the
induction by viruses there may be a need for the expression of
some viral functions, and the cellular metabolism may undergo
profound changes as a result of infection, whereas polynucleotide
inducers generally do not cause such drastic alterations of cellular metabolic activities.

In the work which is reviewed here, attention will be paid
to only some events occurring during the induction of human diploid fibroblast cultures (FS-4 strain) with poly I.poly C. The
details of experiments which are not presented in full here can
be found in a recent publication from this laboratory (1).

Synthesis of Interferon Messenger RNA

The kinetics of interferon mRNA synthesis in rabbit kidney cells or human foreskin cells stimulated with poly I.poly C was studied with the aid of antimetabolites known to inhibit cellular mRNA synthesis. In both cell systems high doses of actinomycin D were found to inhibit interferon production only when added within approximately the first hour of induction. This period of actinomycin D sensitivity was followed by a very short period during which the drug neither inhibited nor enhanced the interferon yield. The addition of actinomycin D 1.5-2 hr after induction, or later, markedly enhanced subsequent interferon production. The results obtained in rabbit kidney cell cultures were published earlier (2), while a summary of similar results obtained in the FS-4 strain of human foreskin cells is shown in Fig. 1.

We believe that the inhibition during the initial period of induction is due to interference by actinomycin D with the process of transcription of interferon mRNA. The dose of actinomycin D employed would, of course, also inhibit the synthesis of other RNA species, including ribosomal RNA. However, we did show earlier that interferon production could go on uninterrupted in rabbit kidney cells treated with toyocamycin-an adenosine analog which preferentially interferes with the maturation of ribosomal RNA. We found that doses of toyocamysin which inhibited the appearance of 18 and 28 S RNA had no inhibitory effect on the interferon yields (3). Thus ribosomal RNA synthesis is apparently not required for interferon induction. These results support the assumption (although they do not prove it) that the early inhibition of interferon production by actinomycin D is the result of interference with interferon mRNA transcription.

Lowering the incubation temperature from 36.5 to 34.5° C
prolonged the time during which interferon production was sensitive to inhibition by actinomycin D (Table 1). This difference is
likely to be the result of slower transcription of interferon
mRNA at 34.5° C. The subsequent enhancement of interferon production by the addition of actinomycin D showed a maximum at 2 hr
after induction in the cultures incubated at 36.5° C, whereas at
the lower temperature this event too was delayed.

Mechanism of Superinduction by Actinomycin D

The literature lists many other examples of increased synthesis of a specific protein after the addition of actinomycin D
at certain times during the induction process (reviewed in ref.4).
Since the understanding of induced protein synthesis in eukaryotic
cells could be as important for the advancement of our knowledge
of the control of gene expression in animal cells as the operator
theory had been for the unraveling of similar processes in
Escherichia coli, it is not surprising that the phenomenon of
superinduction by actinomycin D has attracted a good deal of attention from molecular biologists.

To explain the mechanism of increased synthesis of the enzyme tyrosine aminotransferase after the addition of actinomycin D
to induced rat hepatoma cells, Tomkins et al. (5, 6) postulated
the existence of a posttranscriptional control mechanism. According to this hypothesis, deinduction (which means the decrease in
the rate of enzyme synthesis from the fully induced level to the
level of uninduced cells) is, essentially, the function of a labile regulatory protein, or repressor. The synthesis of this repressor is controlled by a specific gene. The repressor acts by
blocking the translation of the enzyme mRNA, presumably by a di-

rect interaction of the repressor protein with the enzyme mRNA at a cytoplasmic site. Tomkins postulated that this interaction would not only inhibit translation, but it would also promote inactivation of enzyme mRNA, i.e., it would effectively clear the cell from functional enzyme mRNA.

This idea can explain the superinducing effects of actinomycin D, provided that not only the repressor protein, but also the mRNA for the repressor is labile, whereas the enzyme mRNA is relatively stable. In that case the addition of a suitable dose of actinomycin D would rapidly stop the synthesis of the repressor (because the supply of repressor mRNA would be rapidly depleted), thus allowing the continued translation of the more stable enzyme mRNA. In some instances, however, it may not be necessary to invoke the lability of repressor mRNA, provided that the synthesis of the enzyme mRNA precedes that of the repressor mRNA and the treatment with actinomycin D is before the onset of repressor mRNA transcription.

Tomkins' model has not met with universal acceptance. In particular, Schimke et al. (7) suggested that superinduction by actinomycin D can be explained on the basis of differential stabilities of various species of cellular mRNA. According to this idea, once transcription is blocked by actinomycin D, more labile species of mRNA will decay and this will result in a relative enrichment of the stable mRNA which, in turn, can be more efficiently translated. According to this concept, no repressor would have to be involved in the superinduction phenomenon.

We believe that the superinduction of interferon synthesis can be satisfactorily explained by the application of the Tomkins model, postulating the existence of a repressor which inhibits the translation and promotes inactivation of interferon mRNA. Table 1 showed that the addition of actinomycin D at 2 hr after induction produced the greatest accentuation of subsequent interferon production (at 36.5° C), whereas its addition at later times was increasingly less effective. It seems logical to conclude that 2 hr was the optimal time because, by then, enough interferon mRNA had been transcribed, while efficient repressor mRNA synthesis probably did not begin until after this time. The sharp subsequent drop in superinducibility could be due to the gradual accumulation of repressor with the resulting depletion of the intracellular pool of interferon mRNA.

These findings would be more difficult to explain on the basis of Schimke's model. Interferon mRNA is inherently quite stable (see below), and if there were no repressor promoting its inactivation, the addition of actinomycin D at 3.5 hr after induction should result in virtually the same degree of superinduction as its addition at 2 hr. Yet, as shown in Table 1, that is definitely not the case.

Transcription of the Interferon Messenger RNA in the Presence of Inhibitors of Protein Synthesis

Earlier work by Tan et al. (8) and our own data (9) suggested that transcription of the interferon messenger can proceed in the presence of various inhibitors of protein synthesis. In cultures induced with poly I.poly C in the presence of cycloheximide, the removal of cycloheximide at 4-6 hr after induction was followed by a burst of interferon production which coincided with the rapid resumption of protein synthesis in the cultures. The amount of interferon produced after such cycloheximide treatment was significantly greater than in control cultures not incubated with cycloheximide. Many other inhibitors of protein synthesis were

also shown to have a similar enhancing effect on poly I.poly C-
stimulated interferon production (1, 9, 10).

Thus, not only can interferon mRNA transcription proceed in
the presence of inhibitors of protein synthesis, but, actually,
there seems to be more functional interferon mRNA accumulating in
cells in the presence of such inhibitors than in control cells.
This could be the result of either (a) an increased rate of transcription of interferon mRNA or (b) functional stabilization of the
interferon messenger in cells whose protein synthesis is suppressed.

There is no apparent reason why inhibition of protein synthesis should promote transcription. On the other hand, stabilization of the messenger could be predicted on the basis of the Tomkins model: synthesis of the repressor which promotes inactivation
of the interferon mRNA would be suppressed by cycloheximide and
other inhibitors of protein synthesis; the absence of repressor
would thus allow increased accumulation of active interferon mRNA.

It is interesting that no clear-cut demonstrations of enhancing effects of inhibitors of protein synthesis on the synthesis of other induced proteins have been reported. This is all
the more surprising in view of the numerous reported examples of
the superinducing action of actinomycin D (4).

It is by now well known among interferon workers that the
superinducing effects of inhibitors of protein synthesis and of
actinomycin D are additive and that a suitable combination of the
two treatments can often result in a 50- to 100-fold enhancement
of the interferon yield in cultures of rabbit (8, 9, 11) or human
(1, 12-15) cells.

The effect of the addition of cordycepin (3'-deoxyadeno-
sine), at different times during the treatment of cells with
cycloheximide, on the interferon yield measured after the removal
of cycloheximide is shown in Table 2. A marked inhibitory effect
was seen only if the treatment with cordycepin was initiated no
later than 1 hr after the stimulation with poly I.poly C.

Cordycepin is known to inhibit preferentially the appearance of cytoplasmic mRNA, by interfering with the synthesis of
polyadenylate and with the transport of the messenger from the
nucleus to the cytoplasm (16, 17). The results thus suggest,
first of all, that interferon mRNA is likely to contain poly A
sequences. It can also be concluded that transcription of the
interferon messenger in cells induced in the presence of cycloheximide was apparently complete by 2 hr after induction. This
result is similar to the findings in cells induced in the absence of cycloheximide (cf. Fig. 1 and Table 1) and it supports
the notion that inhibition of protein synthesis is unlikely to
promote transcription of the interferon messenger. Finally, it is
noteworthy that in the experiment shown in Table 2, poly I.poly C
was present during the entire first 6-hr period, and yet, transcription was apparently complete by 2 hr. Thus, continued exposure of cells to the inducer after the initial critical interaction also did not seem to result in prolonged transcription of
the interferon mRNA.

The conclusion that the presence of inhibitors of protein
synthesis in cultures during the early period of interferon induction is likely to cause a functional stabilization of interferon
mRNA is a strong argument in favor of the applicability of the
Tomkins model to the control of interferon synthesis.

Independence of Transcription and Translation of Interferon Messenger RNA

Is transcription of interferon mRNA independent of its translation? This question could not be answered satisfactorily on the basis of experiments with cycloheximide alone, because cycloheximide is quite inefficient in inhibiting poly I.poly C-induced interferon production in rabbit (2, 10) or human (1, 12, 14) cells. However, we found that transcription of the interferon messenger in FS-4 cells was apparently also not altered in the presence of puromycin or in the presence of both puromycin and cycloheximide. In the latter group, interferon production during the treatment with inhibitors was suppressed by 98%, yet the amount of interferon produced after the reversal of inhibition of protein·synthesis was comparable to the yield produced after a similar reversal in cells induced in the presence of cycloheximide alone. The amount of interferon made during the treatment with cycloheximide was reduced by only 50%. Thus, transcription of interferon mRNA was apparently not affected when interferon synthesis was suppressed to different degrees by various inhibitors of protein synthesis (1).

Taken together, these results strongly suggest that transcription of the interferon messenger is completely independent from its translation. Stimulation of interferon mRNA transcription is apparently one of the first steps in induction. Unfortunately, the actual mechanism underlying this event remains obscure.

Stability of Interferon Messenger RNA

The fact that in cultures of rabbit or human cells interferon production rises rapidly after induction, reaches a peak in about 3 hr and declines quite quickly thereafter (cf. Fig. 1) sug-

gests that in these systems interferon mRNA functions for only a
very short time. Yet, it is now clear that the interferon messenger is not inherently unstable. The early termination of interferon synthesis is thought to be the function of the repressor
which, as explained earlier, interferes with the translation and
promotes inactivation of the interferon mRNA.

The apparent half-life of the interferon messenger can be
effectively prolonged by treatments which are thought to suppress
repressor synthesis while allowing the synthesis and expression
of interferon mRNA. The results of the following experiment serve
as a particularly good example of such a stabilization of interferon mRNA activity.

Human FS-4 cell cultures were induced with poly I.poly C in
the presence of cycloheximide. Six hours later the cultures were
washed free of cycloheximide and replenished with drug-free medium.
A measurement of the rate of interferon production after the reversal of cycloheximide action showed that a peak of interferon
was attained within 1 hr after the removal of cycloheximide. Subsequently, interferon production decreased at a rate of about 50%
every 70 min. Thus, the apparent half-life of interferon mRNA was
about 70 min.

In the same experiment some cultures were not only treated
with poly I.poly C and cycloheximide as above, but, in addition,
they received actinomycin D at 4 hr, i.e., 2 hr before lifting the
block of protein synthesis. In these latter cultures interferon
production also peaked within 1 hr of the removal of cycloheximide,
but the slope of the subsequent decrease of interferon production
was much less steep than in the first group of cultures. The apparent half-life of the interferon messenger was in the order of

360 min, or about 5 times longer than without the addition of actinomycin D.

    Our interpretation of these results is as follows: In the
former group of cultures interferon mRNA synthesis is stimulated
by poly I.poly C while the presence of cycloheximide inhibits repressor synthesis. The accumulated interferon messenger can be
translated following the removal of cycloheximide at 6 hr. However, the removal of cycloheximide will also allow repressor synthesis and the latter is thought to be responsible for the rapid
turn-off of interferon synthesis. The addition of actinomycin D
to the latter group of cultures would prevent repressor synthesis
after the removal of cycloheximide and thus will allow a more full
expression of the interferon mRNA which had been synthesized prior
to actinomycin D treatment. For further details of this experiment see reference 1. A similar experiment had also been carried
out in rabbit kidney cell cultures - with virtually identical
results (9).

    It has been shown that lowering of the incubation tempera-
ture from 37° C to 32° C during the period of translation of the
interferon messenger also affords a prolongation of its apparent
half-life. The effects of actinomycin D treatment and of lowered
incubation temperature were additive, suggesting that they act
through different mechanisms. We have suggested that the lower incubation temperature might have a direct stabilizing effect on the
interferon mRNA, although stabilization of some other component
that is rate-limiting in protein synthesis could not be ruled out
(1).

Comparison of Some Features of Tyrosine Aminotransferase and Interferon Induction

As pointed out in the preceding discussions, poly I.poly C-induced interferon induction shares some features in common with corticosteroid-induced enzyme synthesis. The latter has been most thoroughly studied on the model of tyrosine aminotransferase in cultures of rat hepatoma cells. Despite the similarities, the two systems also display many important differences.

Induction in the tyrosine aminotransferase system is characterized by about a 2-hr lag period, followed by gradual increase in enzyme synthesis to a plateau level which is about 10 times higher than the basal level of enzyme synthesis in uninduced cells. This induced level of synthesis is maintained for as long as the inducer is present in the cultures (18).

According to the model proposed by Tomkins et al. (5, 6), the steroid inducer binds directly to the repressor in the cytoplasm, thereby causing its inactivation. This event is followed by the stimulation of transcription of enzyme mRNA, which is thought to be caused by the migration of the complex of the steroid inducer with a cytoplasmic receptor protein to the nucleus. The feature of the model which postulates a direct binding of the inducer to the repressor can account for the fact that induced levels of enzyme synthesis are maintained for as long as the inducer is present.

In an earlier publication we proposed that a direct interaction of the polynucleotide inducer with the repressor in the cytoplasm could represent the initial event responsible for setting in motion the process of interferon induction (19). This idea was based on the possible analogy with the Tomkins model for tyrosine

aminotransferase induction as well as on the seemingly logical
conclusion that the repressor which, by definition, has an affinity for mRNA could very possibly also recognize a particular type
of secondary structure on the polynucleotide inducer. Yet, in
hindsight, this part of our model is not entirely convincing.

First of all, unlike in the tyrosine aminotransferase system,
continued presence of the polynucleotide inducer does not result
in sustained induction as one would expect if the repressor were
continually neutralized by the inducer. (On the other hand, there
may not be enough of the polynucleotide inducer to neutralize the
repressor if the synthesis of the latter is markedly stepped up
after induction).

Secondly, recent evidence suggests that with polynucleotide
inducers the triggering event may be taking place at the cell surface, since poly I.poly C covalently bound to solid carriers (20,
21), or firmly attached to the surface of animal cells (22) was
shown to be fully active in inducing interferon. (However, more
work will be needed to rule out the possibility that induction is
the result of the penetration of small quantitites of poly I.poly
C into the intracellular space).

Thirdly, this model does not explain the mechanism underlying the stimulation of transcription of interferon mRNA - an event
whose central significance in the induction process has been emphasized throughout this paper. (It is of little comfort to note
that other authors have also failed to offer an explanation for
this event, except in the most general terms).

Conclusions

Interferon induction represents an attractive model for the study of gene expression in eukaryotic cells. Some features of the control of interferon synthesis seem to be similar in nature to the control of corticosteroid-induced enzyme synthesis whereas other characteristics are unique for each of the two systems. Evidence concerning the posttranscriptional (translational) control of polynucleotide-induced interferon synthesis follows a quite rational pattern and the experimental observations on this particular stage of the induction process can be explained on the basis of a relatively simple hypothesis which owes a great deal to a model proposed by Tomkins to account for the posttranscriptional control of steroid-induced enzyme synthesis.

However, virtually all the evidence in favor of this hypothesis is still indirect and new techniques will have to be developed in order to subject these data to more rigorous experimental scrutiny. It is encouraging to note that interferon mRNA activity from cell extracts can now be assayed directly on the basis of its ability to direct interferon synthesis in uninduced cells of heterologous species (23). This technique, when further developed into a more quantitative assay, could provide a direct method for the testing of the correctness of some conclusions made in this paper.

Acknowledgements

This investigation was supported by United States Public Health Service Grant AI-07057 and Contract Nol-AI-02169. Fermina

Varacalli and Angel Feliciano provided skilled technical assistance, Barbara Dolgonos helped with the preparation of the manuscript.

References

1. Vilček, J. and Havell, E.A. (1973). Proc. Nat. Acad. Sci. U.S.A. 70 (in press).
2. Vilček, J. (1970). Ann. N. Y. Acad. Sci. 173:390.
3. Ng, M.H. and Vilček, J. (1973). Biochim. Biophys. Acta 294:284.
4. Tomkins, G.M., Levinson, B.B., Baxter, J.D. and Dethlefsen, L. (1972). Nature New Biology 239:9.
5. Tomkins, G.M., Thompson, E.B., Hayashi, S., Gelehrter, T., Granner, D. and Peterkofsky, B. (1966). Cold Spring Harb. Symp. Quant. Biol. 31:349.
6. Tomkins, G.M., Gelehrter, T.D., Granner, D., Martin, D., Jr., Samuels, H.H. and Thompson, E.B. (1969). Science 166:1474.
7. Schimke, R.T., Palacios, R., Palmiter, R.D. and Rhoads, R.E. (1973). In: Gene Expression and its Regulation (F. T. Kenney et al., editors), p. 123. Plenum Press, New York-London.
8. Tan, Y.H., Armstrong, J.A., Ke, Y.H. and Ho, M. (1970). Proc. Nat. Acad. Sci. U.S.A. 67:464.
9. Vilček, J. and Ng, M.H. (1971). J. Virol. 7:588.
10. Tan, Y.H., Armstrong, J.A. and Ho, M. (1971). Virology 44:503.
11. Mozes, L.W. and Vilček, J. (1974). J. Virol. 13 (in press).

12. Myers, M.W. and Friedman, R.M. (1971). J. Nat. Cancer Inst. 47:757.

13. Ho, M., Tan, Y.H. and Armstrong, J.A. (1972). Proc. Soc. Exp. Biol. Med. 139:259.

14. Havell, E.A. and Vilček, J. (1972). Antimicrob. Ag. Chemother. 2:476.

15. Billiau, A., Joniau, M. and De Somer, P. (1973). J. Gen. Virol. 19:1.

16. Darnell, J.E., Philipson, L., Wall, R. and Adesnik, M. (1971). Science 174:507.

17. Adesnik, M., Salditt, M., Thomas, W. and Darnell, J.E. (1972). J. Mol. Biol. 71:21.

18. Thompson, E.B., Tomkins, G.M. and Curran, J.F. (1966). Proc. Nat. Acad. Sci. U.S.A. 56:296.

19. Ng, M.H. and Vilček, J. (1972). Adv. Protein Chem. 26:173.

20. Taylor-Papadimitriou, J. and Kallos, J. (1973). Nature New Biology 245:143.

21. Pitha, P.M. and Pitha, J. (1973). J. Gen. Virol. 21:31.

22. De Clercq, E. and De Somer, P. (1972). J. Gen. Virol. 16:435.

23. De Maeyer-Guignard, J., De Maeyer, E. and Montagnier, L. (1972). Proc. Nat. Acad. Sci. U.S.A. 69:1203.

TABLE 1

Effect of incubation temperature on the rate
of interferon mRNA transcription

Hour of actinomycin D treatment[b]	Incubation temperature (^{O}C)[a]			
	34.5		36.5	
	Interferon yield[c]	% control	Interferon yield[c]	% control
None	2,048	(100)	1,365	(100)
1.0	42	2	341	24
1.5	1,365	66	2,730	200
2.0	4,096	200	16,384	1,200
2.5	10,923	533	5,461	400
3.0	10,923	533	5,461	400
3.5	5,461	266	2,730	200

a All cultures were exposed to poly I.poly C (100 μg/ml) for 30 min at 36.5^{O} C, washed and replenished with MEM containing 2% fetal calf serum. After the exposure to poly I.poly C half of the cultures were shifted down to 34.5^{O}, while incubation of the remaining cultures continued at 36.5^{O}.

b At various times after induction, the culture fluids were removed and the cells were treated for 30 min. with actinomycin D (2 μg/ml) at the respective temperature. After this treatment the cultures were washed, replenished with fresh MEM containing 2% fetal calf serum (prewarmed to the appropriate temperature) and incubated at the respective temperature throughout the rest of the experiment.

c The yields indicated are from the end of actinomycin D treatment (or from the end of exposure to poly I.poly C in the control groups) until 24 hr after exposure to poly I.poly C when all culture fluids were harvested.

TABLE 2

Interferon yields from cells treated with
cordycepin during the induction phase[a]

Time of treatment with cordycepin (hr)	Interferon yield
0-6	240
1-6	2,560
2-6	15,360
3-6	30,720
4-6	30,720
5-6	15,360
None	10,240

[a] FS-4 cells were stimulated at 0 hr by the addition of poly
I.poly C (100 µg/ml) in the presence of cycloheximide (50 µg/
ml) in serum-free MEM. Actinomycin D (1 µg/ml) was added to
all cultures at 5 hr. The concentration of cordycepin was 100
µg/ml. At 6 hr, all cultures were washed and replenished with
inhibitor-free MEM containing 2% fetal-calf serum. Interferon
yields were determined in culture fluids collected at 24 hr.

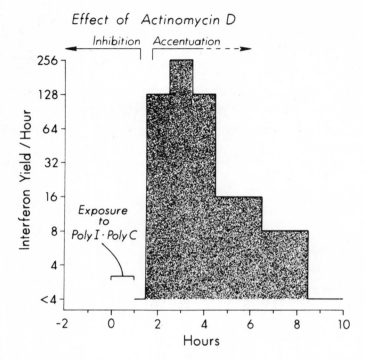

Fig. 1. Kinetics of interferon production in human FS-4 cells and the effects of actinomycin D. Cell cultures were exposed to poly I.poly C (100 μg/ml) for 1 hr as indicated in the graph. The medium was collected from cultures at hourly intervals for interferon assays. At each interval the cultures were replenished with fresh medium which was then kept on the cultures until the next collection time. Although it is not indicated in the graph, the synthesis of intracellular interferon is known to precede its release into the extracellular fluid by about 30 min.

The addition of a high dose of actinomycin D to the cultures until about 1 hr after the exposure to poly I.poly C inhibits interferon production, whereas the same treatment at later intervals leads to enhanced interferon synthesis (see also Table 1).

DISCUSSION

Chany: The post transcriptional blockage appears only after the induction of interferon, so this repressor is not present in the non-induced cells. Am I correct?

Vilcek: I would not really say that it is or is not present in non-induced cells. I think we just don't know.

Chany: That won't fit then with actinomycin data because, if not induced, the actinomycin shouldn't block it.

Vilcek: The reason why actinomycin, added say at 2 hours after poly I:C, causes superinduction, presumably is that at that time you already have interferon messenger RNA transcribed, but the repressor or sufficient quantities of the repressor to block the expression of this messenger would only be made at a later stage. So whether there is any repressor at all present in uninduced cells, I don't know. There may be some but clearly most of it would be made only at a later stage after induction.

Chany: Did you ever study superinduction in mutant cells which have no refractory state to induction? There are constitutive mutants of this type.

Vilcek: We haven't really looked at that. One indication that the repressor may be involved in the refractory state is that if you induce with poly I:C first, and then induce with poly I:C again, say at 6 to 24 hours later, you have a hyporesponsiveness. If you re-induce with poly I:C plus DEAE dextran, there is no hyporesponsiveness; and since I showed that with poly I:C and dextran the repressor is not operative, I think that this would suggest that there may be a correlation.

ASSAY FOR INTERFERON MESSENGER RNA IN HETEROLOGOUS CELLS

E. De Maeyer, L. Montagnier, J. De Maeyer-Guignard
and H. Collandre

Institut du Radium, Université de Paris-Sud,Campus d'ORSAY
and
Unité d'Oncologie Virale, Institut Pasteur,PARIS

Isolation of Mouse Interferon Messenger RNA

About two years ago we developed a biological assay for
interferon messenger RNA (1) and I would like to recapitulate here
the relevant aspects of this assay system.

Interferon induction is characterized by de novo synthesis
of messenger RNA, as indicated by the early work of Wagner and
Huang with metabolic inhibitors (2). It thus seemed theoretically
possible to isolate the interferon messenger from induced cells,
provided a translational system was available. The usual criteria
for determining protein synthesis in cell-free systems such as co-
precipitation, cochromatography or immunological methods could not
be applied in the case of interferon, in view of the very limited
amounts of furthermore highly unpure interferon protein available
as carrier for such assays. Therefore, the end product of our
translational system would have to be a fully functional protein
to be measured by its antiviral activity. It seemed to us that the

This study was supported by the "Fondation pour la Recherche Médicale Française" and the C.N.R.S.

species specificity of the interferon molecule, which on previous occasions had served to gain information concerning the cellular origin of interferon in mice (3) could also be exploited to trace its molecular origin, and we decided to test the possibility of using for messenger translation whole cells, belonging to an animal species different from the species from which the messenger was to be extracted. Under these conditions there could be no doubt as to the origin of the product of translation. At the time we started these experiments, the results of Gurdon et al., with the globin messenger in frog oocytes (4) had not yet been published, but later on these results demonstrated that the choice of whole cells as a translational system was fully justified.

The decision to study mouse mRNA was taken in view of our longstanding experience with mouse interferon. In addition, the existence of antisera directed against mouse interferon, thanks to the work of Fauconnier (5) and of Paucker (6), was an additional asset for the identification of the endproduct. For messenger translation, primary cultures derived from 8 to 9 day old chick embryos were taken, for two reasons: first, and most important, was the lack of cross reactivity between chick and mouse interferon (7), and second, we felt, that embryonic cells might be less restrictive in the translation of a foreign message than would be cells derived from adult tissue.

From our experimental results then it has become evident that chick embryo cells can indeed be used to translate mouse interferon mRNA. However, for this to happen with any degree of reproductivity several conditions are required for the RNA recipient as well as for the RNA donor cells.

Conditions for the RNA recipient cells (the translational system)

1) The cells have to be pretreated with Actinomycin D.
Early experiments, without pretreatment with Act. D, had given
highly irregular results, with evidence for translation in about
one experiment out of four. We then decided to treat the recipient
cells with Actinomycin D, in the hope of reducing endogenous messenger synthesis and thus freeing ribosomes for translation of the
mouse messenger. It was thus found that, when chick embryo cell
cultures are treated with Actinomycin D at a concentration of 0.1
µg per ml for five to six hours before addition of mouse RNA,
translation is obtained with great regularity, and this treatment
is now applied routinely. Whether or not this is due to the theoretical consideration that prompted us to try the treatment is not
known. There is evidence that even relatively low concentrations
of Actinomycin D can affect messenger RNA synthesis; Lindberg and
Persson for example have shown that in KB cells 0.04 µg per ml of
Actinomycin D suppressed the appearance of mRNA on polysomes to
an extent of 50% (8).

2) DEAE-dextran has to be present during incubation of the
chick cells with mouse RNA. It is known that the presence of DEAE-
dextran is required for the efficient uptake of infectious viral
RNA by cells in tissue culture (9). The same requirement was found
to hold for mouse mRNA on chick cells, and when DEAE-dextran was
omitted, no evidence for translation was obtained. Experiments in
which varying concentrations of RNA and dextran were tested indicated that optimal results were obtained when the DEAE-dextran
concentration was roughly equivalent to the RNA concentration, expressed in µg per ml. After removal of the medium containing Act.
D the cells are washed once with PBS and covered with the appropriate solution of dextran in PBS; the mRNA preparation is then

immediately added. The cell cultures are incubated for 45 min at
37°. At this point, the nucleic acid medium is removed and replaced by fresh culture medium. The latter is collected 5 to 16
hours later for interferon determinations.

We have found that chick cells can be replaced as translational system by human diploid or by Vero cells, but in the limited number of experiments in which these cells were compared we
have obtained higher mouse interferon yields from chick cells.

Conditions for the mRNA donor cells

As RNA donor cells we have used mouse cells of three different origins: L cells, secondary cultures of Swiss mouse embryo
fibroblasts and a continuous line of BALB/c embryonic cells. The
only requirements for these cells to yield interferon messenger
activity in the extracted RNA are as follows:

1) they have to be treated with an interferon inducer first
(we have used both poly-IC and Newcastle Disease Virus);
2) the RNA extraction has to take place within a given time
limit after induction (or the cells have to be stored at -70°
within these limits until the RNA can be extracted). Figure 1
gives the relative yield of messenger activity (expressed as mouse
interferon units made by chick cells) obtained from poly-IC-in-
duced mouse embryo fibroblasts as a function of time after addition of the inducer.

What is the evidence that we are dealing with translation of mouse interferon mRNA in chick cells?

Most important of course is the characterisation of the endproduct, proving that the virus inhibitor obtained from the RNA-

treated chick cells really is mouse interferon. The main arguments
in favor of this assumption are: a) it is a protein, since it is
destroyed by pronase and by trypsin, but not by treatment with
pancreatic ribonuclease;

b) it has the species specificity of mouse interferon, since
antiviral activity (inhibition of VSV replication) was only observed in mouse cells, but not in human, monkey, rat, or, most
important, chick cells;

c) it has the broad antiviral activity of interferon, since,
in addition to VSV, it was also tested against herpes simplex,
vaccinia and Sindbis virus and found to be active against these
viruses;

d) the antiviral action can be prevented by pretreatment of
the cells with Actinomycin D. This is an important point, since
it is now well established that interferon exerts its antiviral
activity indirectly, through induction of one or several proteins
(10).

e) it is neutralized by anti-mouse-interferon serum; this
antiserum has no effect on chick interferon. Since there is no
anti-chick-interferon serum available, the effect of such serum
could not be tested;

f) the molecular weights of the inhibitor made by chick
cells correspond to the molecular weights of mouse interferon, as
determined by gel filtration on Sephadex G-75 (see figure 2).

In addition to the foregoing arguments, based upon characterisation of the product obtained from chick cells, there are
other indications that in these cells we are dealing with a translational process, as opposed to interferon induction. The time of
appearance of interferon in the supernatant of the mRNA treated
chick cells is one of them. Four to five hours after addition of
the mRNA, interferon synthesis is essentially finished, whereas

in the case of an induction at least 12 hours are required to obtain maximum interferon synthesis (see figure 3); thus, the kinetics of synthesis in chick cells are clearly in accord with a
translational process. The effect of Actinomycin D is another
point to consider. As discussed earlier, this compound stimulates
the production of mouse interferon by chick cells, and in fact
its presence is a necessary condition to obtain interferon,while,
at the same concentrations it impairs the induction of interferon
in mouse cells (figure 4). Both actions can theoretically be as-
cribed to inhibition of endogenous mRNA synthesis, which in the
chick cells would favor translation of the exogenous messenger,
whereas in the mouse cells less interferon appears as a consequence of inhibition of interferon mRNA synthesis.

Characteristics of mouse interferon mRNA

The fact that a translational system for interferon mRNA has
been developped has made it possible to start purification and
characterisation of mouse interferon mRNA, and the information we
have obtained to date using this system will be published in detail elsewhere (Montagnier et al, in preparation). Early experiments were carried out with total RNA obtained from either the
aqueous phase (A-phase) or the interphase (I-phase) of the first
phenol extraction of induced cells, and the specific activity of
this RNA, expressed as units of mouse interferon obtained per µg
of RNA, was of course quite low, of the order of 0.1 to 0.5 units.
Since then, some of our more purified preparations have yielded
much higher specific activities, up to 40 units per µg of RNA. Sucrose gradient centrifugation of A-phase RNA has consistently
shown a peak of messenger activity in the 8 to 9 S region, the
interesting point being that the interferon, obtained from RNA
this size, also showed the different molecular weights that we

have observed for poly-IC induced interferon in L cells (see figure 2). This then would suggest that the heavier species of interferon are polymers or aggregates of a basic monomeric subunit, of
about 13.000 molecular weight. Such a result is in accordance
with the hypothesis advanced by Carter (11) and this point is now
under further investigation.

Conclusion

The species specificity of the interferon molecule has en-
abled us to develop an assay for its messenger RNA, using Actinomycin D treated heterologous cells as translational system. This
approach is not limited to mouse mRNA translated in chick cells,
since other investigators have been able to confirm our results
in different systems. Human interferon mRNA has been translated
in Actinomycin D treated mouse L cells and, conversely, mouse
interferon mRNA in human cells (A. Wacker, personal communication)
and human interferon mRNA has also been translated very efficiently in Actinomycin D treated chick cells (P. Pitha, personal communication). These translational systems then have proved rather
reliable, and are now being used by several groups to characterize
different interferon messenger RNA's. This will not only provide
specific information concerning the interferon messenger, but it
may also help to gain a better understanding of mRNA's in eukaryotic cells in general.

References

1. De Maeyer-Guignard, J., De Maeyer, E. and Montagnier,
    L. (1972).Proc. Nat. Acad. Sciences USA,69:1203.

2. Wagner, R. and Huang, A.S. (1965). Proc. Nat. Acad. Sciences USA, 54:1112.

3. De Maeyer-Guignard, J., De Maeyer, E. and Jullien, P. (1969). Proc. Nat. Acad. Sciences USA, 63:732.

4. Lane, C.D., Marbaix, G. and Gurdon, J.B. (1971). J. Mol. Biol., 61:73.

5. Fauconnier, B. (1967). Ann. Inst. Pasteur, 113:757.

6. Paucker, K. (1965). J. of Immunology, 94:371.

7. Merigan, T.C. (1964). Science, 145:811.

8. Lindberg, V. and Persson, T. (1972). Eur. J. Biochem., 31:246.

9. Pagano, J.S. (1970). Progress in Medical Virology,12:1.

10. Taylor, J. (1964). Biochem. Biophys. Res. Commun., 14:447.

11. Carter, W.A. (1970). Proc. Nat. Acad. Sciences USA, 67:620.

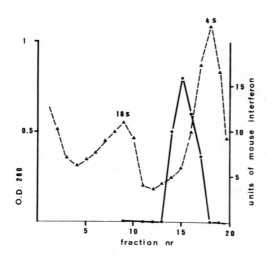

Fig. 5. Sucrose gradient centrifugation of A-phase interferon m-RNA activity. Total A-phase RNA was extracted from I-C induced L cells, 12 hours after induction. Messenger activity of all fractions was measured in chick cells, and interferon assays were carried out in mouse embryo fibroblast cultures.

DISCUSSION

Friedman: Dr. De Maeyer, do you have any experiments which would give you any reason why you have to use Actinomycin in your induction?

De Maeyer: No, actually the reason why we did it was that some time ago, at the beginning, when we started looking for messenger activity, we used just plain chick cells and sometimes it worked a little bit, and sometimes it didn't, and we really didn't know whether we had something or not. Then somebody got the idea that maybe if we used Actinomycin D, we would inhibit the synthesis of endogenous messenger, and thus free ribosomes and they would then be available for the messenger added to the system. Now, this was the reason why we did it, and it worked, but whether that is the explanation why it works, I really don't know.

Friedman: Well, that's true, but there are other manoeuvres you could use which might be at least as effective in freeing ribosomes.

Oxman: Vero cells are less sensitive to Actinomycin D than chick cells. Thus I wonder, Dr. De Maeyer, whether it required higher does of Actinomycin D in Vero cells than in chick cells to obtain an optimum response to exogenous interferon messenger RNA?

De Maeyer: Yes, actually for Vero cells we had to increase the dose of Actinomycin D to get the same effect and we used 0.5 or even 1 microgram per ml and then it worked.

Colby: The Vero cell is interferon negative in that it
doesn't respond either to viral inducers or to (rI)m·(rC)m for
the production of monkey interferon. Have you looked to see
whether or not there is any messenger RNA in the Vero cells in
response to either viral or non viral inducers that could be
translated by chick cells?

De Maeyer: No, we have not. We have used Vero cells as
recipient cells just because we know that there was no possibility for induction, but we have not done the experiment you suggested.

Vilcek: A question about actinomycin D. On that slide you
only used up to 0.25 micrograms. What happens if you increase it
further? Does it then inhibit?

De Maeyer: The chick cells die actually if we use more.
0.25 micrograms/ml is about the maximum we can use.

Baron: Dr. De Maeyer, do the chick cells which you treat
with the messenger RNA in the absence of actinomycin D pre-treatment and which may be making the mouse interferon, become resistant to virus infection?

De Maeyer: Yes, it sometimes does become resistant to
direct challenge. I would like to ask, if I may, a question to
Dr. Vilcek concerning the effect of cordycepin. From your slide
it looked as if you had to add cycloheximide as well. Was I correct?

Vilček: In the experiment which I showed we added both cycloheximide and cordycepin. I should say that we did look at the
effect of cordycepin on "straight" induction with poly I:C in

rabbit kidney cells and under those conditions the effects were not very pronounced. However, it is likely that with cordycepin alone you're looking at the effect of the inhibitor not only on the induction but also you look at the effect of the inhibitor on the control mechanism. That's why, I think, when you use metabolic inhibitors, such as cycloheximide, to delineate transcription from translation, you have a much more exact and accurate picture of what actually is going on. That's what we did in the experiment here where I showed the cordycepin effect.

Levy: The business of the need for actinomycin that you have, could this possibly be related to the fact that, or to the possibility that, when you stimulate the cells with your messenger RNA, it sooner or later turns on, or fairly rapidly turns on, the production of blocker protein, a depression which actinomycin prevents from happening?

De Maeyer: I have no evidence for or against this.

Levy: If blocker protein is made in your semi-synthetic system, actinomycin would prevent its formation.

De Maeyer: It's a possibility, but I have nothing for or against it.

Tan: How many hours prior to the RNA do you treat?

De Maeyer: 6 hours.

Vilček: I think the idea that you are freeing some ribosomes for your exogenous messenger may be a good one, actually, because what is happening in those cells is that the endogenous messenger is being gradually degraded and then you probably have more ribosomes available in these cells.

Revel: I have a question for Dr. Vilček. You mentioned that, as inhibitors of protein synthesis, you have used cyclo-heximide and puromycin. None of these would inhibit initiation of protein synthesis. Accumulation of messenger RNA could be going on despite inhibition of elongation but could be stopped if one inhibits initiation. Have you ever tried any drug which would in-hibit initiation?

Vilček: Yes, we used pactomycin which inhibits primarily initiation, and the effect is essentially the same. Other people have used a number of different inhibitors of protein synthesis and it seems that the effects are essentially the same, no matter what kind of inhibitor of protein synthesis you use.

Kerr: Dr. De Maeyer, can you tell me anything about the kinetics of production of the mouse interferon by the chick cells, when it starts, how long it keeps going, etc? And can you just remind me what controls you do to show it really is interferon you're carrying from the chick cells to the final assay?

De Maeyer: Well, the kinetics were in the slide that was upside down. The mouse interferon appears in the first hour after the RNA is put on the cell and the synthesis, or at least what we measure in the supernatant in the culture fluid of the chick cells is basically finished after 3 hours. You don't get more if you wait longer. So it's between 0 and 3 hours. At concentrations of non-purified RNA, increasing amounts of RNA are inhibitory for A phase RNA. 50 micrograms/ml is the optimal concentration, if you add more, you get less activity.

Kerr: Sorry, I meant at a later time, if you add more at 3 hours, what happens?

De Maeyer: Oh, I don't know. In theory...

Kerr: If you keep adding small doses.

De Maeyer: I don't know, and what would that show? Suppose I do it and I get another batch of mouse interferon. What would one get out of this experiment?

Kerr: Well, I would be more concerned if you didn't get some more and in connection really with the second half of the question?

De Maeyer: Now, what did we do to show that this is mouse interferon and not chick interferon?

Kerr: No, not that it is interferon at all and not some RNA, for example, that's been carried right through.

De Maeyer: Well, the end product is inactivated by proteolytic enzymes but not by RNAse for example. Also it is neutralized by anti-interferon serum, it has the species specificity of mouse interferon, has the same broad antiviral spectrum. We have a molecular weight of about 16, 30 and 72 thousand and a few more arguments I can't think of right now. You know, at least two thirds of this sort of study has really been an exercise in trying to prove that something is mouse interferon and not something else.

Pitha: I just wanted to say that we did a similar kind of experiment and tried to get much better yields. Therefore, we took the mouse cells and induced them with poly IC isolated poly A rich RNA through oligo (dt) column and we didn't get any activity. If we took the whole cytoplasmic RNA, we got some biological activity. We had a different interpretation but this may be the right one.

De Maeyer: Well, I should say that our results on the absence of poly A sequences are very preliminary. They were obtained
only on Millipore membranes, and we are now going over to oligo
(dt) cellulose columns.

De Clercq: I wanted to ask you whether you ever tried priming with interferon either on the recipient cell for the messenger
RNA or on the donor cell. It would be an ideal method, I think, to
see whether priming is affecting a late stage or an early stage in
interferon induction.

De Maeyer: I completely agree. It is something we have been
planning to do for the last two years, but somehow never got around
to doing it.

INTERFERON INDUCTION BY SYNTHETIC POLYNUCLEOTIDES

M. Johnston, M. Eaton, D.W. Hutchinson & D.C. Burke

Department of Biological & Molecular Sciences,
University of Warwick,
Coventry CV4 7AL, England

We wish to report on three aspects of our work on interferon induction by synthetic polynucleotides.

1. Induction by 5-Halogeno substituted poly rC:rI derivatives

We have synthesised a series of 5-halogeno substituted poly rC derivatives, complexed them with poly rI, characterised their physical properties and determined their activity as interferon inducers. Determination of Tm and the ribonuclease resistance of the substituted double-stranded polynucleotides showed that both parameters increased linearly with the volume of the substituent (ie. I>Br>Cl>F>H). However, all four halogeno substituted double-stranded polynucleotides had a similar interferon inducing capacity to poly rI:rC, showing that increase in ribonuclease resistance or Tm in a series of closely related polynucleotides had no effect on their biological activity. It appears from these and other results that the Tm needs to be high enough so that the polynucleotide is in a helical configuration when it interacts with the cell, but that there is no special advantage to be gained in increasing the Tm beyond that point.

We have also synthesised poly (5 hydroxymethyl)rC and attempted to form a complex with poly rI. Several criteria were used
to detect formation of double-stranded polynucleotides (change in
ultra-violet spectra, increase in ribonuclease resistance and elution from a Sephadex column), but no trace of any double-stranded
polynucleotide could be found. However, a mixture of poly (5 hydroxymethyl)rC and poly rI induced interference but not interferon.
This unusual effect is under further investigation.

2.   Requirement of the 2'-hydroxyl group for interferon induction

While the necessity for the 2'-hydroxyl group in the poly-
cytidylic strand of poly rI:rC for antiviral activity is well established, few studies have been done with poly rI modified at the
2'-position. Poly dI:rC is known to be inactive as an interferon
inducer, but the lack of biological activity may be due to strand
separation during the assay, as the Tm in 0.1M No$^+$ solution is
only 35°. We have prepared hybrids from poly dI and poly r(5-halo-
genocytidylic acids) which have Tm's in the region of 60°. These
hybrids are inactive as interferon inducers confirming the requirement for a free 2'-hydroxyl group in both the poly I and poly C
strands of poly rI:rC. We have considered two possible explanations for this effect. The first is that induction involves a
nucleolytic cleavage by an enzyme with similar specificity to pancreatic ribonuclease. However, this does not explain the interferon
inducing activity of (2'-fluoro)polyC:rI, which would not be hydro-
lysed by pancreatic ribonuclease. Such an enzyme would also have to
hydrolyse the poly rI strand by a mechanism similar to that involved
in the cleavage of poly rC and this appears to be unlikely. A more
likely explanation for the absolute requirement for a 2'-OH group
is the stereochemical requirements of the polynucleotide binding

site at the cell surface.

3. Studies of the interaction between poly rI:rC and cells

Interferon was induced in human diploid cells by treatment with poly rI:rC in the absence of DEAE-dextran, and assayed in the same cells using the depression of challenge virus RNA synthesis in order to determine interferon activity. The poly rI:rC was made radioactive by iodination with ^{125}I , and no difficulty was experienced in obtaining poly rC with a specific activity up to 70,000 counts/min/µg RNA. A calculation showed that up to 10% of the cytosine residues were iodinated but this would have no effect on biological activity since poly(5-iodo)rC:rI is known to be as active as poly rI:rC. Iodination did not produce any chain breaks while treatment of the double-stranded polynucleotide with 100µg/ml of ribonuclease for 30 minutes caused complete breakdown. When the fate of such radioactivity labelled poly rI:rC was followed, it was found that 3% of the added radioactivity was bound to the cells but only 1% was ribonuclease-resistant. When cells were treated with poly rI for 18 hours at 37°, and then with radioactively labelled poly rC, 10% of the radioactivity was bound but again only 1% was ribonuclease-resistant. Since the same amount of interferon was formed in each case, it is likely that the small amount of ribonuclease-resistant polynucleotide is of more importance than the total bound material and the fate of this material is now being studied.

INTERFERON INDUCTION BY SYNTHETIC POLYNUCLEOTIDES: COMPETITION BETWEEN INACTIVE AND ACTIVE POLYMERS[x]

Erik De Clercq[*], Paul F. Torrence[+], Bernhard Witkop[+]
and Pierre De Somer[*]

The interferon inducing activity of synthetic polynucleotides is governed by several structural requirements, as outlined in Table 1. These requirements have been derived from com-
parative studies of the antiviral activity of a large number of
polynucleotides. Neither requirement is unique in the sense that
it precludes the necessity of the other parameters. For maximum
interferon inducing capacity, the polynucleotide should possess
all requirements.

It has, however, never been established how or where these
structural prerequisites operate at the cellular level. Do they
play a role in the transfer and binding of the polynucleotide to

---

* Rega Institute for Medical Research
University of Leuven, B-3000 Leuven, Belgium.

+ Laboratory of Chemistry
National Institute of Arthritis, Metabolism and Digestive Dis-
eases, National Institutes of Health, Bethesda, Maryland 20014,
USA.

x The work reported herein was supported by a grant from the Bel-
gian F.G.W.O. (Fonds voor Geneeskundig Wetenschappelijk Onder-
zoek). P.F. Torrence is a National Institutes of Health Senior
Staff Fellow. Details concerning the origin, synthesis and
characterization of the polymers are reported elsewhere (18, P.
F. Torrence & B. Witkop, to be published). The excellent technical assistance of Anita Van Lierde is gratefully acknowledged.

the postulated receptor site for interferon induction? Or, do they specifically regulate the triggering of the interferon induction process at this receptor site? To distinguish between these two possibilities, experiments have been carried out in which cell cultures were first exposed to an inactive polynucleotide (lacking one of the structural parameters listed above) and then incubated with the active polynucleotide [either poly(I).poly(C), poly(A).poly(U) or poly(A).poly(rT)]. It can be assumed that an inactive polynucleotide that does not bind to the receptor site would not prevent the interaction of the active polynucleotide with this receptor site, hence would not compete with the antiviral activity of this active polynucleotide. On the other hand, one may postulate that an inactive polynucleotide that competes with the activity of the active duplex, would do so by preventing the receptor sites' interaction with the active polymer. Thus, competition experiments in which cell cultures are successively exposed to inactive and active polynucleotide may allow differentiation between inactive polynucleotides and the reasons for their inactivity.

Most competition experiments were carried out in primary rabbit kidney (PRK) cells. Confluent PRK cell monolayers in plastic (60 mm) petri dishes were exposed to 10 µg/ml of the inactive polynucleotide in MEM (1 ml/petri dish) for 1 hr at 37°, washed (3 x with MEM), and immediately thereafter exposed to 10 µg/ml of the active polynucleotide in MEM (1 ml/petri dish) for another hour at 37°. The cells were washed again (3 x with MEM) and then treated with metabolic inhibitors (31) to potentiate their interferon producing capacity ('superinduction'). Therefore, the cells were incubated with cycloheximide (2 µg/ml in MEM + 3% calf serum) (2 ml/petri dish) for 3 hr at 37°, washed again (3 x with MEM) and

incubated with actinomycin D (3 μg/ml in MEM + 3% calf serum)
(2 ml/petri dish) for 30 min at 37°, washed again (3 x with MEM)
and further incubated with MEM + 3% calf serum (4 ml/petri dish)
for 20 hr at 37°. The supernatant fluids of the cell cultures
were then withdrawn and titrated for interferon. For interferon
titration, serial (1:3:10:30:...) dilutions of the samples, prepared in MEM + 3% calf serum, were brought on PRK cells in tubes
(1 ml/tube) for 20 hr at 37°. The supernatant fluids were then removed and the cells challenged with vesicular stomatitis virus
(VSV) (80 plaque forming units/0.2 ml/tube) for 1 hr at 37°, and
further incubated with MEM + 3% calf serum (1 ml/tube). Viral
cytopathogenicity was read one or two days later. The interferon
titers were defined as the reciprocal of the highest dilution of
sample that reduced viral cytopathogenicity by 50%. The N.I.H.
reference standard of rabbit interferon, defined as 20.000 units/
ml, titrated 6000 to 10.000 units/ml in this assay system.

The inactive polynucleotides tested for their competitive
effects in this assay system were (1^O) single homopolyribonucleotides, (2^O) triple-stranded complexes and (3°) poly(7-deaza) duplexes. As shown in Table 2, the homopolymers poly(U), poly(A),
poly(I) and poly(C) did not compete with the interferon inducing
activity of the corresponding duplexes poly(A).poly(U) and poly
(I).poly(C). Yeast RNA also failed to inhibit interferon induction by poly(A).poly(U) and poly(I).poly(C), even if it was applied to the cells at extraordinary high concentrations (up to 1
mg/ml) (data not shown). Experiments, now in progress have revealed that some 2'-OH substituted complexes [e.g. poly(A) com-
pexed to poly(dUz) (poly 2'-azido-2'-deoxyuridine)] are also unable to block the interferon response to poly(A).poly(U).

The triple-stranded complexes poly(U).poly(A).poly(U) and poly(rT).poly(A).poly(rT) partially inhibited the activity of their double-stranded counterparts (Table 3). A marked reduction in interferon production was also observed in cell cultures successively exposed to poly(c^7A).poly(U) and poly(A).poly(U), or poly(c^7A).poly(rT) and poly(A).poly(rT) (Table 4).

According to the results presented above, single-stranded polynucleotides and 2'-OH substituted complexes, on one hand, and triple-stranded complexes and poly(c^7A) duplexes, on the other hand, may owe their lack of activity to different causes. Single-stranded polynucleotides and 2'-OH substituted complexes do not prevent interferon induction by the active double-stranded complexes, most probably because they do not interact with the receptor site for interferon induction. Triple-stranded complexes and poly(c^7A) duplexes, although inactive themselves, may bind to the receptor site. Apparently, the conformation of the triple-stranded complexes and poly (c^7A) duplexes are such that a suboptimal interaction with the receptor site occurs, sufficient to block at least partially the receptor sites' affinity for the active complexes, but insufficient to switch on the interferon response.

That triple-stranded structures, in contrast with single-stranded structures compete with double-stranded complexes for the same receptor site, is not surprising in view of the similarities that have been noted in the conformation of double- and triple-stranded poly(U)/poly(A) complexes (32).

To establish unequivocally that the inhibitory effect of triple-stranded and poly(c^7A) duplexes on the antiviral activity of the active double-stranded complexes is due to competition for the same receptor sites, more trivial explanations should be ruled out, e.g. cell damage, caused by the inactive polynucleotide and eventually potentiated upon addition of the active complex, or decrease in overall binding of the active complex to the cell. These possibilities are currently being examined.

If the competitive effects obtained with triple strands and poly(c^7A) duplexes are really due to an occupation of the specific receptor sites for interferon induction, the most pronounced competition might be expected with the active double-stranded complexes themselves. Therefore, a second series of competition experiments was initiated in mouse L-929 cells. L-929 cells do not respond to the interferon inducing activity of poly(I).poly(C) unless they have been treated ('primed') with homologous interferon (33). This system offers the opportunity to determine whether poly (I).poly(C) applied before interferon priming interferes with the activity of poly(I).poly(C) applied after priming.

Confluent L-929 cell monolayers in plastic (60 mm) petri dishes were exposed to 10 µg/ml of poly(I).poly(C) in MEM (1 ml/ petri dish) for 1 hr at 37°, washed (3 x with MEM), and treated with mouse interferon (10 U/ml in MEM + 3% calf serum) (2 ml/petri dish) for 24 hr at 37°, washed again (3 x with MEM) and exposed to a second dose of 10 µg/ml of poly(I).poly(C) in MEM (1 ml/petri dish) for 1 hr at 37°. The cells were then washed again (3 x with MEM) and incubated with MEM + 3% calf serum (4 ml/petri dish) for 20 hr at 37°. The supernatant fluids of the cell cultures were then withdrawn and titrated for interferon. These titrations were performed in a plaque reduction assay in L-929 cells with VSV as challenge virus. The interferon titers corresponded to the reciprocal of the highest dilution of sample that reduced VSV plaque formation by 50%.

As shown in Table 5, poly(I).poly(C) did not stimulate interferon production in L-929 cells unless the cells had been primed with mouse interferon. However, this priming effect of interferon was completely annihilated if the cells were exposed to an identical dose (10 µg/ml) of poly(I).poly(C) before interferon treatment. This competitive effect between poly(I).poly(C) before and poly(I).poly(C) after interferon priming appeared to be specific for the double-stranded complex. Neither poly(I) nor poly(C) alone, even if they were applied at 100 µg/ml, proved capable of reversing the priming effect of interferon on interferon induction by poly(I).poly(C) (data not shown).

From Table 5 the following (tentative) conclusions can be drawn: (1°) the receptor sites for interferon induction in L-929 cells are specifically altered by treatment with homologous interferon so that they become able to recognize the particular conformation of poly(I).poly(C) and other double helical polyribonucleotides; (2°) poly(I).poly(C) interacts perfectly well with the receptor sites on L-cells, even before these have been adapted by interferon treatment. However, once poly(I).poly(C) has interacted with the receptors in their inactive state, it will prevent interferon from adapting them and/or another dose of poly(I).poly (C) from transmitting the message for interferon production.

According to their pattern of interaction with the cell, polynucleotides may be divided in three classes (Table 6): (1°) a first class of polynucleotides that do not bind to the receptor site for interferon induction, or do only bind reversibly. In this sense they would be displaced easily by the active inducers, because they do not compete with the activity of these inducers; (2°) a second class of polynucleotides that bind to the receptor site, do not induce interferon but prevent interferon induction

and interaction with the receptor site of the active complexes;
(3°) a third class of polynucleotides that bind to the receptor
site and trigger interferon production. Some polynucleotides have
already been designated to one or another group of this classification model. Where other polynucleotides should be accommodated
into this model is being studied.

How the interaction between the inducer molecule and the
receptor site leads to the transmission of the message for interferon production is a matter of conjecture. Whether the postulated
receptor site is intracellular or located at the outer cell membrane is also open for discussion (14,23,34-40). However, there is
growing evidence that the receptor for interferon induction by
synthetic polynucleotides is situated at a superficial cell site
(23,34-38).

References

1. Wacker, A., Singh, A., Svec, J. and Lodemann, E. (1969).
    Naturwissenschaften 56, 638.
2. Lampson, G.P., Field, A.K., Tytell, A.A., Nemes, M.M.
    and Hilleman, M.R. (1970). Proc. Soc. Exp. Biol. Med.
    135, 911.
3. Tytell, A.A., Lampson, G.P., Field, A.K., Nemes, M.M.
    and Hilleman, M.R. (1970). Proc. Soc. Exp. Biol. Med.
    135, 917.
4. Niblack, J.F. and McCreary, M.B. (1971). Nature 233, 52.
5. Morahan, P.S., Munson, A.E., Regelson, W., Commerford,
    S.L. and Hamilton, L.D. (1972). Proc. Nat. Acad. Sci.
    USA 69, 842.

6. Shiokawa, K. and Yaoi, H. (1972). Arch. Ges. Virusforsch. 38, 109.

7. Carter, W.A., Pitha, P.M., Marshal, L.W., Tazawa, I., Tazawa, S. and Ts'O, P.O.P. (1972). J.Mol.Biol.70,567.

8. Mohr, S.J., Brown, D.G. and Coffey, D.S. (1972). Nature New Biol. 240, 250.

9. Black, D.R., Eckstein, F., De Clercq, E. and Merigan, T.C. (1973). Antimicrob. Ag. Chemother. 3, 198.

10. Stewart, W.E. II and De Clercq, E. (1973). In preparation.

11. Field, A.K., Tytell, A.A., Lampson, G.P. and Hilleman, M.R. (1967). Proc. Nat. Acad. Sci. USA 58, 1004.

12. Field, A.K., Tytell, A.A., Lampson, G.P. and Hilleman, M.R. (1968). Proc. Nat. Acad. Sci. USA 61, 340.

13. Baron, S., Bogomolova, N.N., Billiau, A., Levy, H.B., Buckler, C.E., Stern, R. and Naylor, R. (1969). Proc. Nat. Acad. Sci. USA 64, 67.

14. Colby, C. and Chamberlin, M.J. (1969). Proc. Nat. Acad. Sci. USA 63, 160.

15. De Clercq, E. and Merigan, T.C. (1969). Nature 222,1148.

16. De Clercq, E., Eckstein, F. and Merigan, T.C. (1970). Ann. N.Y. Acad. Sci. 173, 444.

17. De Clercq, E., Nuwer, M.R. and Merigan, T.C. (1970). J. Clin. Invest. 49, 1565.

18. De Clercq, E., Torrence, P. and Witkop, B. (1973). Proc. Nat. Acad. Sci USA, in press.

19. Matsuda, S., Kida, M., Shirafuji, H., Yoneda, M. and Yaoi, H. (1971). Arch. Ges. Virusforsch. 34, 105.

20. De Clercq, E., Eckstein, F. and Merigan, T.C. (1969). Science 165, 1137.

21. De Clercq, E., Eckstein, F., Sternbach, H. and Merigan, T.C. (1970). Virology 42, 421.

22. De Clercq, E., Wells, R.D. and Merigan, T.C. (1970).
     Nature 226, 364.

23. De Clercq, E., Wells, R.D., Grant, R.C. and Merigan,
     T.C. (1971). J. Mol. Biol. 56, 83.

24. Vilcek, J., Ng, M.H., Friedman-Kien, A.E. and Krawciw,
     T. (1968). J. Virol. 2, 648.

25. Black, D.R., Eckstein, F., Hobbs, J.B., Sternbach, H.
     and Merigan, T.C. (1972). Virology 48, 537.

26. De Clercq, E., Zmudzka, B. and Shugar, D. (1972). FEBS
     Letters 24, 137.

27. Steward, D.L., Herndon, W.C. Jr. and Schell, K.R.
     (1972). Biochim. Biophys. Acta 262, 227.

28. Torrence, P.F., Waters, J.A., Buckler, C.E. and Witkop,
     B. (1973). Biochem. Biophys. Res. Commun. 52, 890.

29. De Clercq, E. and Janik, B. (1973). Biochim. Biophys.
     Acta 324, 50.

30. De Clercq, E. and Shugar, D. (1973). Unpublished data.

31. Vilček, J. and Ng, M.H. (1971). J. Virol. 7, 588.

32. Arnott, S. and Bond, P.J. (1973). Nature, New Biol.
     244, 99.

33. De Clercq, E., Stewart, W.E. II and De Somer, P.(1973).
     Infect. Immun. 8, 309.

34. De Clercq, E., Wells, R.D. and Merigan, T.C. (1972).
     Virology 47, 405.

35. De Clercq, E. and De Somer, P. (1972). J. Gen. Virol.
     16, 435.

36. De Clercq, E. and De Somer, P. (1973). J. Gen. Virol.
     19, 113.

37. De Clercq, E. and De Somer, P. (1973). Submitted for
     publication.

38. Taylor-Papadimitriou, J. and Kallos, J. (1973). Nature,
     New Biol. 245, 143.

39. Pitha, J. and Pitha, P.M. (1971). Science 172, 1146.
40. Pitha, P.M. and Pitha, J. (1973). J. Gen. Virol., in
     press.

TABLE 1

Structural requirements for interferon
induction by synthetic polynucleotides

1. Sufficiently high molecular size (superior to 5S for demon-
    stration of full antiviral activity) (1-10).

2. Double-strandedness (double-stranded complexes significantly
    more active than single- and triple-stranded complexes)(11-18).

3. Requirements of strand continuity (high molecular size) and
    base pairing (double-strandedness) more stringent for the
    purine strand than for the pyrimidine strand, as established
    with poly(I).poly(C) (3, 7, 8, 10, 19).

4. Sufficiently high thermal stability (superior to 60° for demon-
    stration of full antiviral activity (14-16, 18, 20, 21).

5. Adequate (not necessarily complete) resistance to degradation
    by nucleases (viz. pancreatic ribonuclease)(9, 20-23).

6. Presence of 2'-hydroxyl groups [substitution of 2'-H, 2'-N_3,
    2'-F, 2'-Cl, 2'-O-CH_3, 2'-O-CH_2-CH_3 or 2'-O-CO-CH_3 for 2'-OH
    in one of the strands, viz. the pyrimidine strand, of either
    poly(I).poly(C) or poly(A).poly(U) leads to a marked reduction
    in antiviral activity] (14, 22, 24-30).

7. Presence of an intact purine ring [double-stranded complexes
    of poly(U), poly(rT) and poly(br^{5}U) with poly(A) in which the
    N-7 is replaced by CH are all inactive](18).

TABLE 2

Competition between single homopolyribonucleotides
and homopolyribonucleotide duplexes[*]

Inactive polynucleotide	Active polynucleotide	Interferon production (U/ml)
-	Poly(A).poly(U)	800
Poly(U)	-	< 3
Poly(A)	-	< 3
Poly(U)	Poly(A).poly(U)	1200
Poly(A)	Poly(A).poly(U)	600
-	Poly(I).poly(C)	6000
Poly(I)	-	< 3
Poly(C)	-	< 3
Poly(I)	Poly(I).poly(C)	6000
Poly(C)	Poly(I).poly(C)	4800

[*] Assay system: PRK cells superinduced with cycloheximide and actinomycin D.

TABLE 3

Competition between triple-stranded homopolyribonucleotide
and double-stranded homopolyribonucleotide complexes[*]

Inactive polynucleotide	Active polynucleotide	Interferon production (U/ml)
-	Poly(A).poly(U)	3000
Poly(U).poly(A).poly(U)	-	20
Poly(U).poly(A).poly(U)	Poly(A).poly(U)	200
-	Poly(A).poly(rT)	3000
Poly(rT).poly(A).poly(rT)	-	15
Poly(rT).poly(A).poly(rT)	Poly(A).poly(rT)	600

[*]

Assay system: PRK cells superinduced with cycloheximide and
actinomycin D.

TABLE 4

Competition between 7-DEAZA-homopolyribonucleotide
and regular N-7 homopolyribonucleotide duplexes[*]

Inactive polynucleotide	Active polynucleotide	Interferon production (U/ml)
–	Poly(A).poly(U)	3000
Poly(c^{7}A).poly(U)	–	6
Poly(c^{7}A).poly(U)	Poly(A).poly(U)	20
–	Poly(A).poly(rT)	3000
Poly(c^{7}A).poly(rT)	–	10
Poly(c^{7}A).poly(rT)	Poly(A).poly(rT)	300

[*]

Assay system: PRK cells superinduced with cycloheximide and
actinomycin D.

TABLE 5

Competition between poly(I).poly(C) before and
poly(I).poly(C) after interferon priming[*]

First dose	Interferon priming	Second dose	Interferon production (U/ml)
-	-	Poly(I).poly(C)	5
-	+	Poly(I).poly(C)	160
Poly(I).poly(C)	-	Poly(I).poly(C)	2
Poly(I).poly(C)	+	Poly(I).poly(C)	3

[*]
Assay system: L-929 cells.

TABLE 6

Patterns of interaction of polynucleotides with the cell

1°   Single-stranded polyribonucleotides [e.g. poly(U), poly(C),
     ...], 2'-OH substituted complexes [e.g. poly(A).poly(dUz),
     ...], ... bind to the cell,
     do not bind (or only reversibly) to the receptor site for
     interferon induction,
     do not induce interferon.

2°   Triple-stranded polyribonucleotide complexes
     [e.g. poly(U).poly(A).poly(U), ...],
     poly(7-deaza) duplexes [e.g. poly(c⁷A).poly(U),...], ...
     bind (partly irreversibly) to the receptor site for inter-
     feron induction,
     yet fail to induce interferon.

3°   Double-stranded polyribonucleotide complexes
     [e.g. poly(I).poly(C), ...]
     bind (irreversibly) to the receptor site for interferon
     induction,
     induce interferon.

DISCUSSION

Oxman: Dr. De Clercq, have you done any experiments in which you exposed cells to poly I:C or poly A:U for a short time before adding the inactive polynucleotide competitor?

De Clercq: In rabbit kidney cells you may not be able to suppress the activity of the regularly active polynucleotides by applying the inactive polymers afterwards, because the message for interferon induction may have been transmitted at the time you add the inactive polymer. However, we might be able to do it in mouse L-cells which are not sensitive to the regularly active polynucleotides such as poly I:C, unless they have been primed with interferon. Maybe it is a good suggestion to perform these experiments in L-cells. The point is that the polynucleotide applied first should be inactive, because if it is fully active you would never see the effect of the second one.

Oxman: I ask this question because the evidence for receptor competition is still indirect, and it seems quite possible that the inactive polymers may actually affect a later step. For example, they might act intracellularly to reduce the cell's capacity to synthesize interferon. The addition of the inactive polymer after poly I:C might distinguish between these possibilities. If it does act by competing for receptors, it should have little effect when added after the poly I:C. On the other hand, if it acts at some later step, it might still inhibit the cells' response when added after the poly I:C.

De Clercq: I'm nearly absolutely sure, I would say, that as soon as you put on the active polynucleotide for, let's say one hour, you cannot reverse its activity anymore by putting on an inactive afterwards, but I agree it would be a control experiment that's worth doing.

De Maeyer: It's nice to be able to be absolutely sure. It doesn't happen very often to me.

De Clercq: I said: nearly absolutely sure.

Vilček: Can you answer the question whether the receptor site for poly I:C, poly A:U and A:T is the same or whether you are dealing with different receptors for each polymer on the basis of your results? Did you use heterologous non-inducing polymers?

De Clercq: Recently, I have initiated these experiments in the system that I described at the end (interferon-primed L-cells). These cells were first exposed to a certain ds-RNA, e.g. mycophage ds-RNA, then treated with interferon, and then exposed to another ds-RNA, e.g. poly I:C. It is as yet premature to state unequivocally whether we get competition with all ds-RNAs.

Colby: Have you looked for competition with the helical polynucleotides which are substituted on the two prime hydroxyls?

De Clercq: This work is now in progress. At the moment, the data are not clear-cut to be discussed in public, but there is certainly work going on with a lot of 2'-OH substituted polynucleotides (both single- and double-stranded polynucleotides with 2'-OH substituted by either 2'-fluoro, 2'-chloro, 2'-azido, 2'-O-methyl or 2'-O-ethyl groups).

De Maeyer: This is not really a public discussion!

De Clercq: The results are not in definite form yet.

Merigan: Right. We published that with the two prime cloro polymers and there was no competition in either binding or biological induction activity.

De Clercq: Well, I may just point out that in connection with these competition experiments, I have also looked at the uptake of radiolabeled polymer by the cell and, even in the cases where we got competition, there was no change in the uptake of radiolabeled material by the cells. This shows again that the uptake of the polynucleotide by the cell as measured by radioactivity is very aspecific.

Ankel: I was wondering, has anybody ever looked whether you have to have a free 3' end on the poly I:C? Is that known? Do you have to have a phosphate, or is it a free ribose which is necessary for induction?

De Clercq: I don't think it has ever been done.

Ankel: How about the 5' end?

De Clercq: I don't think either of those have been done.

Ankel: I think this would be an easy experiment to do. One could just treat with phosphatase or periodate and see whether the activity remains.

Burke: I would just like to ask. Do you suggest that the priming is an alteration in the receptor for polynucleotides that increases its binding to the receptor?

De Clercq: It's a working hypothesis that, at least for the interferon inducing capacity of polynucleotides, priming with interferon results in an unmasking or specific adaptation of the

receptor site so that the polynucleotide would interact with it
in an optimal way. It is a working hypothesis that would accomodate quite well the results I have obtained in interferon-primed
L-cells.

De Maeyer: I would put a question also to both of you: the
fact that now there is poly I:C available bound to Sepharose,
couldn't that be used as a tool for trying to isolate the hypothetical receptor for poly I:C? Because you're talking about the
receptor, but what is the hard evidence that there is such a thing
as a specific receptor for poly I:C for interferon induction?

Burke: It shows that lots of people have thought about it.
I think this is the secondary aim in binding polynucleotides to
columns. We've thought of it and lots of other people have thought
of it, I'm sure. I don't know any results. We did some experiments
looking for materials in cytoplasmic fractions that bound to double-stranded polynucleotides which had been fixed on to nitrocellulose filters. I think other people have also done such experiments. There is a vast amount of material in cells which will bind
to the double-stranded RNA, far more than could possibly explain
the interferon phenomenon. We decided we just didn't have a negative control and it was hopeless to proceed.

Colby: Exactly. The problem is getting an appropriate negative control. One can envision not only that there are many, many
proteins that will interact in a relatively nonspecific way with
all sorts of nucleic acids just on the basis of ionic charge.
There also is the very likely possibility that if there is a receptor protein then it most likely would be in the membrane matrix.
With most of the enzymology that has been done with proteins that
are in a membrane matrix, people have found that as soon as one
destroys the structural integrity of the membrane matrix the bio-

logical activity of the enzyme is simultaneously destroyed. Thus, simply cracking open cells and throwing away all the lipid and pouring all the proteins through columns made with poly I· poly C Sepharose is at best an optimistic thing to do.

De Maeyer: So, would you conclude that present day technology is not sufficient to isolate this receptor?

Colby: I don't know where to start.

Burke: The analogous situation would be the isolation of the binding proteins in bacteria for enzyme induction and there they had to construct negative mutants, and look for a difference in binding between the positive and the negative mutants. And, of course, we are hoping that people will be able to find some way of getting a negative mutant for this system, but what you're looking for is a mutant which won't interact with poly I:C, at the specific binding site, although one can think of ways of selecting mutants that don't interact with poly I:C, but maybe they fail to interact for all sorts of trivial reasons which would not necessarily be an interaction with the binding site.

Colby: This was really the direction of my earlier question about whether or not there is any interferon messenger RNA in Vero cells. If there is interferon messenger in the Vero cells under induced conditions that would suggest that the hypothetical repressor may be constitutive in that cell. On the other hand, if there is no interferon mRNA in the Vero cell, either that cell cannot recognize the inducer molecule because of an absent or modified receptor site or something in the chain between the initial recognition of the inducer molecule and the stimulation of a functional messenger is affected. In either way, that's a potentially very interesting mutant.

Chany: We have some evidence that is preliminary, that the
Vero cells do not carry the chromosome responsible for monkey
interferon induction. In spite of the fact that an antiviral state
can be obtained with a virus. The messenger is not present in the
Vero cells because the genetic information is probably missing.

INDUCTION OF VIRAL RIBONUCLEIC ACIDS
IN NON-PERMISSIVE MSV-IF[+] CELLS
(PRODUCERS OF INTERFERON)INFECTED WITH NDV

M.F. Dubois and J. Huppert

Institut National de la Santé et de la Recherche Médicale
U.43 de Recherches sur les Infections Virales
Hôpital St.-Vincent-de-Paul
74,ave.Denfert-Rochereau, 75014 Paris, France

and

Institut Gustave Roussy
Groupe de Recherches N? 8 du CNRS
Villejuif 94, France

Newcastle disease virus in an efficient inducer of interferon in many cell strains, and retains its properties of induction when irradiated by UV light (1, 2, 3, 4). In permissive cells,
such as chick embryo cells, infection by irradiated NDV results
in a synthesis of a single-stranded RNA, which is complementary
to viral RNA, without viral production, as shown by Huppert (5).
In contrast, Gandhi and Burke were unable to detect any viral RNA
synthesis in interferon-producing cells (4).

In some non-permissive cells, NDV does not replicate; but
can, nonetheless, still induce interferon synthesis (6), as in
the case of MSV-IF[+] cells.

MSV-IF[+] cells (murine sarcoma virus - interferon) are a
continuous line of Balb/C mouse cells, transformed by murine sarcoma virus, selected in the presence of interferon. These cells

do not reproduce NDV at all, as shown in Table 1. Total virus produced was assayed for hemagglutination of guinea pig red blood
cells and for infectivity in embryonated eggs at 1, 10 and 24 h
after infection.

This virus does not cause any cytopathic effect and infection with NDV (at the m.o.i. = 100) induces interferon production
with titers as high as 5000 units/ml.

These properties of MSV-IF[+] cells stimulated us to investigate the following question: Is there any synthesis of viral RNA
in completely non-permissive cells; and, if so, what happens to
this RNA during cellular multiplication?

RNA labeled by tritiated uridine was extracted from MSV-IF[+]
cells infected with NDV for 8 h at $40^{\circ}C$, in the presence of 4 µg/
ml of actinomycin D, and analyzed by sucrose gradient centrifugation. No 57 S RNA (viral RNA) was detectable in the infected cells
after 8 h of infection, but a large amount of radioactivity sedimented at a lower S value (Figure 1). Under the same experimental
conditions, in chick embryo cells (CEC), permissive to NDV, we
observed peaks sedimenting at 57 S ("plus" strand), 30 S and 18 S
("minus" strands).

To study the synthesis of viral RNA in infected MSV-IF[+]
cells, we subjected RNA to a centrifugation for a longer period
of time on a similar type of gradient (Figure 2). We observed a
pattern of incorporation of tritiated uridine into 18 S RNA,
which was different from that of RNA extracted from uninfected
cells. In parallel experiments, chick embryo cells infected with
NDV synthesized more 18 S RNA and 30 S RNA than MSV-IF[+] cells.

To identify the RNA synthesized in the infected MSV-IF[+]
cells, the fractions corresponding to the 18 S peak (Pool B) and

the 30 S peak (Pool A) were mixed. RNA was precipitated by ethanol at $-20^{\circ}C$, dissolved in SSC buffer (0.15 M NaCl, 0.015 M Na citrate), and then annealed with (and without) NDV "plus" strand RNA prepared from virions (Table 2). According to the experiments, 56 to 97% of the RNA extracted from MSV-IF⁺ cells, infected by NDV for 8 h, became resistant to RNAse after annealing with NDV "plus" strand. In non-infected cells, the percentage of annealing was never higher than 20%. Thus, MSV-IF⁺ cells produced NDV "minus" strand RNA in a much smaller quantity than chick embryo cells, although infection was completely abortive. The quantity of acid insoluble radioactivity before annealing was no higher in the infected cells than in the control cells. This indicates that no "plus" strand viral RNA is synthesized during infection. The relatively high self-annealing of RNA from non-infected, actinomycin D-treated control cells may be the result of a symetric transcription of some cellular RNA.

These results show the presence of "minus" strand RNA synthesis in the MSV-IF⁺ cells. The following experiments were performed in order to verify how long the synthesis of this RNA persisted in the cells during cell divisions. We extracted labeled RNA from the cells 24 and 48 h after infection; that is, after at least 1 and 2 cellular divisions. Actinomycin D and tritiated uridine were added to the culture medium 2 h before the extraction of RNA. We observed that 24 h after infection, the synthesis of viral "minus" strand RNA was still detectable (Table 3); and 48 h after infection, the synthesis of viral RNA could not be detected by annealing. Neither double-stranded, nor "plus" strand, viral RNA were detected.

Discussion

Our results show that MSV-IF[+] cells are completely non-permissive to NDV, but that they synthesize single-stranded "minus"
RNA for several hours. This RNA can be identified by annealing
with "plus" strand NDV RNA. In contrast to permissive cells, one
does not observe viral "plus" strand synthesis by gradient analysis of the RNA from infected cells: self-annealing, without the
addition of "plus" viral RNA, was no higher than in control cells.
The synthesis of NDV "minus" strand RNA seems to diminish with
time and cell growth; and 48 h after infection, no viral RNA
could be detected.

In our experiments, we have not detected any double-stranded RNA, but the synthesis of a "minus" strand involved the presence of at least a transient complex containing the two strands.
The failure to detect double-stranded RNA may be due either to
the fact that each cell contains very few molecules, or to a
rapid turnover of viral precursors. Moreover, we know that labelled double-stranded RNA represents only a small proportion of
intracellular viral RNA.

Concerning the induction of interferon, the role of double-
stranded viral RNA is not definitely established, but is the most
frequently suggested mechanism. However, synthetic single-stranded polynucleotides, as shown by Baron et al (7), and single-
stranded viral RNA (4, 8, 9) are also weakly active as interferon
inducers.

In this system, we cannot conclude that single-stranded RNA
(viral or complementary RNA) is the inducer of interferon. However, if double-stranded RNA were the inducer, a very small quantity would be necessary for the induction of very high amounts of

interferon.

This is in contrast with the findings in chick embryo cells, where double-stranded RNA is detectable, but no interferon is produced. This discrepancy could be due either to the blocking which appears in the permissive cycle before interferon synthesis, or to the fact that double-stranded RNA is not really responsible for interferon induction.

References

1. Youngner,J.S., Scott, A.W., Hallum, J.V. and Stinebring, W.R. (1966). J. of Bacteriology, 92:862-868.
2. Bratt, M.A. and Rubin, H. (1968). Virology, 35:381-394.
3. Youngner, J.S. and Scott, A.W. (1968). J. of Virology, 2:81-82.
4. Gandhi, S.S. and Burke, D.C. (1969). J. of Gen. Virology, 6:95-103.
5. Huppert, J., Hillova, J. and Gresland, L.J. (1969). Nature, 223:1015-1017.
6. Chany, C. and Vignal, M. (1968). C.R.A.S. Paris, 267: 1798-1800.
7. Baron, S., Bogomolova, N.N., Billiau, A., Levy, H.B., Buckler, C.E., Stern, R. and Naylor, R. (1969). Proc. Nat. Acad. Sci., 64:67-74.
8. Huppert, J., Gresland, L. and Hillova, J. (1970). In "The Biology of Large RNA Viruses" (R.D. Barry and B.W.J. Mahy. eds.), p. 482. Academic Press, London.
9. Clavell, L.A. and Bratt, M.A. (1971). J. of Virology, 8:500-508.

TABLE 1

NDV Production by MSV-IF$^+$ cells

Duration of Infection	H.A.U.	I.D.$_{50}$ in Embryonated Eggs
1 hour	1	$10^{6.24}$/ml
10 hours	0	10^{6}/ml
24 hours	0	$10^{5.9}$/ml

NDV production by MSV-IF$^+$cells. The infected cultures were frozen at -80°C and thawed. The medium and cell extract were then assayed for hemagglutination (H.A.U.) and infectivity in embryonnated eggs.

TABLE 2

Expt. No	Fractions	Acid Insoluble C.P.M.	% Acid Insoluble Counts After RNAse Digestion		
			Before Annealing	After Annealing	
				Without Added + Strand	With + Strand
Infected Cells					
1	A	2400	8.1	21	56
	B	1900	7.9	15	63
2	B	1460	7.7	15	97
3	B	1950	5.7	9.8	57.8
Control Cells					
1	A	2200	11	16.3	14.5
	B	1800	9	12	20
3	B	2960	7.5	15	17

Annealing of labelled RNA from MSV-IF$^+$ cells infected for 8 h with NDV. RNA-RNA annealing was performed, as described by Huppert et al (5).

TABLE 3

Duration of Infection	Expt. No.	Fractions	C.P.M.	% Acid Insoluble Counts After RNAse Digestion		
				Before Annealing	After Annealing	
					Without Added + Strand	With + Strand
8 hours	1	B	1950	5.7	9.8	57.8
24 hours	1	B	4000	11	14	17.5
	2	A+B	1460	12.2	31	73
48 hours	1	B	1190	5.5	6.4	8.3
	2	A+B	2360	10.8	10	13.3
	3	A	1130	12	14	15

Annealing of labelled RNA from MSV-IF$^+$ cells infected by NDV and incubated at 37°C for 8, 24 and 48 h. Labelling with ^{3}H-uridine for 2 h at 40°C before RNA extraction.

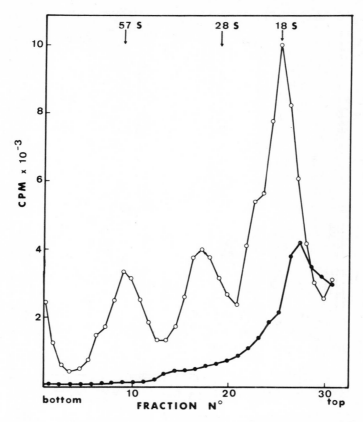

Fig. 1.   Sucrose gradient (5-20%) sedimentation of RNA from
NDV infected cells. Centrifuging for 5 h at 24000 rpm in a SW 25
rotor at 4°C. ●——● MSV-IF[+] cells; ○——○ CEC.

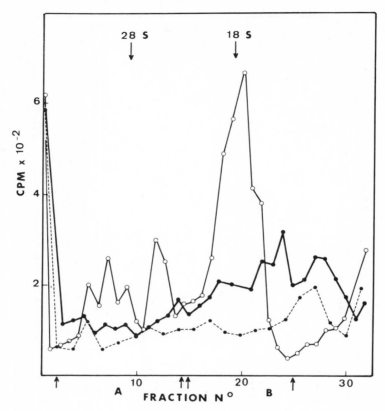

Fig. 2. Sucrose gradient (5-20%) sedimentation of RNA from NDV infected cells. Centrifuging for 17 h at 24000 rpm in a SW 25 rotor at 4°C. ●——● MSV-IF⁺ cells infected by NDV; ●---● MSV-IF⁺ control cells; ○——○ CEC infected by NDV.

DISCUSSION

Pereira: You show that there is no hemagglutinin produced. Have you looked for other viral proteins?

Dubois: No, we have not tried.

INDUCTION OF INTERFERON BY A NONREPLICATING
SINGLE-STRANDED RNA VIRUS[*]

F. Dianzani, A. Pugliese and S. Baron

Institute of Microbiology,University of Turin,Turin,Italy
and
National Institute of Allergy & Infectious Diseases
National Institutes of Health,Bethesda,Maryland 20014

The event(s) during viral infection which is the stimulus for cellular production of interferon has not been determined finally. Also undetermined is whether the viral stimulus or inducer is the same for all viral infections. Isaacs et al. (1, 2) presented evidence that viral or nonviral nucleic acids could be a stimulus. The finding by Field et al. (3) that double-stranded ribonucleic acids (RNA) were the most effective among the isolated nucleic acid inducers raised the possibility that double-stranded viral RNA is the common stimulating factor (4). On the other hand isolated single-stranded nucleic acid can be stimulatory (5, 6) and it may be one of the viral stimulatory substances. Additional stimulating and controlling mechanisms are likely since the production of intracellular viral nucleic acids is sometimes inadequate to act as a stimulus (7).

In a previous study (8) mouse L cells stimulated with the single-stranded RNA virus, Newcastle disease virus (NDV), produced

---

[*] This work was supported by Consiglio Nazionale delle Richerche, Italy.

messenger RNA for interferon during inhibition of protein synthesis and in the absence of formation of detectable viral double-
stranded RNA. Since there was no detectable synthesis of viral
RNAs, it was suggested that a component of the input NDV was the
stimulus for interferon production. However, the subsequent
demonstration of a small quantity of RNA transcriptase associated
with NDV virions (9) raised the possibility that undetectable
amounts of double-stranded NDV RNA could have been produced by
the input virion and thus have stimulated interferon. To eliminate this possibility we repeated the study using a stimulating
virus (chikungunya virus, group A arbovirus) which does not contain a virion-associated RNA transcriptase (10). The findings
again indicate that some fraction of the input virus can stimulate
interferon production.

Materials and Methods

Cycloheximide (Sigma) was used at a final concentration of
100 µg per ml, and DL-p-fluorophenylalanine (FPA, Sigma) at 800
µg per ml. These drugs were purchased from Sigma Chemical Co.
Their activity and/or reversibility was controlled by measuring
their effect on the incorporation of labeled precursors. Actinomycin D was used at a concentration of 10 µg/ml.

Chikungunya virus, grown in the brains of newborn mice or
in BHK-21 cells, was used as the inducer of interferon at an input multiplicity of 50 ID_{50} per cell unless otherwise specified.
This multiplicity of infection was obtained by diluting the 10%
mouse brain pool of virus 1 to 3. Primary or passaged cultures of
rat embryo (RE) cells were prepared by standard methods. Culture
medium for experiments was Eagle's medium plus 2% fetal bovine
serum. Interferon was assayed by the single cycle, Sindbis virus
yield reduction assay as previously described (11). Interferon

samples were maintained at pH 2 for 24-48 hours before assay to inactivate virus. In every experiment an additional aliquot of the virus which was used as inducer was maintained at pH 2 and tested to ensure its loss of interfering activity after acidification. The absence of interference eliminated the possible presence of residual interfering virus, interferon activity, or extraneous interferon-inducing nucleic acids in the preparation of chikungunya virus.

Purification of chikungunya virus was performed as previously described (12) for the experiments in which viral RNA was extracted. Chikungunya virus was titrated by the CPE endpoint method in BHK-21 cells and the titers expressed as $TCID_{50}$.

Results

Induction of mRNA for interferon by chikungunya virus during inhibition of protein synthesis. The experimental design was to permit production of mRNA for interferon in rat embryo cells induced with chikungunya virus during inhibition of protein synthesis (8). In this way it could be determined whether interferon mRNA could be induced during the time that viral replication and synthesis of viral components were blocked by the inhibition of formation of viral specific proteins such as RNA polymerase. Rat embryo cells were pretreated with cycloheximide for 30 minutes and then stimulated with chikungunya virus. The block to protein synthesis was maintained by the presence of cycloheximide and FPA. After 4 1/2 hours at 37°C actinomycin D was added to inhibit any further transcription of mRNA for interferon. After incubation for another hour the cultures were washed 4 times (to reverse the inhibition of protein synthesis by cycloheximide and FPA but not the inhibition of transcription of RNA by actinomycin D) and refed with inhibitor-free medium. After overnight incubation the culture fluids were harvested and assayed for interferon content.

As was previously found in mouse cells (8), protein synthesis (as measured by incorporation of ^{14}C proline) in the rat cells was inhibited >98% but RNA synthesis was unaffected (as measured by incorporation of ^{3}H uridine) during the 5 1/2 hours of treatment with cycloheximide and FPA. After removal of cycloheximide and FPA, protein synthesis resumed fully within 1/2 hour, indicating the reversibility of the inhibition of protein synthesis. In comparison, transcription was irreversibly blocked (96% decrease) by the added actinomycin D. Additional controls for inhibitor effectiveness demonstrated that rat cell cultures which were stimulated with chikungunya virus in the continued presence of cycloheximide and FPA did not produce the interferon protein when tested at 5 1/2 hours or 20 hours. Cultures treated with actinomycin D for 1 hour and then washed before stimulation with chikungunya virus did not produce any interferon, indicating the irreversibility of this inhibition of transcription.

Table 1 and figure 1 show the yield of interferon in rat embryo cultures which were stimulated with chikungunya virus in the presence or absence of the metabolic inhibitors. It may be seen that full interferon production occurs under the conditions of sequential metabolic inhibition. This finding indicates that the mRNA for interferon is stimulated by chikungunya virus during inhibition of protein synthesis since the mRNA could not have been transcribed after the later addition of actinomycin D.

To determine whether a lower multiplicity of infection would give a similar result the experiments were repeated using an input multiplicity of 5. Again interferon production occurred (150 units/ml) under the conditions of the metabolic inhibition but it was somewhat reduced as compared with an input multiplicity of 50.

Examination for possible replication of chikungunya virus or its RNA during inhibition of protein synthesis. Experiments were done to determine if synthesis of virus or double-stranded viral RNA had occurred in the inhibitor-treated cultures. Infectivity titrations demonstrated absence of virus replication in the presence of cycloheximide and FPA for 5 1/2 hours or 20 hours. Experiments were performed to determine whether partial replication of the viral RNA occurred under the experimental inhibitory conditions. Monolayers of rat embryo cells (10 cells/culture) were treated with 10μg/ml actinomycin D for 1 hour to reduce the background of cellular RNA synthesis. The cultures were then infected with an input multiplicity of 50 pfu of chikungunya virus in the presence or absence of cycloheximide plus FPA. After 30 minutes of incubation 20 μC/ml of tritiated uridine and 20 μC/ml of tritiated adenine (Amersham) were added. Five hours later the medium was decanted and the cultures washed with cold phosphate buffered saline containing cycloheximide. Then the cells were suspended with a rubber policeman and the RNA was extracted through the use of phenol (13).

The amount of radioactivity incorporated into RNA from infected cells treated with cycloheximide and FPA was less than 1/10 of that from infected cells not treated with these inhibitors. Analysis of both RNA preparations in a 15-30% sucrose gradient for 90 minutes (12) (Fig. 2) showed that labelled RNA from the infected cells treated with actinomycin D had 2 peaks as previously reported (12). One of the peaks (presumably single-stranded RNA) corresponds to the single peak of RNA extracted from purified virions. In comparison, the radioactivity from infected cells treated with cycloheximide and FPA in addition to actinomycin D was found only at the top of the gradient. This finding confirms the prediction that inhibition of protein synthesis prevents detectable synthesis of chikungunya virus RNA.

Biological assay for the presence of double-stranded RNA.
To test further the possibility that interferon was stimulated
by amounts of double-stranded RNA which were undetectable by iso-
topic techniques, the extracted RNA from (a) infected cells
treated with cycloheximide and FPA, (b) infected control cells
and (c) purified virions were tested for their ability to induce
interferon. This experiment is based on the previous findings
that isolated double-stranded RNA is a potent inducer of interferon (3) and isolated single-stranded RNA is a weak inducer(5).
To digest single-stranded RNA but preserve double-stranded RNA
half of each RNA preparation (RNA extracted from 10^8 cells or
from 10^{11} TCID$_{50}$ of virus) was treated with 2 µg/ml of purified
RNase (Worthington) for 20 minutes at 37C in 0.15M buffered saline. 0.2 ml was inoculated into each of 2 tube cultures of rat
embryo cells containing medium and 200 µg/ml DEAE-dextran to enhance the action of any active RNA (14). Twelve hours later the
culture fluids were harvested and assayed for interferon.   The
results are shown in table 2 . It may be seen that neither the
RNA from cells infected in the presence of cycloheximide and FPA
nor the RNA from purified virions stimulated the production of
interferon. This finding indicates that neither preparation contained sufficient quantities of double-stranded RNA to induce
interferon.

In comparison, the RNA from productively infected cells did
stimulate the production of interferon (table 2). The expected
findings of RNase-resistant (double-stranded) RNA in cells infected in the absence of inhibitors of protein synthesis (table
2) indicates that chikungunya virus does produce double-stranded RNA during its normal replicative cycle and it validates the
usefulness of this method to detect double-stranded RNA under the
present experimental conditions.

Discussion

The present results indicate that even when the syntheses of detectable viral components are blocked by cycloheximide and FPA full yields of interferon may be produced. It is reasonable to conclude that the input virion or some component of it can be an effective interferon inducer. If the effective component of the virus is RNA, the present data suggest that single-stranded RNA can be the effective inducer during some viral infections. Although single-stranded viral RNA may have some double-stranded regions or regions of homology with cellular nucleic acids, they would not be expected to stimulate as much interferon as the replicative form of RNA. The finding that nonreplicating virus can induce as much interferon as replicating virus argues against this possibility. Thus it is possible that in some cases, the input, virion-associated, single-stranded viral RNA may be as effective as replicated double-stranded RNA. The reason that isolated single-stranded RNA is a less effective stimulator than is isolated double-stranded RNA may be its greater sensitivity to degradation by intracellular and extracellular RNases.

A recent study showing enhanced interferon production by chicken cells pretreated with interferon and then stimulated with chikungunya virus also indicated that nonreplicating chikungunya virus can induce interferon (15).

Although viral nucleic acid is the most likely virion component responsible for induction of interferon, other substances associated with the input virion could induce interferon. The small fraction of double-stranded RNA detected in some viral preparations (16) is not likely to have been the stimulus for interferon under the present conditions because (a) purified chikungunya virions contained no detectable double-stranded RNA when tested chemically and biologically; (b) only concentrated pre-

parations of virus have been reported to contain detectable
quantities of double-stranded RNA (16). The present experiments
employed as little as 5 pfu per cell (1 to 30 dilution) to obtain consistent yields of interferon—not nearly enough to contain sufficient double-stranded RNA to stimulate the cells.

The virion lipids and proteins are other possible stimuli
under the present conditions. Lipid or protein is less likely
than nucleic acid to be the inducing substance since those few
lipids or proteins which stimulate interferon production in vivo
are ineffective in the type of cell culture used in the present
study (17, 18). There is not enough information available to assess the possible stimulating roles of viral attachment, penetration, uncoating events or cellular enzymatic factions.

Summary

A study was undertaken to help determine whether the input
virions of a nonreplicating, single-stranded RNA virus could
stimulate interferon production. Rat embryo cells were treated
with inhibitors of protein synthesis during infection with
chikungunya virus. After 4 1/2 hours incubation, RNA synthesis
was inhibited with actinomycin D and 1 hour later the inhibition
of protein synthesis was reversed by washing. Thereafter the culture fluids were tested for production of interferon. Since not
even partial replication of chikungunya virus or its components
was demonstrable under the conditions of inhibition of protein
synthesis, the finding of full yields of interferon indicated
that a component of the input virion stimulated production of the
interferon. The results of control experiments make it unlikely
that contaminating double-stranded RNA was the stimulus for interferon production. Since viral and other nucleic acids are the
most general inducers of interferon and since the input chikun-

gunya virion contains single-stranded RNA, it seems probable that
at least certain single-stranded viral RNAs can stimulate interferon production.

Acknowledgement

The authors wish to acknowledge the helpful suggestions
and criticisms made by Dr. H. B. Levy.

References

1. Isaacs, A., Baron, S. and Allison, A.C. (1961). As
    referred in Sci. Am. 204:51.

2. Isaacs, A., Cox, R.A. and Rotem, Z. (1963). Lancet 2:
    113.

3. Field, A.K., Tytell, A.A., Lampson, G.P. and Hilleman,
    M.R. (1967). Proc. Natl. Acad. Sci. USA 58:100.

4. Colby, C. Jr. (1971). Prog. Nuc. Acid. Res. Mol. Biol.
    11:1.

5. Baron, S., Bogomolova, N.N., Billiau, A., Levy, H.B.,
    Buckler, C.E., Stern, R., Naylor, R. (1969). Proc.
    Natl. Acad. Sci. USA 64:67.

6. Fukada, T., Kawade, Y., Ujihara, M., Shin, C. and
    Shima, T. (1968). Jap. J. Microbiol. 12:329.

7. Lockart, J.Z. Jr., Bayliss, N.L. and Yin, F.H. (1968).
    J. Virol. 2:962.

8. Dianzani, F., Gagnoni, S., Buckler, C.E. and Baron, S.
    (1970). Proc. Soc. Exp. Biol. Med. 133:324.

9. Huang, A.S., Baltimore, D. and Bratt, M.A. (1971). J.
    Virol. 7:389.

10. Baltimore, D. (1971). Bacteriol. Rev. 35:235.

11. Oie, H.K., Buckler, C.E., Uhlendorf, C.P., Hill, D.A. and Baron, S. (1972). Proc. Soc. Exp. Biol. Med. 140: 1178.

12. Yoshinaka, Y. and Hotta, S. (1971). Virology 45:524.

13. Sherrer, K. and Darnell, J.R. (1962). Biochem. Biophys. Res. Commun. 7:1178.

14. Dianzani, F., Cantagalli, P., Gagnoni, S. and Rita, G. (1968). Proc. Soc. Exp. Biol. Med. 128:708.

15. Levy, H.B. and Wheeler, J. (1973). Arch. Ges. Virusforsch, in press.

16. Field, A.K., Lampson, G.P., Tytell, A.A. and Hilleman, M.R. (1972). Proc. Soc. Exp. Biol. Med. 141:440.

17. Ferngold, R.S., Youngner, J.S. and Chen, J. (1970). Ann. N. Y. Acad. Sci. 173:249.

18. Grossberg, S.E. (1972). New Eng. J. Med. 287:13.

TABLE 1

Interferon Production by Rat Embryo Cells Stimulated With
Chikungunya Virus During Inhibition of Protein Synthesis

Treatment of cultures before addition of actinomycin D at 4 1/2 hours	Interferon Production (units/ml)		
	Experiment		
	1	2	3
Chikungunya virus[a]	320	320	1000
Cycloheximide + Chikungunya virus + FPA[b]	320	320	1000

[a] Multiplicity of infection = 50

[b] See text for details of sequential treatment

TABLE 2

Interferon Inducing Activity of RNA Extracted from Cells
Infected with Chikungunya Virus or from Purified Virions

Source of RNA	Treatment	Interferon Production (units/ml)
Cells infected in the presence of inhibitors	None	<3
	RNase	<3
Cells infected in the absence of inhibitors	None	32
	RNase	32
Purified virions	None	<3
	RNase	<3

Cells were treated with 200 µg/ml of DEAE-dextran.

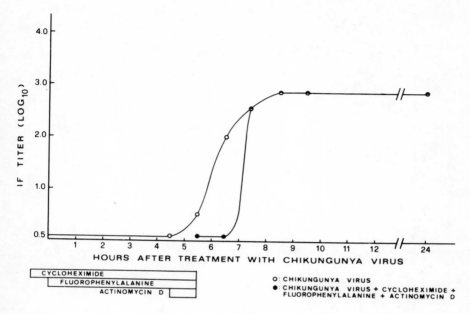

Fig. 1. Kinetics of interferon production in rat embryo cells induced with chikungunya virus in the presence or absence of inhibition of protein synthesis.

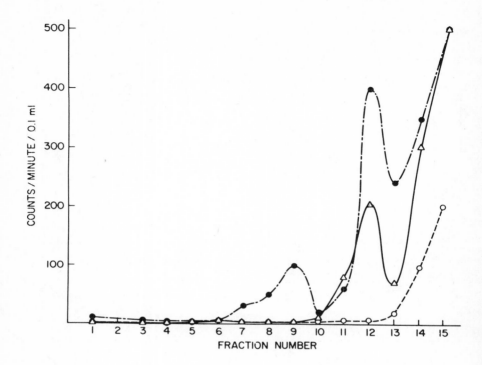

Fig. 2. Sucrose density gradient (15-30%) centrifugation of H labelled RNA extracted from (a) rat embryo cells pretreated with actinomycin D and infected with chikungunya virus in the presence (o----o) or absence (●·—·—●) of inhibition of protein synthesis and (b) purified chikungunya virus (△——△).

DISCUSSION

Burke: We have been in the same difficulty as you have. Can you be sure that there is no synthesis of any viral RNA in the presence of cycloheximide? I think this is the very hard question and it is still not absolutely certainly resolved.

Dianzani: Well, this virus needs newly synthesized polymerase to make RNA.

Burke: Yes, indeed. But I'm saying, can you exclude the possibility that there is a small amount of protein synthesis and that this escapes the cycloheximide effect?

Dianzani: I think so. In our system the inhibition of protein synthesis is obtained by combining two different compounds, cycloheximide and FPA. As you know, these two inhibitors have a different mechanism of action. Cycloheximide inhibits translation of messenger RNA, FPA inhibits elongation of polypeptides. Under these conditions even if some protein molecule could escape to the inhibition by cycloheximide, it would not be properly translated due to the presence of FPA. I agree that this is not an evidence, but the possibility that some functional protein could be synthesized in such conditions is quite slight. Anyway, if some double-stranded RNA would have been produced in the system, it should have been able to induce interferon, while on the contrary, the RNA extracted from cells treated with Chikungunya virus in the presence of the inhibitors did not induce any interferon.

Burke: I think there are three possibilities and one is that the viral RNA, if it's a single-stranded RNA, is adequate to act as an inducer. Secondly, that one produces double-strand-

ed RNA, and the third possibility is that there is some process
connected with or flowing from the actual viral RNA synthesis
which triggers the induction mechanism, and that would explain
your results and would be consistent with what Dr. Dubois just
told us. I'm not able to choose between them. We spent 2 years
using the Reo system in an attempt to decide between them - without success. I've got no data to present, but I think that whatever happens it is clear that there must be another receptor
which is distinct from the polynucleotide receptor because I
think the viral systems must work in cytoplasm, while the polynucleotides may well work from the surface.

Dianzani: I agree.

Levy: It may be of course as Derek Burke pointed out in
the past, that different viruses work in somewhat different ways,
but we have evidence with the Chikungunya system which is, as
you know, quite in agreement with yours. If you treat cells,
chick cells, with good quantities of interferon and then infect
with Chikungunya virus, you can block the formation of all detectable single-stranded and double-stranded RNA determined in
gel electrophoresis analysis. Under those conditions not only do
you not get just as much interferon made, but you actually get
more interferon made. It is true that this is not a rigid exclusion of the possibility of making one or two molecules of
double-stranded RNA. It seems to me that if one strongly depresses the formation of new RNA, you would anticipate getting less
interferon induced, at least it appears to me that that would be
the reasonable expectation, not an equal amount or more.

Dianzani: Of course, I agree.

III - INTERFERON ACTION AT THE CELLULAR LEVEL; ANTAGONISTS

ISOLATION AND PRELIMINARY CHARACTERIZATION OF
VIRUS-RESISTANT MUTANT MOUSE EMBRYO FIBROBLASTS

C. Colby, M.J. Morgan, J.L.N. Hulse and T. Loza

Microbiology Section
University of Connecticut
Storrs, Connecticut, USA

The IF system may be thought of as composed of three basic units: the induction of interferon, the establishment of the antiviral state and the expression of the antiviral activity. Each of these units contain a number of sophisticated and diverse molecular control mechanisms.

A. The induction of IF involves a series of interactions of various regulatory components and may be outlined as follows:

1. The inducer molecule. There is now a large body of experimental evidence supporting the original observation of Field et al (1) that exogenously presented double-stranded ribonucleic acid (ds-RNA) is an efficient inducer of interferon. Much of the experimental evidence obtained with virus-infected cells is consistent with ds-RNA being the inducer molecule, however, there are some conflicting reports. Unambiguous results with virus-infected cells can not be obtained until the other molecular components of the induction system are identified and characterized.

2. The mechanism of recognition of the inducer molecule. If there is a unique set of physical and chemical properties of the inducer molecule required for interferon induction,

then there must be a mechanism for recognizing it. Accordingly, a proteinaceous receptor site has been postulated (2). Initially the receptor site was postulated to have an intracellular location. However, recent evidence (3) concerning the interaction of helical polyribonucleotides with the cell surface suggests that the receptor site may be a membrane-associated protein and that it may exist in both intracellular and surface membrane fractions.

3. Synthesis of interferon m-RNA. The synthesis and release of interferon is blocked in actinomycin D treated cells (4) suggesting that DNA-dependent RNA synthesis is a necessary intermediate. The existence of an interferon m-RNA has recently been demonstrated (5) and confirmed (6).

4. Translation of IF m-RNA. Experiments with various metabolic inhibitors indicate that translation of the IF m-RNA is a necessary event and that there may be a regulatory protein induced by interferon that inhibits prolonged translation of IF m-RNA (7, 8).

5. Processing and release of interferon. At some point during or after its synthesis the interferon polypeptide chain is modified by carbohydrate attachment and then released. The latter process appears to be related to the physiological state of the cell since much high titers of IF are found in the media of virus-infected cells than in that from cells treated with dsRNA.

B. The series of events occuring during the establishment of the antiviral state are:

1. The interaction of interferon molecules with the cell. This reaction is a species specific one and as such suggests the

existance of another receptor molecule. As in the case of
the receptor site for the IF inducing molecule, the receptor of IF itself is likely to be found in a membrane matrix.

2. A nuclear transcriptional event. Two lines of published
experimental evidence suggest that a nuclear transcriptional event is required for the establishment of the AVS. The
first is the well confirmed observation that cells are unable to develop the AVS if treated with actinomycin D before, during or immediately after interferon treatment. The
second is the observation by Cassingena et al (9) that in
populations of intersomatic hybrids of rodent-primate origin (which randomly lose primate chromosomes) clones may
be isolated which can synthesize, but not respond to primate interferon and vice versa. These results suggest that
there is a repository of genetic information required for
the AVS and that such information resides on a chromosome
different from the one carrying the structural gene for the
IF molecule itself.

3. A translational event. The AVS is not established in interferon-treated cells simultaneously treated with cycloheximide (10) suggesting the requirement for a translational
event.

4. Pleiotypic response. The physical and chemical properties
of the interferon molecule are quite similar to those of
some of the growth hormones and apparently only a very few
number of IF molecules are required to elicit the antiviral
response (11). Also, at higher doses, many authors have reported inhibitions of cellular functions by interferon
treatment (12, 13). Accordingly, there is the possibility
that interferon-treatment results in a number of physiological responses (14) one of which may be the establish-

ment of the AVS.

C. The mechanism of the antiviral activity of interferon is not
    known. The block in viral replication is after adsorption
    and penetration of the virus and before the assembly of ma-
    ture virions. Therefore the bulk of the experimental work
    has been directed towards examining an interferon-mediated
    block on viral transcription and/or translation. Experimental
    evidence is available supporting both possibilities.

    1. Inhibition of viral transcription. A marked decrease in
       the appearance of viral RNA in infected cells pretreated
       with interferon has been reported for SV40 (15), vesicular
       stomatitis virus (16, 17), vaccinia virus (18) and reo-
       virus (19). Investigators have been unable to show an ef-
       fect on in vitro virion-bound transcriptase reactions.

    2. Inhibition of viral translation. An inhibition of the in
       vitro translation of picorna virus virion-RNA by components
       isolated from IF-treated cells (20) and IF-treated, virus-
       infected cells (21) has been reported recently.

    One of the most effective and productive approaches to de-
lineating the molecular basis of regulatory mechanisms has been
the biochemical and genetic analysis of regulatory mutants. We
believe that the regulatory mechanisms governing the induction
and action of interferon are no exception. Interferon is an inducible protein whose synthesis results from presenting cells
with a specific class of molecules whose physical and chemical
properties are known, viz double-stranded RNA. The antiviral
state is also inducible and is the basis for the assay of interferon, this assay being one of the most sensitive currently available in animal cell biology.

We reasoned that regulatory mutants of the interferon system that constitutively synthesize either interferon or the molecule(s) required for establishing the antiviral state would be resistant to viral infections. Furthermore, this common phenotype would provide the basis for the selective pressure necessary for the isolation of such mutants. Finally, the formation of heterocaryons, and subsequently of hybrid cell lines, mediated by inactivated paramyxoviruses offers the means for a genetic analysis of such mutants. Thus, we could ask whether these control mechanisms utilize a diffusible molecule and whether or not the wild type is dominant or recessive.

Isolation of Virus Resistant Mutants

We have successfully isolated virus-resistant mutants of mouse embryo fibroblasts. Cells were subjected to the mutagenic action of nitrosoguanidine at a concentration and for a period of time such that 50% of the cells survived. The mutagenized population of cells was then infected with a temperature-sensitive, RNA$^-$ mutant of Sindbis virus, ts-15 (22). Incubation at the permissive temperature for a period of time sufficient to allow the synthesis of viral RNA was followed by a period of incubation at the nonpermissive temperature during which time viral replication and the cytopathic effects of the infection occurred. The virus produced, however, could not initiate continuing rounds of infection due to their temperature sensitivity. Survivors were grown out and the selection procedure was repeated, this time yielding many more survivors that again were allowed to multiply. The application of the selection procedure for the third time yielded negligible cell death. This population of mutant cells was found to be resistant to the growth of vesicular stomatitis virus (VSV), Mengo virus and Semliki forest virus (SFV) as well as temperature-sensitive and wild-type Sindbis virus (See Table 1).

We then isolated a number of clones from this mutant population. One of the clones was found to be resistant to six different classes of viruses; picorna (mengo), arbo (Sindbis, SFV),
rhabdo (VSV), paramyxo (NDV), pox (vaccinia) and herpes (HSV);
(See Table 2). The magnitude of virus-resistance varies among
these viruses and is multiplicity dependent.

Tests for Persistent Infection

Since infectious virus was used to select these mutants,
it is possible that a persistent infection was established and is
responsible for the virus-resistant phenotype. We therefore performed a variety of experiments to test for persistant infection
of these cells with Sindbis ts-15:

1. Clonal populations were incubated for 14 days at $29^{\circ}C$.
    No cytopathology was observed.

2. Growth medium was harvested from clonal populations
    grown at $29^{\circ}C$ and plaqued on CEC monolayers at $29^{\circ}C$.
    No plaques were observed.

3. Cells from individual clones were plaqued as potential
    infective centers on CEC monolayers and incubated for
    7 days at $29^{\circ}C$. No plaques were observed.

4. Cells from individual clones were mixed with an equal
    number of CEC, plated as monolayers and incubated for
    11 days at $29^{\circ}C$. No cytopathology was observed.

These results indicate that the virus-resistant mutant
cells are not shedding infectious Sindbis virus. A second possibility is that the temperature-sensitive mutant of Sindbis
established a latent infection in these cells, i.e., that the
cells are carrying but not producing the virus. To test this

possibility we employed ts-mutants of Sindbis virus that belong
to other complementation groups. (There are three ts-RNA⁻ complementation groups represented here by ts-15, ts-11 and ts-6). The
temperature-sensitive phenotype of all three are maintained in
both wild type and virus-resistant cells, as shown in Table 3,
indicating that there is no viral genetic information in the
mutant cell that can rescue other ts-mutant Sindbis viruses.

Adsorption and Penetration of Viruses

It seems unlikely to us that our cells are resistant to
virus infection as the result of an alteration in their cell membrane such that viral adsorbance or penetration is blocked. We
find no detectable differences in the adsorption of any of the
viruses tested to original 3T6 and mutant S3A5 cells. In these
experiments adsorption of the viruses by both 3T6 and S3A5 cells
was measured by assaying the infectivities of the input virus
suspensions before and after the period of adsorption.

The possibility that the viruses could not adsorb to or
penetrate resistant cells was investigated further by measuring
the uptake of radioactively labelled Sindbis virus. Monolayers
of 3T6, S3A5, S3E11 and S3G1 cells were infected with ^3H -
uridine labelled Sindbis virus (4×10^6 p.f.u./dish; 7250 cpm/
dish) for 0.5 H and the amount of virus taken up measured. The
growth of Sindbis virus was also determined. The results (Table
4) show that Sindbis virus was taken up by all four cell monolayers. The virus grew best in 3T6 cells and most poorly in S3A5
cells. Thus, there was a 2.5 log unit reduction in the yield of
Sindbis virus grown in S3A5 cells, but only a 38% reduction in
the uptake of Sindbis virus by these cells.

Finally, we have preliminary evidence that Mengo virus RNA
is less infectious in virus-resistant mutant cells than in their

wild-type parents (See Table 5). We are currently preparing infectious Sindbis virus RNA since the mutant cells are far more resistant to Sindbis than to Mengo virus.

Is the Interferon System Involved?

None of the mutant clones thus far examined secretes measureable amounts of mouse interferon into the growth medium. This, of course, does not rule out the possibility that the mutant cells are constituitively synthesizing a small amount of intracellular interferon. Experiments are in progress to test the possibility that the mutants are constituitively synthesizing the product(s) required for the establishment of the antiviral state.

Further Genetic Manipulations

We have recently isolated a virus-resistant mutant from a population of mouse L-cells deficient in thymidine kinase (TK^-). We are also selecting for TK^- and $HGPRT^-$ mutants of our virus-resistant MEF cells. Thus, we anticipate being able to determine whether the virus-resistant phenotype is dominant or recessive.

Acknowledgements

We are grateful for the excellent technical assistance of Ms. McLeod. The research was supported by grants from NIH-NIAID, Damon Runyon Memorial Fund and University of Connecticut Research Foundation. Individual support was derived from NIAID Research Career Development Award, Harkness Foundation, NIH Postdoctoral Fellowship and the University of Mexico Medical School Fellowship.

References

1. Field, A.K., Lampson, G.P., Tytell, A.A., Nemes, M.M. and Hilleman, M.R. (1967). Proc. Nat. Acad. Sci. USA 58: 2102-8.

2. Colby, C. and Chamberlin, M.J. (1969). Proc. Nat. Acad. Sci. USA, 63: 160-67.

3. De Clercq, E. and De Somer, P. (1972). J. Virol. 9: 721-731.

4. Burke, D.C. (1966). In Interferons, ed. N.B. Finter, 55-86, Amsterdam.

5. De Maeyer-Guignard, J., De Maeyer, E. and Montagnier, L. (1972). Proc.Nat.Acad.Sci.USA, 69:1203-1207.

6. Lodeman, E., Diederich, J., Orinda, D., Drahovsky, D. and Wacker, A., personal communication, January 1973.

7. Vilcek, J. (1970).Ann. NY Acad. Sci., 173:390-403.

8. Tan, Y.H., Armstrong, J.A. and Ho, M. (1971). Virology, 44:503-509.

9. Cassingena, R., Chany, C., Vignal, M., Estrade, S., Suarez, H.-G.(1970).C.R.Acad.Sci.Paris,270:1189-91.

10. Friedman, R.M. and Sonnabend, J.A. (1964). Nature, 203:366-367.

11. Colby, C. and Morgan, M.J. (1971). Ann. Rev. Microbiol, 25:333-360.

12. Johnson, T.C., Lerner, M.P. and Lancz, G.M.(1968). J. Cell.Biol., 36:617-624.

13. Gresser, I., Brouty-Boyé, D., Thomas, M.T. and Macieira-Coelho, A.(1970). Proc. Nat. Acad. Sci. USA, 66:1052-1058.

14. Hershko, A., Mamont, P., Shields, R. and Tomkins, G. M. (1971). Nature New Biol., 232:206-211.

15. Oxman, M.N. and Levine, M.J. (1971). Proc. Nat. Acad. Sci. USA, 68:299-302.

16. Marcus, P.I., Engelhardt, D.L., Hunt, J.M. and Sekellick, M.K. (1971). Science, 174:593-598.

17. Manders, E.K., Tilles, J.G. and Huang, A.S. (1972). Virology, 49:573-581.

18. Bialy, H.S. and Colby, C. (1972). J. Virol., 9:286-289.

19. Gauntt, C.J. (1972). Biochem. Biophys. Res. Comm., 47: 1228-1236.

20. Falcoff, E., Lebleu, B., Falcoff, R. and Revel, M. (1972). Nature New Biol, 240:145-147.

21. Friedman, R.M., Metz, D.H., Esteban, R.M., Tovel, D. R., Ball, L.A. and Kerr, I.M. (1972). J. Virol., 10: 1184-1198.

TABLE 1

Virus Yield After Infection of Normal (3T6) and
Mutant (3T6MS3) Mouse Embryo Fibroblasts

Viruses assayed

Cells	Sindbis virus (p.f.u./ml)	SFV (p.f.u./ml)	VSV (p.f.u./ml)	Mengo virus (p.f.u./ml)
3T6	3.4×10^9	2.5×10^8	1.3×10^8	6.3×10^8
3T6MS3	2.0×10^5	1.8×10^7	5.0×10^6	1.6×10^8

TABLE 2

Growth of viruses in normal (3T6) and mutant (3T6S3A5) mouse embryo fibroblasts

Virus	Cells	p.f.u./cell	Virus yield p.f.u./10^6 cells	Log_{10} Unit reduction
Sindbis virus	3T6	3.0	6 x 10^7	2.4
	3T6S3A5	3.0	2.5 x 10^5	
	3T6	0.3	1.4 x 10^7	2.4
	3T6S3A5	0.3	6 x 10^4	
SFV	3T6	0.03	1.7 x 10^6	3.3
	3T6S3A5	0.03	8 x 10^2	
	3T6	0.25	4 x 10^8	2.1
	3T6S3A5	0.35	3 x 10^6	
VSV	3T6	0.02	8.5 x 10^8	4.6
	3T6S3A5	0.02	2 x 10^4	
	3T6	2.0	1.85 x 10^8	0.9
	3T6S3A5	2.0	1.9 x 10^7	
	3T6	0.01	1.25x10^8	3.4
	3T6S3A5	0.01	5 x 10^4	

Virus	Cells	p.f.u./cell	Virus yield p.f.u./10^6 cells	Log_{10} Unit reduction
Mengo virus	3T6	2.0	5 x 10^3	0.85
	3T6S3A5	2.0	6 x 10^2	
	3T6S3A5	0.2	1.2 x 10^4	1.7
	3T6S3A5	0.1	2.5 x 10^2	
NDV	3T6	0.03	1.5 x 10^7	2.8
	3T6S3A5	0.02	2.5 x 10^4	
Vaccinia virus	3T6	1.5	3.1 x 10^6	
	3T6S3A5	1.5	2.5 x 10^6	1.2
	3T6	0.2	1.2 x 10^6	
	3T6S3A5	0.2	7 x 10^4	
Herpes Simplex virus	3T6	2.5	6 x 10^6	1.4
	3T6S3A5	2.5	2.5 x 10^5	
	3T6	0.1	6.5 x 10^5	2.2
	3T6S3A5	0.1	4.1 x 10^3	

Cells were infected at the indicated multiplicities; 18-22 h after infection the yield of viruses was determined by plaque assay on CE cells (Sindbis virus, SFV, VSV, NDV and vaccinia virus), L cells (Mengo virus) and HeLa cells (Herpes Simplex virus).

TABLE 3

Complementation of Sindbis ts RNA⁻ Mutants

Cells	Temperature of incubation	Temperature sensitive mutant of Sindbis virus assayed		
		ts6 (p.f.u./ml)	ts11 (p.f.u./ml)	ts15 (p.f.u./ml)
3T6	29°	1.4×10^7	3.6×10^6	3.0×10^6
	40°	1.8×10^3	0.5×10^2	1.7×10^3
S3A5	29°	1.2×10^6	2.5×10^5	1.0×10^6
	40°	1.8×10^3	0.5×10^2	1.8×10^3

TABLE 4

Adsorption, Penetration and Growth of Sindbis
Virus in 3T6 Original and Mutant Cells

Cell Line	Virus Yield p.f.u./10^6 Cells	Extracellular $[^3H]$-cpm/10^6 Cells	Intracellular $[^3H]$-cpm/10^6 Cells
3T6	7.5×10^7	1940	1210
3T6S3A5	4.1×10^5	3560	750
3T6S3E11	6.5×10^5	1810	1290
3T6S3G1	3.2×10^6	2800	635

TABLE 5

Cell Line	Infected With	Virus Yield PFU/10^6 cells
3T3	Mengo	4×10^7
3T3	Mengo RNA	2×10^7
3T6-VR	Mengo	3.4×10^6
3T6-VR	Mengo RNA	1.9×10^6

DISCUSSION

Friedman: I have two questions. One is technical: in that
last slide, you had really excellent yields from infectious RNA.
How do you manage to get such high yields of virus using infectious RNA? The other question is: in giving the spectrum of viruses to which the cells are resistant, you mentioned several
but you left out the last one you had on that table, Herpes Simplex, which is usually relatively resistant to interferon. Yet,
it was fairly sensitive in your cell line, and I wondered if
that doesn't count possibly against your notion. In other words,
does any of this have anything to do with interferon?

Colby: I haven't done the interferon-Herpes experiments
in these cells, but Herpes is classically very resistant in
mouse lines to the interferon system. With respect to the high
yield of Mengo virus, all I can do is describe what I did. The
cultures were infected with a multiplicity around a hundred plaque forming units per 5×10^5 cells. The cells were pretreated
for 10 minutes with a hundred micrograms per ml of DEAE dextran
and the RNA was added in DEAE dextran usually for 35 minutes.
Much more than 45 minutes and 3T3 cells crump under that much
dextran. The cells were washed 3 times and the yield was taken
at 18 hours and was associated with 2 cycles of freeze thaw. So
it's not a single cycle.

Friedman: You were measuring not only the yield from infectious RNA, but also the yield from the first round of infection with the progeny of the infectious RNA?

Colby: Exactly.

Friedman: That just might modify your conclusions somewhat. After the first growth cycle you may catch up because the
growth cycle of that virus is about 7 hours; so you probably
have gone through more than one cycle. I just want to point out
the fact that it would be interesting to see what it looks like
after one growth cycle. It would help even if the yields are low;
just the comparison would be important.

Levy: You said you were planning to follow each of the
various steps in virus replication. The interferon system would
be implicated if there was an inhibition of either viral RNA
production or viral proteins. Did you check to see whether viral
RNA synthesis is decreased in these cells?

Colby: Yes, we've done that. We looked initially at viral
protein synthesis and viral RNA synthesis and I'm really not in a
position to put any numbers on the board. I've done the experiments now 3 times. 2 of the times there was a significant inhibition of Sindbis RNA synthesis and a less significant inhibition
of VSV RNA synthesis, suggesting that, since Sindbis requires
protein synthesis in order to get its RNA synthesis, the block
may have something to do with protein synthesis. I stress that
this result is preliminary.

Revel: You mentioned that in the mutant line, cell density
was changed and that cells have contact inhibition at a much lower density. This would suggest maybe that cyclic AMP levels would
be changed in those cells. Have you tried the effect of cyclic
AMP?

Colby: No, I'm looking forward to doing it this winter.

Ankel: I was wondering if it was the interferon system
which interferes with the multiplication of the virus. Wouldn't
it be possible to test an antagonist of interferon to see whether

that blocks the antiviral effect in these cells?

Colby: I would like to have some. Someone will give it to me surely.

Morahan: Are your mutant cells more sensitive to the action of interferon? You said they don't produce interferon, but are they more sensitive to the action?

Colby: I don't know whether or not they produce it in response to an inducer just under normal conditions. The sensitivity to interferon again is an incomplete story. That is, I have not done the experiments enough times to really convince myself that what I have is absolutely right. In the case of both Sindbis virus and VSV virus, one can reach a saturation plateau level of interferon inhibition of one cycle growth step in the wild type 3T3 cells. That level is reached in the mutant cell with the same amount of interferon, albeit that you're starting at a much lower level. So if you look at virus yield from the wild type with increasing doses of interferon, it goes down. If you look in the mutant, it starts very much lower but it goes to the same level. However, in the case of both Mengo virus and Vaccinia virus, the one time I've done that experiment, I could not really significantly reduce the yield below what I was getting from the resistance of the mutant per se by treating with interferon. So in this case, I really can't say one way or another what's going on. These experimental results are too preliminary for me to answer your question.

INTERFERON ANTAGONISTS IN EMBRYONIC TISSUES

Page S. Morahan

Medical College of Virginia
Virginia Commonwealth University
Richmond,Virginia 23298

Introduction

An age-related increase in resistance to many viruses occurs from embryonic life to neonatal life to adulthood. For example, the young chicken embryo (first week of incubation) is
more susceptible to certain virus infections than is the older
chicken embryo (second week of incubation) (21, 26, 27). This increased resistance of the intact embryo toward viruses is also
observed in cell cultures prepared from embryos of different ages
of embryogenesis, and is correlated with increased sensitivity
of cells from older embryos to the action of interferon (21, 26).
We have previously reported that a small proportion of cells from
young embryos will decrease the action of interferon in a culture of predominantly older cells (17). These observations led
us to postulate that an "antagonist" of interferon action was
present in young chicken embryos and in cell cultures prepared
from these embryos. Interferon antagonists have been reported
from various sources, including human placental tissue, normal
allantoic fluid of the chicken embryo, and fetal bovine serum (5,
8, 10, 29). In this paper, we report the presence of interferon
antagonist activity in tissues of young chicken embryos. This
antagonist activity appears to decrease with embryonic development in parallel to the increase in sensitivity to interferon of

older chicken embryo cells.

Materials and Methods

Cell cultures. Specific pathogen free and COFAL-negative
chicken embryos were obtained from Spafas, Inc., Biglersville,
Penn. Primary cell cultures were prepared from 6-day old (CEC-6)
and 13-day old (CEC-13) chicken embryos as previously described
(26). Mouse fibroblast cells, strain L929, were obtained from
Microbiological Associates Inc., Bethesda, Md., and grown in
Eagle's minimal essential medium with Hanks' balanced salt solution (HMEM) and 10% fetal calf serum.

Viruses. Pools of Newcastle disease virus CG strain (NDV),
Sindbis virus strain Ar1055, vesicular stomatitis virus Indiana
strain (VSV-Indiana) and New Jersey strain (VSV-NJ) were cultured
in chicken embryo cells. These viruses were titrated by plaque
formation on primary chicken embryo cell cultures, using an overlay medium consisting of 5% calf serum, HMEM, 1.5% Difco agar,
150 µg/ml DEAE-dextran, 100 µg/ml penicillin and 100 µg/ml streptomycin. Mouse poliovirus (GD-7) was cultured in BHK-21 cells and
the virus hemagglutinin titrated according to the methods of Oie
et al. (28).

Interferon antagonists. Chicken embryos with amniotic membranes were collected at various gestational ages, washed with
Hanks' balanced salt solution, frozen at -70°C, and lyophilized.
The lyophilized tissue was rapidly homogenized in a Waring blender with HMEM to a 2-10% w/v concentration, and stirred overnight
at 4°C. The suspension was centrifuged at 5,000 rpm for 20 minutes at 4°C, and the supernatant fluid was centrifuged at 30,000
rpm at 4°C overnight. The supernatant fluid, usually containing
some lipid, was recovered and, if necessary, filtered through a
0.22 nm Millipore filter for sterilization. The material was kept

frozen at -70°C, or stored at 4°C for up to two months. The antagonists were relatively unstable, and lost considerable activity
on storage. The usual yield of antagonist from 6-day old chicken
embryos was 3 to 6 grams per 100 embryos. Interferon antagonists
were also prepared by similar procedures from human placental
membranes obtained through the courtesy of the Department of
Obstetrics and Gynecology, Medical College of Virginia.

Interferon assays. Assays for interferon by plaque reduction procedures involved incubating cell cultures overnight at 36
°C with 1 ml of 2- or 3-fold interferon dilutions prepared in
maintainance medium consisting of 2% fetal calf serum, HMEM,
antibiotics. The cells were washed twice with Hanks' balanced
salt solution, the appropriate dilution of virus adsorbed for 1
hour at 36°C, and the overlay medium added. A minimum of seven
dilutions of interferon were adsorbed to duplicate cell cultures
in each experiment. Plaques were counted after three days incubation at 36°C, and a dose response curve was calculated by the
method of least squares. The titer of interferon (units/ml) is
expressed as the reciprocal of the greatest dilution of interferon resulting in 50% inhibition of plaque formation as compared
to virus control cultures.

Assay for interferon by yield reduction of virus involved
incubating cell cultures overnight with 1 ml of interferon dilutions at 36°C, washing the cells twice, adsorbing the appropriate dilution of virus to give 1.0 multiplicity of infection
(m.o.i.). After virus adsorption for 1 hour at 36°C, the cells
were washed twice and maintainance solution added. After additio-
al incubation for 18-24 hours at 36°C, cells were observed for
cytopathic effect, and cells plus supernatant fluid were frozen
at -70°C. The yields of VSV or Sindbis viruses were measured by
titration of plaque forming units of virus in CEC-13 cells. The
yield of GD-7 virus hemagglutinin was measured by the procedure

of Oie et al. (28). Dose response curves were calculated by the method of least squares. The titer of interferon (units/ml) is expressed as the reciprocal of greatest dilution of interferon which reduced the virus yield by 0.5 $\log_{10}$ from the yield in virus control cultures.

Assays for interferon antagonist activity. Essentially, the procedure for interferon assays was followed, except that cells were treated with the interferon antagonist preparation (2% w/v in maintenance medium) for 4 hours at 36°C before interferon dilutions were added to the cultures. Thus, for most experiments, cells were in contact with the antagonist both before and during the interferon incubation period. For some experiments, the cells were washed free of antagonist before addition of interferon. The presence of the antagonists did not markedly affect growth of viruses, and toxicity was only seldom observed in antagonist treated cell culture controls. Dose response curves were calculated as previously described, and the slopes and the titers of experimental groups with antagonists plus interferon were compared statistically by analysis of variance to slopes and titers of groups with interferon alone.

Results

Decrease of interferon activity by small proportions of CEC-6. Cells were dispersed by trypsin from 6-day old and 13-day old specific pathogen free chicken embryos, the number of viable cells determined by trypan blue exclusion, and primary cell cultures prepared with various ratios of 6 and 13-day old cells. Plaque reduction assays for interferon using VSV-Indiana were performed on each of these cell populations and the interferon titer was determined for each cell mixture. A small proportion of CEC-6 cells in the mixed population was able to reduce profoundly the interferon titer observed in a culture of CEC-13 cells alone (Fig. 1). The reduction in titer was greater than that which would have been expected if the CEC-6 cells did not possess receptors for interferon or were unable to develop the antiviral state. The observations were consistent with the proposal that the CEC-6 cells from chicken embryos free of latent viruses produced a natural substance ("antagonist") that inhibited the action of interferon in the CEC-13 cells.

Interferon assay maximizing differences between CEC-6 and CEC-13. Various interferon assay systems were studied in order to develop the most sensitive assay for detection of interferon antagonist activity in the 6-day old chicken embryo cells. Plaque reduction and yield reduction assays for interferon using several different viruses were performed in 6 and 13-day old chicken embryo cell cultures in order to determine in which virus-assay system the greatest difference in sensitivity to interferon occurred between 6 and 13 day cells. While plaque reduction assays using Sindbis virus did not show a significant difference in interferon titers between CEC-6 and CEC-13 cells, similar assays using vesicular stomatitis virus (either Indiana or New Jersey serotypes) or Newcastle disease virus showed significant reduction (62-220 fold) in interferon titers between CEC-6 and CEC-13 (Table 1). Thus, the insensitivity of CEC-6 cells toward interferon could be demonstrated with viruses from at least two groups - Paramyxoviruses and Rhabdoviruses.

When plaque reduction assays with VSV-Indiana were compared to yield reduction assays for interferon using the same virus, only the plaque reduction assays demonstrated the large differences in interferon titers between CEC-6 and CEC-13 cells (Table 2). It was possible that an interferon antagonist might not have been active in the yield reduction assay in which cells were infected at 1 m.o.i. and virus yields harvested only 24 hours later. Conditions in the plaque reduction assay involved infection at a

very low m.o.i. and measuring virus growth after multiple cycles
of viral replication. The sensitivity of CEC-6 and CEC-13 cells
to interferon was compared in yield reduction assays in which
cells were infected at a very low m.o.i. (3×10^{-5}) and virus
yields harvested either after a single cycle of virus replication or after multiple cycles of virus growth and development of
complete cytopathic effect. There was little difference in interferon titer between the CEC-6 and CEC-13 cells in either yield
reduction assay, even in the assay in which conditions approxi-
mated those in the plaque reduction assay. Thus, the plaque reduction assay for interferon using vesicular stomatitis virus
Indiana strain was selected as a sensitive and reproducible assay to detect natural antagonist activity in 6-day old chicken
embryos or cell cultures.

Assay of interferon antagonists. In order to determine the
optimum method for detecting interferon antagonist activity, the
chicken or human antagonists were added to CEC-13 cells at different times during interferon adsorption, and interferon assayed
by plaque reduction of VSV-Indiana. Interferon titers were reduced consistently in experimental groups in which antagonists
were present before addition of interferon, or in which interferon antagonists were present both before and during adsorption
of interferon. The antagonist prepared from 6-day old chicken embryos reduced the interferon titer 2-6 fold in general, while the
human antagonist reduced the titer 3-16 fold. The embryonic antagonist preparations were not as effective as live CEC-6 cells, in
which the interferon titer could be reduced up to 220 fold from
the titer observed in CEC-13 cells (Table 1). The low level of
inhibition of interferon activity by the antagonist may be related to instability of the antagonist substance; we have observed
repeatedly the loss of antagonist activity that occurs on limited
storage of the material at either 4°C or -70°C.

The chicken embryo antagonist was also reduced from 2-5 fold the activity of mouse interferon, although the human amniotic antagonist was again more active. In some experiments with the human antagonist, interferon titers were reduced as much as 73-fold (Fig. 2). The human antagonist reduced the interferon titer equally well in two different yield reduction assays, and was also effective in reducing the titer of interferon measured by the plaque reduction assay. These results indicate that antagonist activity is a general phenomenon and not dependent upon the interferon assay procedure. The slopes of the dose response curves for interferon were similar whether the cells were treated with interferon alone, or with the interferon and the human amniotic antagonist. These observations suggest the possibility that both interferon and the antagonist may act at the same site.

Ontogeny of chicken embryo antagonist activity. Extracts from chicken embryos of different ages of incubation were tested for natural interferon antagonist activity, using the interferon assay of plaque reduction of VSV-Indiana in CEC-13 cells (Fig. 3). Cell cultures were treated with 2% (w/v) chicken embryonic extracts or maintenance medium for 4 hours at 36°C, were washed twice, interferon dilutions adsorbed for 4 hours, the cells washed again, and maintenance medium added for an additional 20 hours. Virus was then adsorbed to the cells, and plaques were counted 3 days later. Extracts from 6- or 7-day old embryos significantly reduced the interferon titer obtained in cells treated with maintenance medium alone ($p < 0.05$). The extract from the 8-day old embryo had slight activity, while extracts from 11- and 13-day old embryos possessed no antagonist activity.

Discussion

Cells prepared from young 6-day old chicken embryos (CEC-6) were insensitive to the action of interferon as measured by plaque reduction assay against several viruses. Addition of CEC-6 cells to cell cultures from 13-day old chicken embryos (CEC-13) profoundly reduced the sensitivity to interferon of the CEC-13 cells. Interferon antagonist prepared from extracts of 6-day old embryos also reduced significantly the titer of interferon in CEC-13 cells; however, the extracts were not active to the same extent as were live CEC-6 cells cocultivated with CEC-13 cells.

The embryonic antagonist appears to be a natural substance(s) occurring in chicken embryos. Certain viruses are known to produce antagonists of interferon action. These viruses include both DNA or RNA containing nononcogenic viruses such as parainfluenza viruses, tick-borne encephalitis virus, frog virus 3, Sindbis virus, poliovirus, cowpox virus, and Newcastle disease virus, and DNA or RNA oncogenic viruses such as murine sarcoma virus and SV-40 virus (1, 3, 6, 13, 14, 22, 25, 30, 31, 32). Although some of these viruses may infect chicken embryos, the embryos used for the present experiments were specific pathogen free and COFAL-negative. However, the majority of chicken embryos carry certain functions characteristic of avian leukosis-sarcoma viruses, and there is considerable evidence that all chicken embryos may contain the genetic information for the helper function of these viruses (18). However, if this virus genome is responsible for production of the endogenous embryonic antagonist, its activity is age related. The interferon antagonist activity disappeared with embryonic development, indicating that the production or expression of antagonist activity is under autogenetic regulatory control.

The mode of activity of the chicken embryo antagonist is still under investigation. The chicken embryonic antagonist is

similar to the human amniotic antagonist in that its action is
not species specific (10). However, time course studies to determine whether the chicken embryonic antagonist is more active before, during, or after interferon adsorption have been equivocal.
Examination of the slopes of the dose-effect curves suggested
that the antagonist and interferon may have the same site of action. The observation that live CEC-6 cells possessed a much
greater antagonist activity than did extracts from these embryos
may indicate that the antagonist is labile, or is active on other
cells only in a local environmental milieu.

The correlation of the disappearance of interferon antagonist activity with acquisition of sensitivity to interferon of
chicken embryonic cells is a provocative finding. Interferon was
first described because of its antiviral activity. However, recent investigations have indicated that other activities appear
to be closely linked to the antiviral activity of interferon.
These activities include inhibition of: growth of tumor cells,
leukemia virus activation in graft versus host disease, growth
of rapidly dividing cells such as regenerating liver cells, humoral or cell mediated immune reactions where interferon may be inhibiting proliferation of lymphocytic cells (2, 7, 11, 15, 16,
20, 24). This range of activities leads to the speculation that
interferon (or substances that are purified along with interferon) may exert growth regulatory functions in vertebrate cells.
This regulation of cell division and growth may occur through a
natural inhibition of gene expression effected by interferon.The
mechanism is unknown, although in many regards the inhibitory
action of interferon on protein and RNA synthesis resembles that
of hormones. The interferon antagonist might be postulated to
counteract the interferon-mediated inhibition of gene expression,
in order to permit macromolecular synthesis required for cell
division functions. The mechanism of interferon antagonist activity is also obscure, although it might involve selective dere-

pression of the genome (12). In support of a general concept of a normal inhibition of gene expression by interferon which is counteracted by the interferon antagonist, Fournier and Leauté have recently demonstrated that treatment of cells with interferon led to decreased synthesis of RNA, while the murine interferon antagonists appeared to stimulate RNA synthesis (9). It is intriguing to speculate that interferon is prominent in regulation of normal differentiated cell growth, while an embryonic antagonist of interferon action may be necessary for normal chemical and morphologic differentiation processes to occur during embryonic development.

Acknowledgements

The excellent technical assistance of Rose Ragland and Charles Fleming is appreciated. This research was supported by Public Health Service Research Grant No. CA12689 from the National Cancer Institute.

References

1. Brailovsky, C.A., L.D. Berman and C. Chany (1969). Int. J. Cancer 4:194-203.
2. Braun, W. and H.B. Levy (1972). Proc. Soc. Exp. Biol. Med. 141:769-773.
3. Canivet, M., J. Peries, M. Olivie and M. Boiron (1972). C.R. Acad. Sc. Paris 274:1106-1108.
4. Chany, C., A. Gregoire and J. Lemaitre (1969). C.R. Acad. Sc. Paris 269:1236-1237.

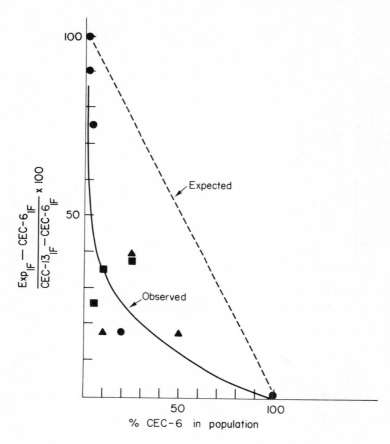

Fig. 1. Reduction of sensitivity to interferon of CEC-13 cells cocultivated in the presence of small percentages of CEC-6 cells. The inhibition index (% inhibition) =

$$\frac{\text{interferon titer in cell mixture} - \text{interferon titer in CEC-6}}{\text{interferon titer in CEC-13} - \text{interferon titer in CEC-6}} \times 100$$

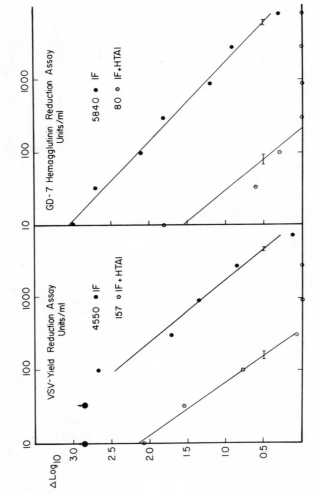

Fig. 2. Reduction in mouse interferon titer by treatment of L929 cells with 2% human amniotic membrane antagonist for 4 hours before and during the 18 hour interferon adsorption period. VSV-yield reduction = interferon assay by measuring the yield of plaque forming units of VSV. GD-7 = interferon assay by measuring the hemagglutinin yield of GD-7 virus.

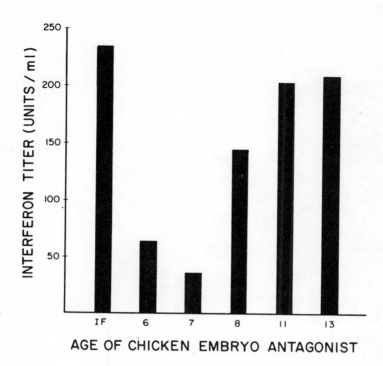

Fig. 3. Age-related reduction in chicken interferon titer by treatment of CEC-13 cells with 2% embryonic antagonists prepared from 6-, 7-, 8-, 11-, and 13-day old chicken embryos.

DISCUSSION

Pitha: Have you looked for these antagonists in other rapidly growing tissue like regenerating liver?

Morahan: No, we have not. We have been looking in certain
tumors and have assayed for antagonistic activity in the B 16
melanoma tumor and Lewis Long carcinoma. We do find antagonist
activity, but this is just one preliminary experiment.

Pitha: But I think with tumors, one should be very careful
to be sure they don't carry viruses.

Morahan: They do.

Chany: Do you have any idea about the chemical nature of
these substances?

Morahan: No, we have done no tests yet.

De Maeyer: Does some of the antagonist appear into the
supernatant of the culture medium of six day old embryo cells?

Morahan: I've not been able to detect significant amounts
of activity.

De Maeyer: And have you any idea about its size?

Morahan: No.

Levy: As you know, when you add serum, spent medium, tissue juices or anything else to a tissue culture and then measure
the effect on RNA or protein synthesis, there are frequently profound effects. Could this just be that when you preincubate your
cells with this extract that you really turn off RNA synthesis or
something like this, sort of like an actinomycin or cycloheximide

effect, namely inhibiting the production of interferon or the antiviral substance just because you're turning down the metabolism of the cell?

Morahan: The mechanism of action of these substances is not known. Dr. Fournier will be talking about this later on. I feel that since the older extracts from embryos does not have this ability, there has to be some sort of specific factor present in the younger embryonic tissues.

Colby: May I ask you, is the antagonist from any of these tissues able to survive the initial purification procedures that we normally use with interferon, such as low pH?

Morahan: I have not done a great deal of this. These materials are relatively labile to purification procedures.

Colby: Could you do the experiment of simply combining directly the antagonist and an interferon preparation, allowing them to interact, then purifying the interferon from that and seeing if the antagonist is still active?

Morahan: I've done this mixture type of experiment and did not find any inactivation of interferon in it. These experiments were done by mixing a concentrated interferon preparation with an antagonist for 2 hours at room temperature, and then making dilutions of the interferon and assaying it; there was no decrease in interferon titer under those conditions.

Planterose: I might have missed the point but have you looked at different tissues for these antagonists? Does it preferentially come from any one particular tissue within the embryo?

Morahan: No, I have not looked. The six day embryos are quite small, and we're using the entire embryo and the amniotic membrane.

REGULATION OF THE ANTIVIRAL STATE
INDUCED BY INTERFERON

F. Fournier and J.B. Léauté

Institut National de la Santé et
de la Recherche Médicale
U. 43 de Recherches sur les Infections Virales
74, Avenue Denfert-Rochereau, 75014 Paris,France

Summary

We have previously reported that actinomycin D, when added
4-6 h after interferon to sensitive cells, significantly increases the antiviral effect of this substance (1). Similar findings were published by Lab, using both cycloheximide and actinomycin D (2). On this basis, we have postulated the existence of
a regulatory protein of the antiviral state which appears in the
cell when the antiviral protein (s) reaches a critical concentration.

On the other hand, when during the same critical period
(4-6 h after interferon), tissue antagonists, extracted from
normal (3) or tumor tissues (4), are added to the cells, the
antiviral effect of interferon decreases significantly.

These antagonists are mainly located in the fundamental
tissue. Their physical-chemical properties seem to indicate that
they are glycoproteins.

In our attempt to correlate these two phenomena, we have
studied the effect of the tissue antagonist on cellular ribosomal RNA synthesis. Experiments based on the use of antimeta-

bolites, such as actinomycin D and toyocamycin, seem to indicate
that these antagonists act at least partially by affecting ribosomal RNA synthesis, thus decreasing indirectly the effect of
the antiviral protein.

Interferon induces the cellular synthesis of protein (s)
probably responsible for conferring the antiviral state to the
cell. These antiviral proteins have never been isolated nor
identified, but their existence is based on the integrity of the
cellular apparatus necessary to the induction of the antiviral
state, and the asynteny of chromosomal location of genes responsible for the interferon synthesis or for the antiviral state
induced by this substance.

On the basis of these arguments, we have postulated that
the synthesis of interferon, the induction of the antiviral
state and its maintenance are governed by distinct regulatory
machanisms (5).

During our investigations on the antiviral state, we have
noted two remarkable phenomena: firstly, an unexpected potentiation of the antiviral action of interferon in the presence of
actinomycin D; secondly, the decrease of the established antiviral state by antagonist factors isolated from normal tissues
or tumors.

Effect of actinomycin D on the interferon-induced antiviral state

Actinomycin D, when added _after_ interferon, might increase
its antiviral action about 10 times. This potentiating effect is
observed only during a well-defined period of 4 to 6 h after the
addition of interferon to the cells.

In Figure 1 is summarized the experimental procedure where,
in parallel series, actinomycin is added to the cells either be-

fore interferon (2 h) or at selected time intervals after interferon (1, 2, 3, 4 and 6 h). In every set, after a 3-h incubation
period, the actinomycin D is discarded, replaced by fresh medium;
and the L cells are infected with vesicular stomatitis virus
(VSV) at the multiplicity of infection (m.o.i.) = 1 PFU/cell.

The results obtained are presented in Figure 2. It is
clearly shown that actinomycin (at the concentration of 1 μg/ml),
when added 2 h before interferon, blocks its antiviral action.
When added 1, 2, 3 and 4 h after interferon, its inhibitory effect on interferon decreases linearly and disappears completely
at 4 h. On the contrary, when actinomycin D is added 6 h after
interferon, an increase of about 10-fold of the antiviral state
can be obtained. In control cells (not treated with interferon),
incubated for parallel time intervals with actinomycin D, no significant effect on the yield of VSV can be observed.

These results were confirmed by Lab and Koehren who used
cycloheximide in chick embryo fibroblasts (2).

On the basis of these data, we suggest that the potentiating effect of actinomycin D or cycloheximide on the antiviral
state after 4 h could result from their inhibitory effect on the
synthesis of a cellular control protein of the antiviral state.
The synthesis of this control protein could be induced as soon
as the antiviral protein (s) reaches a suitable concentration in
the cell.

Tissue antagonists of interferon (T.A.I.)

We have previously extracted substances present in human
amniotic or chorionic membranes, which decrease the antiviral
state when added 4 to 7 h after interferon (3). More recently,
similar antagonists were isolated from mouse muscles and mouse
cartilage (6). It is of interest that interferon antagonists,like

actinomycin D, act only when added 4 to 6 h after interferon to
the cells. This has been shown by a careful and detailed kinetic
analysis performed by Dr. D. Sergiescu (unpublished data).

In a new series of investigations, we have studied the possible relationship which might exist between control protein (s)
of the antiviral state and tissue antagonist (s). We have previously shown (7) that these tissue antagonists accumulate outside of the cells in the fundamental substance. It can be suggested, therefore, that they might act from the outside through
the cell membrane and might affect the control protein either
directly, or indirectly, via another cellular metabolic chain.

We have, therefore, studied the combined effect of actinomycin D and the tissue antagonist (s) on the antiviral state in
the presence of a constant amount of interferon or antagonist
(s), but using increasing concentrations of actinomycin D. The
dose-response relationship between the yield of VSV and increasing concentrations of actinomycin D are presented in Figure 3.
The analysis of the results shows that i) the antiviral state induced by interferon is significantly potentiated by increasing
amounts of actinomycin D between 0.125 and 2 μg/ml; ii) these
different concentrations, which inhibit the cellular RNA synthesis from 65% to 90% (Profile E) have, nevertheless, no effect on
viral replication itself (as shown in the control series C and
D); and iii) the effect of the antagonist (s), which decreases
the interferon action about 40 times, is abolished by the small-
est dose of actinomycin D: 0.125 μg.

With antagonist (s) extracted from mouse cartilage, similar
results were obtained. The concentrations of actinomycin D used
in this case were 0.06 to 0.5 μg and inhibited 70% to 90% of
cellular RNA synthesis (Figure 4).

Perry and Kelly have previously shown that small doses of actinomycin D affect primarily the synthesis of ribosomal RNAs, since the DNA template for ribosomal RNAs has a particularly high G.C. content (for which actinomycin D has a well-known affinity) (8). Therefore, in a new series of experiments, we explored the effect of toyocamycin on the biological action of T. A.I. Tavitian reported that toyocamycin (an adenosin analogue) inhibits, at low concentrations, the maturation of the ribosomal RNAs (18 and 28 S components) without affecting the synthesis of other cellular RNA species (9).

In a preliminary study, the effect of toyocamycin on ribosomal RNA synthesis in L cells was studied. At the concentration of 0.250 µg, toyocamycin inhibits in 3 h mainly the two mature components with an inhibition of about 50%, but also affects slightly the synthesis of ribosomal precursors, especially the 32 S precursor (Figure 5).

In another preliminary study, 0.06 and 0.125 µg of toyocamycin were used since at these two concentrations, toyocamycin had no effect on VSV replication (although 60% to 75% of the total RNA synthesis was inhibited). In Figure 6 are summarized these experiments on the effect of toyocamycin (0.06 and 0.125µg) on the antiviral state induced by interferon and on the effect of antagonist (s). Toyocamycin (as well as actinomycin D in previous experiments) was added 5 h after interferon, in the presence or absence of antagonists prepared either from mouse muscles or from mouse cartilage. The results are presented as the ratio of the amount of VSV yield in control cells and in treated cells, expressed in log 10.

In the absence of antagonists, toyocamycin does not affect the action of interferon. Occasionally the antiviral effect is even increased. This observation is in favor of the hypothesis that toyocamycin (just like actinomycin D) might interfere with

the synthesis of the control protein. In the presence of both
antagonists (muscle and cartilage extracts), the antiviral state
induced by interferon decreased about 10 times. In both cases,
however, their effect is completely abolished by 0.125 µg of
toyocamycin.

We have postulated, therefore, that these antagonists might
not act directly on the control protein but might affect the
antiviral state indirectly by increasing the ribosomal RNA synthesis needed when the control protein is synthesized.

Finally we have studied the effect of tissue antagonists
on cellular RNA synthesis after an incubation of 18 h. Antagonists extracted either from muscle or from cartilage do not affect the cellular multiplication but increase about 3-fold the
incorporation of tritiated uridine in the insoluble fraction, as
well as in the soluble fraction.

This stimulation seems to indicate a change in the permeability of the cell membrane for uridine and increasing incorporation in the acido-precipitable fraction. The here presented
results are, therefore, of a yet preliminary character.

Conclusion

The presently available data seem to indicate that muscle
or cartilage extracts of murine origin decrease (or occasionally
suppress completely) the antiviral state induced by interferon.
The effect is blocked by small doses of actinomycin D and toyocamycin. This is consistent with the idea that tissue antagonists
might interfere with ribosomal RNA synthesis, but an increase in
the uptake of labelled uridine seems to indicate parallel changes
in cell membrane permeability to uridine. Since amniotic antagonists were mainly found in the fundamental layer (7), it can be
postulated that these substances act on the cell membrane by in-

ducing metabolic changes sensitive to inhibitors.

References

1. Chany, C., F. Fournier and S. Rousset (1971). Nature (New Biol.) 230:113.
2. Lab, M. and F. Koerhen (1972). Ann. Inst. Pasteur 122: 569.
3. Fournier, F., S. Rousset and C. Chany (1969). Proc. Soc. Exp. Biol. Med. 132:943.
4. Chany, C., J. Lemaitre and A. Grégoire (1969). C.R. Acad. Sci (Paris) 269:223.
5. Chany, C., F. Fournier and S. Rousset (1970). Ann. New York Acad. Sci. 173:505.
6. Fournier, F., M. Sarragne, A. Rouffet, J.B. Léauté and C. Chany (1974). (In print.) C.R. Acad. Sci. (Paris).
7. Fournier, F., C. Chany and M. Sarragne (1972). Nature (New Biol.) 235:47.
8. Perry, R.P. and D.E. Kelley (1968). J. Cellular Physiology 72:235.
9. Tavitian, A., C. Stanley, S.C. Uretsky and G. Acs(1968). Biochem. Biophys. Acta 157:33.

TABLE 1

Action of tissue extracts (muscle or cartilage
preparations) on cellular RNA synthesis

L-Cells	Uridine-^{3}H 60 minutes cpm/1.5 x 10^6	
	soluble TCA	insoluble TCA
Control medium 18h	1,500	1,000
Treated by Tissue extract for 18h	4,600	3,700

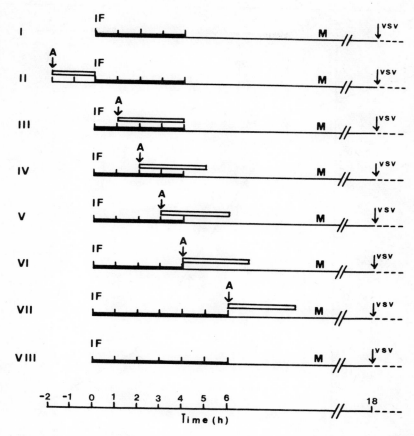

Fig. 1. Experimental procedure summarizing the different time intervals of the addition of actinomycin D (1 µg/ml) <u>before</u> and <u>after</u> interferon.

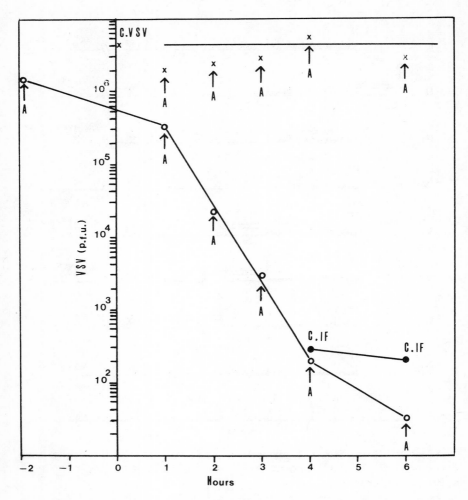

Fig. 2. Details of the experimental protocol are described in the legend of Fig. 1. At hourly intervals, when actinomycin D is added, its blocking effect decreases progressively to zero at 4 h. After 4 h, actinomycin D potentiates the antiviral effect of interferon.

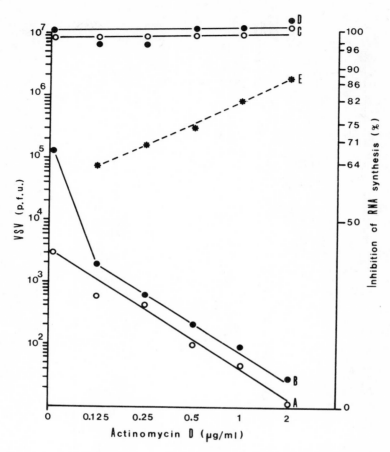

Fig. 3. Dose-response relationship between the yield of VSV and increasing concentrations of actinomycin D. A, L cells are treated with mouse interferon for 5 h and then with actinomycin D; B, in addition to interferon and actinomycin D, a tissue antagonist of interferon (TAI) is added; C, VSV control + TAI + actinomycin D; D, same viral control without TAI; E, this scale represents the inhibition of RNA synthesis by actinomycin D added to the cells 5 h after interferon treatment. 3H-Uridine is added 30 min after actinomycin D, and its incorporation in the acido-precipitable fraction is measured 2 h later.

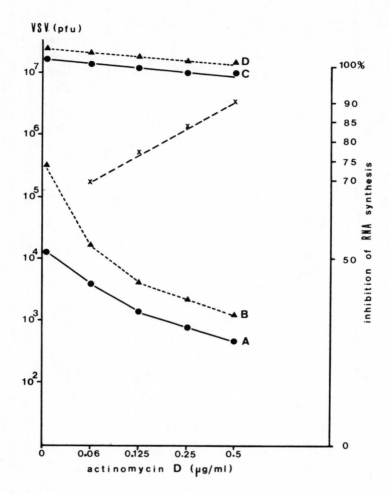

Fig. 4.   See legend for Fig. 3.

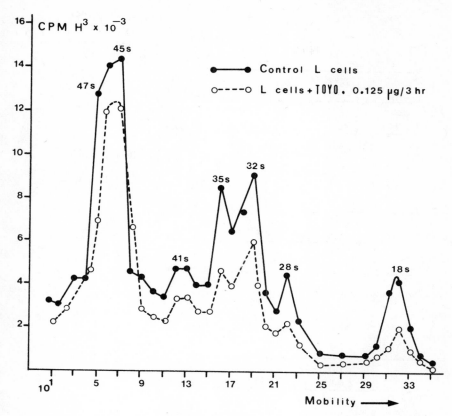

Fig. 5. Effect of toyocamycin on RNA synthesis in L cells. Two cell preparations, 8×10^6 cells, (one is previously treated with 0.125 µg of toyocamycin for 3 h) are labelled with 10 µCi/ ml of tritiated uridine for 1 h. The RNA of these two preparations is extracted and analyzed in polyacrylamide gels (1.7%, 180-200 V., 5 mA/gel, migration 5 h).

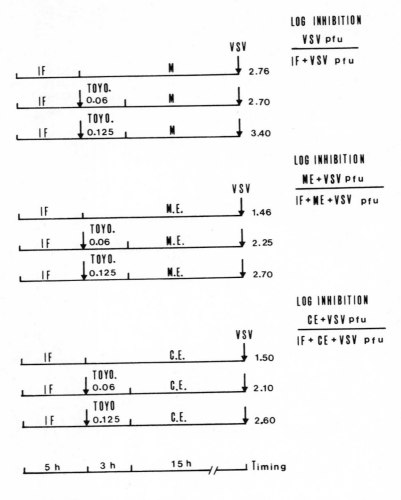

Fig. 6. Effect of toyocamycin on the: i) antiviral action of interferon; ii) antagonist action of tissue extracts.

DISCUSSION

Tan: In your last slide describing the inception of the
control protein for AVP, what if cycloheximide was added with
interferon and at the sixth hour adding in actinomycin D. Would
you not get a superinduction (in order of magnitude of 100-fold)
like the kind previously described in the regulation of interferon synthesis.

Fournier: I haven't been successful in getting a superinduction with cycloheximide because of its toxicity for VSV replication at the doses used (3 to 10 µg). Lab and Koerhen (Stras-
bourg), however, obtained in another cell system a potentializa-
tion of 10 to 20 times when adding cycloheximide 6 h after interferon. On the other hand, they obtained a decrease of the antiviral state when adding cycloheximide at the same time as interferon.

Tan: If you observe potentiation of AVP with cycloheximide
and actinomycin D or cycloheximide alone, then in the presence
cycloheximide there should be no AVP or at least very little of
it is made. Could it not be that something other than AVP perhaps interferon that is turning on control protein for AVP.

Fournier: I would like to insist on the fact that in the
experiments here presented, actinomycin or cycloheximide are added to cells 4 to 5 h after interferon, when the antiviral state
has already been well established. The participation of interferon itself in turning on control protein for AVP seems unlikely because of its removal after a 5-h induction period.

Came: Dr. Vilček has constructed a model describing the
blocking of a hypothetical inhibitor as being responsible for
superinduction. Are the kinetics of the blocking of his hypothe-

tical inhibitor consistent with actinomycin D or cycloheximide
blocking of the tissue antagonist you describe, or perhaps, consistent with the antagonist which Dr. Morahan described earlier
today?

Fournier: There could be a relationship between this
hypothetical inhibitor (proposed by Dr. Vilček) and the tissue
antagonist that we have isolated. Indeed, during a study on the
correlation between a refractory state and interferon synthesis,
it has been shown that tissue antagonists decrease the refractory state of primary induced cells and thus allow iterative
inductions.

Chany: Maybe I can give a partial explanation to your
question. If I understand you clearly, the problem is: Does the
antiviral state feedback on interferon induction and does this
fit with the model proposed by Dr. Vilček? Dr. Rousset in our
laboratory has shown that a tissue antagonist which decreases the
antiviral state induced by interferon decreases also the refractory state in normal and in hybrid cells to interferon induction. This is in favor of the hypothesis that at least partial
induction is dependent on the antiviral state.

Came: Is the analysis consistent?

Chany: Yes, it is.

Vilček: On that last model which you showed you postulated
that the tissue antagonist acts on ribosomal RNA synthesis; and
if I followed your reasoning correctly, the reason for this postulate is that toyocamycin inhibited the action of your tissue
antagonist. Is that correct?

Fournier: This hypothesis is not only based on indirect
arguments when using antimetabolites, but also on a direct study
of the effect of the tissue antagonist on cellular RNA synthesis.

Vilček: I would just like to point out that low doses of toyocamycin also increased interferon production stimulated with poly I:C in rabbit kidney cells. Although it is true that toyocamycin primarily inhibits the maturation of ribosomal RNA synthesis, some other species of RNA may also be inhibited, like some messenger RNAs . So I just don't know whether the conclusion that ribosomal RNA synthesis is the factor which mediates the action of a tissue antagonist is entirely valid on this basis.

Fournier: It is well known that actinomycin or toyocamycin act primarily on the transcription of ribosomal RNA, but it is possible that they act elsewhere, too.

Chany: I think Jan Vilček is right. It is always difficult to interpret results only based on the use of antimetabolites. The small doses of toyocamycin employed act primarily on ribosomal RNA and do not affect the antiviral state induced previously by interferon. However, toyocamycin could perhaps act somewhere else, too. But there is also direct evidence on increased ribosomal RNA synthesis, since T.A.I. in untreated cells increases by 30% the 45 S ribosomal RNA and subsequently all the other fractions. The mechanism of this increase is now under study.

Revel: Have you considered the possibility that the effect of T.A.I. on ribosomal RNA is really indirect and that it controls the rate of cell division since it takes 18 hours until you can see the effect. As soon as you change the rate of ribosomal RNA and ribosome synthesis in the cell, you are going to change all the parameters of growth. Have you considered then that the effect on interferon sensitivity would be due to this change in growth of cells?

Fournier: A treatment of cells by tissue antagonists for 18-20 hours doesn't seem to affect either the growth rate or the sensitivity of cells to interferon.

Grossberg: I must say that I am full of admiration for the beautiful results that you have. Dr. Sedmak in our laboratory has been trying for a year and a half to repeat the experiment showing the increased antiviral effect, using a whole range of doses of actinomycin D in the same fashion that you described to try to get an enhanced effect, but we have been unsuccessful, both in L cells, or in chicken embryo cells where actinomycin D dose-response curves **cover a** much lower range. Could you or anyone explain why only low doses of actinomycin D should be effective and why, if you work at the concentration range where you inhibit 80 to 95% inhibition or RNA synthesis, you do not see this effect?

Colby: Quite a good deal of evidence has come out within the last two or three years. I know of work done in Sheldon Penman's Lab at MIT that very high doses of actinomycin not only interact with the cell in a way to reduce RNA synthesis but also apparently directly affect the rate of initiation of protein synthesis. However, very low doses of actinomycin D, down around a tenth of a microgram per ml, appear to selectively inhibit ribosomal RNA synthesis and apparently do not affect the synthesis of messenger RNA nor noticeably affect the rate of initiation of protein synthesis.

Grossberg: Could you redefine that in terms of percentage of inhibition of RNA synthesis, that is, overall incorporation of uridine and not in terms of micrograms since the effective doses may vary with different cell cultures used?

Colby: Yes. Just the straight incorporation of tritiated uridine into acid insoluble RNA is not a very descriptive way to talk about RNA species since the gross majority of total RNA that is made in the cell is ribosomal. The heterogeneous nuclear RNA turn over very rapidly and so, just looking at percentage inhibition of acid precipitable counts really does not reflect the details of what's going on inside the cell. One can find 95% inhibition of total apparent RNA synthesis using very low and very high concentrations of actinomycin. But very different things are going on inside the cell. It simply reflects the differences in the way the cell processes its RNA.

Grossberg: The question I am raising does not only relate to the percentage. I am aware of the work you mention. I am really interested in what class of functions are inhibited in relation to the dose given in the particular cells being studied. I think it is not proper to attribute effects seen in one cell system with the same concentrations of actinomycin D used in another system unless your system is defined, both in terms of effect of synthetic activity and in terms of the species or sub-species of RNA inhibited or still functional. Why is this effect only seen at 30 to 50% inhibitory concentrations that were reported I think by Dr. Chany, rather than at other concentrations that are normally used if it is thought to be an effect only on ribosomal RNA?

Baron: If interferon induces both antiviral protein and a regulator of antiviral protein, then in a cell which has reacted with interferon subsequent addition of increased interferon concentrations should have a diminished effect as compared with cells previously unreacted with interferon. In our hands cells first reacting with small amounts of interferon, subsequently developed the same level of resistance to a high dose of interferon. We think this may argue against the idea of regulatory protein. Have you performed such experiments?

Chany: Similar experiments have been published by Dr. Besançon about a year ago (F. Besançon, M. Vignal, C. Chany, C.R.A. S. Paris, 1971, 273, 2694-2697). They are in disagreement with Sam Baron's observations, maybe because of the differences in the

time course of the experiments. When cells are treated with low
doses of interferon, a new dose, added 4 h later, increases the
antiviral state; however, the slope of the dose-response curve
changes and becomes more horizontal. These results do not argue
against the idea of a regulatory protein of the antiviral state.

Colby: I would like to re-emphasize Dr. Chany's point. I
believe it was Szent Giorgi who said that "only the uninhibited
draw their conclusions exclusively from studies with inhibitors".

EFFECT OF OUABAIN ON THE ACTION
AND PRODUCTION OF INTERFERON

P. Lebon and M.-C. Moreau

Institut National de la Santé et
de la Recherche Médicale
U. 43 de Recherches sur les Infections Virales
Hôpital de St.Vincent de Paul
74, Avenue Denfert-Rochereau, 75014 Paris,France

The antiviral action of interferon is indirect and is related to the synthesis of a protein responsible for the antiviral state. The existence of specific receptor sites on the cell
membrane has already been shown (1)(2). Interferon attaches to
these receptors and induces a series of events which lead to an
antiviral state. The aim of this present study is to determine
the role of the cell membrane ATPase in the interaction of interferon and its receptor sites. Ouabain inhibits mainly the function of this enzyme and is employed in our experiments.

The sensitivity of monkey BSC cells and mouse L cells to
different concentrations of ouabain has been previously tested
(3). When monkey BSC cells were treated with increasing amounts
of ouabain up to 0.1 µg/ml, the intracellular concentration of
Na^+ increased, while that of K^+ decreased. Under similar experimental conditions, mouse L cells were not affected (Table 1). It
can be concluded, therefore, that ouabain blocks the Na^+ K^+ dependent ATPase in monkey BSC cell membranes, but not in mouse L
cell membranes.

The action of ouabain on the antiviral effect of interferon
was studied in these two cell species. Monkey BSC cells were in-

cubated at 37° C simultaneously with human interferon and different concentrations of ouabain for 5 h. Ouabain was then removed
and minimum essential medium (MEM) was added to the cells for 18
h. The cells were then infected with vesicular stomatitis virus
(VSV) at a multiplicity of infection (m.o.i.) of 1 (Figure 1).
After one replicative cycle, the viral yield was measured by plaque titration. The antiviral activity of interferon was completely inhibited with 0.25 µg/ml of ouabain. Even amounts of ouabain
one hundred times higher did not change the activity of murine
interferon in L cells (3).

The effect of ouabain on the membrane Na^+ K^+ dependent
ATPase was reversed only with K^+ ions (4)(5). Increasing K^+ concentrations in the medium suppressed the anti-interferon activity of ouabain. This was observed for 40 Meq/l K^+ concentrations
(Figure 2). Maximal inhibitory action of ouabain was obtained
when interferon was assayed simultaneously with ouabain in monkey
BSC cells.

BSC cells were incubated for 7 h with interferon and ouabain was then added at selected time intervals. Ouabain had no
effect on the antiviral state 5 h after the addition of interferon (Figure 3).

The activity of ouabain was probably not the result of a
competition with interferon for the same cellular receptor. As
shown in Figure 4, BSC cells were incubated at 4°C for 5 h with
interferon and ouabain. Interferon and ouabain were then removed
and the cells incubated for 18 h with MEM at 37°C. Under these
conditions, ouabain did not block the antiviral activity of
interferon.

Even a possible indirect inhibitory effect of ouabain on
cellular protein synthesis could not explain its anti-interferon
properties. The antiviral effect of interferon was totally in-

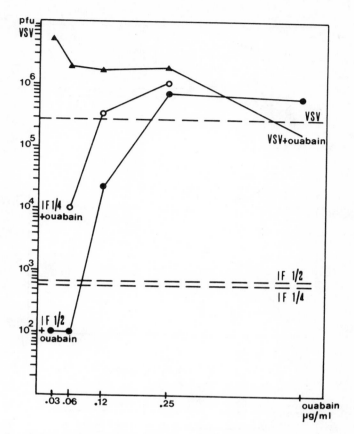

Fig. 1.   Effect of ouabain on the action of human interferon in BSC cells. IF=interferon; VSV=vesicular stomatitis virus; $IF^{1/2}$= 1000 units of interferon/ml.

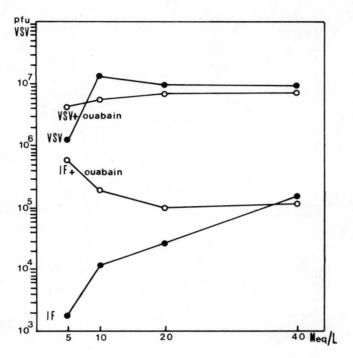

Fig. 2.   Effect of K-ion concentrations in the medium on the anti-interferon activity of ouabain.

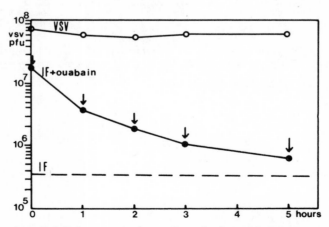

Fig. 3.   Inhibitory action of ouabain added between 1 and 5 h after interferon on the antiviral state.

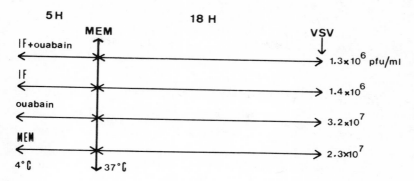

Fig. 4. Action of ouabain on human interferon in BSC cells at 4° C.

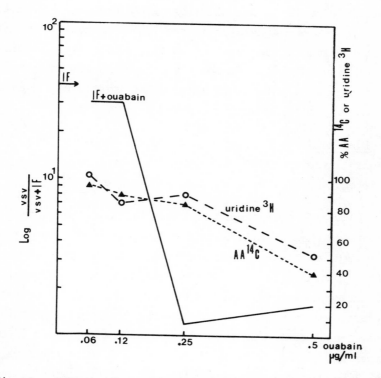

Fig. 5. Effect of ouabain on the action of interferon and on the incorporation of ^{14}C-amino acids and ^{3}H-uridine in the acido-insoluble fraction of BSC cells.

DISCUSSION

Dianzani: Do you know or does anybody here know, whether
ouabain can increase the level of cyclic AMP in the cells? In
fact we have obtained about the same results with adrenaline.

Lebon: We have not tried to measure cyclic AMP in the system. I don't think that the cyclic AMP system is related to the
action of interferon. The action of ouabain on interferon could
be explained either by the blocking of the membrane ATPase activity or by the decrease of an intracellular potassium concentration which might inhibit the activity of protein (s) responsible
for the antiviral state. Ouabain is only active on interferon
when it is in the presence of interferon. Interferon is not inhibited when the cells are pretreated with ouabain.

Dianzani: If I understood correctly, the contact of ouabain with interferon does not alter interferon as a molecule.
Then it must react with the cells. Am I correct?

Chany: I should like to comment briefly on the findings
of Dr. Lebon which relate to yesterday's discussion between Dr.
Stewart and Dr. Ankel. The findings on ouabain, together with
the fact that interferon covalently attached to sepharose is
still active, demonstrate analogies which might exist between
interferon and hormones. As known, ouabain affects the sodium-
potassium-dependent membrane ATPase. This analogy is an interesting approach to the study of the nature of interferon. Interferon, like hormones is a molecule which diffuses widely, acts
on membrane receptors, and is blocked by ouabain. The difference between interferon and hormones is that interferon is not
produced by specialized cells.

Tan: Do you think that the inhibition by ouabain might be due to a consequence of a secondary effect such as morphologic changes in the ouabain treated cells?

Lebon: Not at this concentration.

Oxman: The only reservation one might have is that a reduction in the cell's capacity to replicate VSV is a rather insensitive index of toxicity.

Chany: I think it is unlikely that an intoxicated cell produces viruses normally. For instance, actinomycin D, added at a toxic dose level, blocks the replication of VSV, too.

Oxman: Of course it is possible to damage a cell so that it cannot support the replication of VSV. However, we have observed many instances in which cellular RNA and protein synthesis have been markedly inhibited without any reduction in the cells capacity to replicate VSV. In fact it is quite easy to render cells incapable of responding to exogenous interferon without affecting their capacity to replicate VSV.

Chany: As a matter of fact, another argument against cell intoxication is that at the doses employed in control experiments, ouabain does not affect the production of interferon.

Ankel: Do you remember if in the case of insulin ouabain works at the same time only, or does it work afterwards?

Lebon: When ouabain is added after, it doesn't inhibit interferon.

Ankel: But with insulin?

Lebon: Insulin is blocked only when it is in the presence of ouabain.

Ankel: Because I think the analogy between insulin and
interferon is quite interesting, although it might not be real.
However, with many hormones people have found that cyclic AMP is
involved. I suppose many people have thought about this system
in the case of interferon. Recent work has shown that in the case
of insulin it is really the level of cyclic GMP which is raised.
So maybe that would be something to look at.

TISSUE ANTAGONISTS OF INTERFERON IN PRIMATE BRAIN

P. Brown[1,2], M. Sarragne[1], C. Chany[1],
C.J. Gibbs, Jr.[2] and D.C. Gajdusek[2]

During the course of investigations on slow virus infections of the central nervous system, we examined 25 specimens of
brain tissue - human, chimpanzee and monkey - infected by either
Kuru or Creutzfeldt-Jacob (C-J) disease, as well as 19 specimens
of normal, uninfected brain tissue, for the presence of an interferon antagonist.

Tissue specimens were obtained under sterile conditions at
autopsy and stored at -80° until extracted. After thawing, they
were ground in a mortar and pestle using sterile sand, diluted
to a 5 g per cent suspension in Eagle's medium containing penicillin and streptomycin, and magnetically stirred for 24 h at 4°.
The suspension was then centrifuged at 2000 rpm for 15 min, the
supernate removed and re-centrifuged at 27,000 rpm for 1 h. This
final clear supernate was aliquoted and stored in glass vials at
-80° until use.

Mouse interferon was induced in BALB/c cells (MSV-IA
strain) by infection with Newcastle disease virus (3). This stock
preparation contained 640 units of interferon per 0.5 ml, and
was diluted to contain 50 units per 0.5 ml for the tests.

---

[1] Institut National de la Santé et de la Recherche Médicale, U.43
de Recherches sur les Infections Virales, Hôpital St. Vincent
de Paul, 74, Avenue Denfert-Rochereau, 75014 Paris, France.

[2] National Institute of Neurological Disease and Stroke, National
Institutes of Health, Bethesda, Maryland, U.S.A.

The Indian strain of vesicular stomatitis virus (VSV) grown in L cells, and with a titer of 2×10^7 PFU/ml, was used to challenge L cells at a multiplicity of infection (m.o.i.)=0.1.

Tubes containing confluent L cells were incubated with interferon for 4 h. The medium was then replaced by brain extract dilution and incubated for 24 h. The extract was discarded and the cells challenged with VSV at a m.o.i. = 0.1. Cytopatic effect was read after 18 h (2 growth cycles) and the tubes frozen at -80°. Virus yields were determined by a routine plaque method, using a final 0.8% agarose-medium overlay on L cells in covered petri dishes. Cell, interferon, specimen extract and virus controls were included in all tests.

Several preliminary experiments defined optimal conditions for demonstration of interferon antagonist activity. Extracts that were centrifuged at 2000 rpm, but not 27,000 rpm before use, were frequently toxic for the tissue culture cells. Neither lyophilization nor several freeze-thaw cycles had any effect on their antagonist activity. In a range of 2-fold dilution steps from 4 to 0.25 g per cent, the higher concentrations consistently showed more activity than the lower concentrations, but the 4% concentration tended to be cytotoxic. Filtration of the ultracentrifuged specimens through a 100 mμ Millipore filter (through which kuru and C-J virus infectivity does not pass) had no effect on their activity.

Brain extracts from 41 animals were assayed for antagonist activity in a single test. Twenty-three of the animals had died of either kuru or C-J disease, and 18 were normal. In addition to chimpanzees, brain extracts from 6 species of old and new world monkeys were included (Rhesus, African Green, spider, squirrel, woolly and capuchin). The results are shown in Table 1. Antagonist activity of approximately 1/2 log was demonstrated in extracts from all groups, whether from infected or normal chimpanzees or monkeys.

An additional test was made using extracts from 3 human brains: one from a kuru patient, one from a C-J patient, and one from a normal person. These extracts showed antagonist activity of 0.96, 0.55 and 0.46 logs, respectively.

Since the amount of antagonist activity was similar in all brain extracts tested, an attempt was made to distinguish normal from infected extracts by their behavior in cells treated with the metabolic inhibitor, actinomycin D. In this experiment, L cell cultures were treated with varying doses of actinomycin D for a period of 1 h, following incubation of the cultures with interferon, and before addition of the brain extracts. The results are shown in Table 2. In the absence of actinomycin D, the brain extracts diminished interferon activity by about 0.7 logs. This antagonist effect was partly blocked by a dose of actinomycin D as low as 0.0625 µg/ml and was abolished by doses of 0.125 and 0.25 µg/ml. Both the infected and normal brain extracts behaved similarly under the influence of this metabolic inhibitor.

The results presented in this paper establish the presence in extracts of human, chimpanzee and monkey brain tissue of a substance which antagonizes the action of interferon on the replication of VSV in L cells. Although a systematic effort to characterize the substance has not yet been made, those biological properties already known suggest that it is similar to the tissue antagonist of interferon (TAI) previously demonstrated in extracts of human amniotic and chorionic membranes (4), embryonic egg allantoic fluid (5), and normal muscle and sarcoma tissue from hamsters (6), and humans (7). Thus, the increasing activity over a range of 0.125 to 4 g per cent of the extract concentrations, the activity against interferon of a different species than those from which the extracts were made, and the abolition of its activity by relatively low doses of actinomycin D are all comparable to that shown for TAI. This represents the first time such a substance has been identified in brain tissue.

Its biological similarity to TAI and the fact that it is present in comparable amounts in normal, kuru, and C-J disease brain tissue suggest that it is rather a normal tissue constituent than a consequence of "slow virus" infections. However, the experiments have so far been carried out using only crude extracts of brain tissue. Current investigations in this laboratory of interferon antagonists present in neonatal mouse muscle and mouse sarcoma tissue have shown that although the activity of crude extracts is similar, purification and fractionation of the extracts reveal a peak of activity in sarcomateous tissue that is not present in normal mouse muscle. These same techniques have not yet been used to search for a possible qualitative difference between the antagonist in normal and infected brain tissue.

Acknowledgements

This work was supported in part by a fellowship award (PB) from the National Multiple Sclerosis Society (USA).

References

1. Katz, M. and Koprowski, H.(1968). Nature 219:639.
2. Baron, S., Gibbs, Jr., C.J. and Gajdusek, D.C. (unpublished observations).
3. Chany, C. and Vignal, M. (1968). C.R. Acad. Sci.(Paris) 267:1798.
4. Fournier, F., Rousset, S. and Chany, C. (1969). Proc. Soc. Exp. Biol. Med. 132:943.

5. Chany, C., Galliot, B., Renard, N. and Moreau, M.C. (1970). C.R. Acad. Sci. (Paris) 270:3000.

6. Chany, C., Grégoire, A. and Lemaître, J. (1969). C.R. Acad. Sci. (Paris) 269:1236.

7. Chany, C., Lemaître, J. and Grégoire, A. (1969). C.R. Acad. Sci. (Paris) 269:2628.

TABLE 1

	Number in group	Reduction of $\log_{10}$ inhibition (mean)
C-J Chimpanzees	8	0.60
Kuru Chimpanzees	7	0.60
Normal Chimpanzees	7	0.46
C-J Monkeys	2	0.41
Kuru Monkeys	6	0.52
Normal Monkeys	11	0.54
All C-J and Kuru Animals	23	0.56
All Normal Animals	18	0.51

Comparison of interferon-antagonist activity in brain extracts from 41 normal and kuru or C-J disease infected animals. Results are expressed as the reduction in the inhibition by interferon of VSV replication in L cells (interferon alone inhibited viral yield by 3.49 logs). Details of the experimental protocol are found in the text.

TABLE 2

	Actinomycin D (µg/ml)			
	0	0.0625	0.125	0.25
Interferon Alone	1.88	2.31	2.17	2.25
Interferon + Normal Brain	1.25	2.01	2.17	2.13
Interferon + C-J Brain	1.13	2.05	1.98	2.29

Comparison of anti-interferon activity in brain extracts of a normal and a C-J infected chimpanzee, in L cell cultures treated with varying doses of actinomycin D. The figures represent $\log_{10}$ inhibition of VSV replication. Details of the experimental protocol are found in the text.

IV - INTERACTIONS WITH THE IMMUNE SYSTEM

SUPPRESSION OF ANTIBODY PRODUCING SPLEEN CELLS IN MICE BY VARIOUS INTERFERON PREAPRATIONS VERSUS ENHANCEMENT BY DOUBLE-STRANDED RNA[*]

T. C. Merigan, T. J. Chester
Division of Infectious Diseases
Department of Medicine, Stanford University
School of Medicine, Stanford California 94305

and

K. Paucker
Department of Microbiology
Medical College of Pennsylvania
Philadelphia, Pennsylvania 19129

The relationship of interferon to immunity has received more and more attention in recent years. Interferon has been identified both as a product of immunocompetent cells and as a naturally occurring material which can inhibit or influence lymphocyte function, particularly T-lymphocytes.

Our laboratory has recently completed a study which strengthens this association. We were not expecting or planning for such results; instead, we were aiming to investigate the mechanism by which synthetic, double-stranded RNA Poly(rI). Poly(rC) injections achieved its adjuvant effect on antibody production. Because of improvements in our facilities and methods for production of mouse interferon in tissue culture, we are able to simulate serum levels of interferon produced by doses of poly (rI).poly(rC) with exogenous interferon. When this dosage regimen of interferon was given to mice 2 days prior to antigen (sheep red blood cells), we were quite surprised to find significant inhibition of antibody forming spleen cells as measured in vitro

_____

[*] Supported by a grant from the U.S. Public Health Service (AI-05629).

at 6 days after primary immunization. This sharply contrasted
with the 200% increase in such cells seen in animals who were
given 100 μg of poly (rI).poly (rC) when studied at the same time
after immunization (and after circulating interferon).

Since that time we have put our effort into defining the
dosage optimum for this effect and verifying that the interferon
in our interferon preparations appeared to underlie the effect.
These studies are reported in detail elsewhere (1). The extent
of the inhibitory effect required increased with increasing dosage of interferon (over 100,000 units). It was noted with a wide
variety of interferon preparations produced by Newcastle disease
virus stimulation, including mouse serum and tissue culture
(L929 and C243-3C) preparations. Most significantly, it was observed with an L cell interferon preparation which was purified
with anti-interferon antibody to a purity of 1.96×10^8 units/mg
protein. A number of control preparations were inactive, including normal mouse serum, uninfected tissue culture supernatant,
human leukocyte interferon and trypsin or heat (56°C) inactivated
mouse interferon. These findings all supported the basic observation that mouse interferon at this dosage and time prior to antigen administration has an immunosuppressive effect on humoral immunity.

The mechanism of this immunosuppressive effect remains to
be clarified. It is tempting to speculate that these results are
related to the observation of Gresser and associates that interferon will inhibit DNA synthesis in mouse lymphocyte preparations
stimulated by phytohemagglutinin (2) and inhibit proliferation
of transferred spleen cells as well as the ability of these transferred lymphocytes to become sensitized to host alloantigens as
assayed by an in vitro cytotoxic assay system (3). It is likely
with this antigen at this time of spleen cell assay we are studying primarily an IgM response which is B-lymphocyte mediated.

Hence, an effect could either be on macrophages involved in antigen trapping or on the B-lymphocyte itself.

Our results may form grounds for concern with regard to the
use of interferon preparations in the treatment of viral infections in humans. It should be noted, however, that circulating
interferon titers of the level required to produce these effects
are produced transiently during a variety of systemic viral infections in the mouse. Also, concerning the possible clinical
usefulness of exogenous interferon, it is important to compare
the doses which we find to inhibit antibody producing cells in
the spleen with that required to prevent various viral infections.
The immunosuppressive doses are approximately 10 to 100-fold
greater than that required to prevent a lethal cytocidal virus
infection (4) or virus induced neoplasm (5) in the same species.

Others (6) have reported variable (inhibitory or stimulatory) effects of in vivo administration of interferon on antibody
formation by murine spleen cells. The inhibitory effect in these
studies were observed at considerable lower interferon dosage,
and it is not clear whether their observations are related to
ours. However, we have studied viral humoral immunity in 12 patients given large doses of interferon during acute viral infection and have noted no immunosuppression (7). These individuals
had serum interferon titers up to 1500 units without any evidence
of a delay in antibody kinetics. However, only further observations will tell whether this sort of immunosuppression might be
a limit to interferon clinical utilization.

Summary

The pattern of i.v. injections and the dosage of mouse
interferon was determined which produces serum interferon levels
in mice similar to those following a 100 µg injection of poly(rI).
poly(rC). This was 120,000 units divided into 4 doses and given

over 4 hours. The Jerne plaque assay was employed to measure the number of cells in the spleen of mice producing antibody to sheep red blood cells 6 days after primary antigenic stimulation. In contrast to the immune enhancement observed consistently with prior administration of double-stranded RNA, a significant (p=<.001) immunodepression was observed following 120,000 units of mouse interferon made in L929 cells. The same immunodepressent effect was observed on administration of equivalent doses of C243-3C cell interferon, mouse serum interferon and L cell interferon purified by affinity chromatography using anti-mouse interferon antibody to a purity of 1.96×10^8 units/mg protein. However, this splenic response could not be influenced by prior administration of various appropriately prepared "mock" interferon or trypsin or heat (56°C) inactivated interferons.

References

1. Chester, T.J., Paucker, K. and Merigan, T.C. (1973). Nature 246:92.

2. Lindahl, P., Leary, P. and Gresser, I. (1972). Nature New Biol. 237:120.

3. Cerottini, J.C., Brunner, K.T., Lindahl, P. and Gresser, I. (1973). Nature New Biol. 242:152.

4. De Clercq, E., Nuwer, M.R. and Merigan, T.C. (1970). J. Clin. Invest. 49:1565.

5. De Clercq, E. and De Somer, P. (1971). J. Nat. Cancer Inst. 6:1345.

6. Braun, W. and Levy, H.B. (1972). Proc. Soc. Exptl. Biol. Med. 141:769.

7. Jordan, G.W., Fried, R.P. and Merigan, T.C. (1973). Submitted for publication.

DISCUSSION

Lindahl: I would like to comment on Dr. Merigan's talk by saying a few words about our own studies on antibody synthesis and the effect of interferon. This work was done in collaboration with Dr. Roland Gisler in Basel utilizing "three cell mosaic cultures" with purified mouse macrophage, T or B cells in an in vitro system with sheep red blood cells as an antigen. By pre-treating with interferon or by addition of interferon within 40 hours after administration of the antigen to such cultures, you'll get a virtually total suppression of the antibody synthesis. When pre-treating the individual cell populations, we found that the effect was exclusively on the B lymphocytes, whereas pre-treatment of either the T cells or the macrophages had no effect whatsoever on the antibody response. This would thus confirm your results and indicates, because of the time period, that it may be due to an effect on cell division. On the other hand, when utilizing "three cell mosaic cultures" in a certain number of experiments you will get "low responder" cultures, giving only about 20% of the response of "high responder" cultures. When pre-treating the individual cell populations of such "low responder" cultures, low doses of interferon will act on the B lymphocytes to restore the antibody response back to normal levels; that is, you will actually get an enhancement over the response of the interferon control, whereas with higher doses of interferon again you can see a suppression of the response. We would, therefore, caution that the effect of interferon on the immune response may not be that of a simple immune depression, but depending on a variety of factors, perhaps especially the individual responsiveness of the host, you may find either depression or enhancement. This might explain why, in your patients that may be already immuno depressed, you may have seen the enhancing part of the response.

Merigan: There are the suppressor T cells as well, I
guess. One has to consider that an enhancement could be affected
by killing or inhibiting a suppressor T cell.

Levy: Your results, Dr. Lindahl, sound quite like the ones
that Dr. Braun and I reported. I would just be curious to know
how low did you use your interferon levels when you got enhancement? We really had to go quite low to get enhancement. Just a
few units per mouse gave us enhancement.

Lindahl: I think it may be hard to compare as our study
was done in vitro, but the order is 10 units of interferon per
ml with about 10 million lymphocytes per ml.

Paucker: May I recall at this time a study we published
a number of years ago on the treatment of mouse spleen cells
with interferon preparations. We did indeed notice that the number of antibody-producing spleen cells was increased when non-
purified, crude interferon preparations were used for pre-treatment. However, this effect was abolished when the cells were exposed to partially purified interferon. Because of this finding,
I would like to ask Dr. Lindahl about the quality of interferon
she has used in her studies.

Lindahl: We have used several different semi or purified
preparations, among them your early materials. We have also used
purified material from Dr. Tovey.

Tovey: Yes, this has a specific activity of about 10^7
units per mg.

Vilček: Just to add to the complexity of the picture, I
would like to mention briefly some experiments we have performed
recently with Drs. Thorbecke and Friedman-Kien at N.Y.U. In rabbits, giving up to 750,000 units of interferon daily did not inhibit the primary antibody response against sheep red blood

cells in vivo. In the secondary antibody response in cell cultures using lymph node cells from animals previously immunized with diphtheria toxoid, there was no inhibition and no stimulation of antibody response with doses up to 20,000 units per ml. However, the proliferative response, the stimulation of DNA synthesis by either antigen or by phytohemagglutinin, was partially suppressed by the same preparations of interferon. The conclusion was that possibly there may be a differential effect on B cell and T cell functions, but, more likely, it looked like those responses which require cell proliferation may be suppressed by interferon, and the responses where cell proliferation is not so limiting a factor may not be affected.

De Clercq: I'm wondering whether interferon given after the antigen would not stimulate instead of inhibit the antibody response in the system used by Dr. Merigan. It has been described with many other interferon inducers (e.g., endotoxin, poly I:C) that they have a two-sided effect on antibody production, depending on the time that they are administered. Interferon itself may also have a two-sided effect, depending on the time that is given in relation to the antigen.

Merigan: We are studying the kinetics in much more detail now as well as studying T independent antigens. This is most likely a T dependent antigen, that is, sheep red blood cell in the conventional mouse. But, we will study this response in much more detail in the future.

Morahan: What strain of mice were you using for this work? I noticed that you had in your abstract that you looked six days after antigen administration, which is somewhat late in most mouse strains for peak of antibody titer in the Jerne plaque system.

Merigan: Swiss, and we know it to be primarily an IgM response in the spleen at this time.

Morahan: And six days is your peak antibody response under these conditions?

Merigan: It's just before the peak. We are planning to look at the effect of interferon on the course of appearance of circulating antibodies as well, in the future.

SUPPRESSION OF LYMPHOCYTE STIMULATION IN MOUSE SPLEEN CELLS BY INTERFERON PREPARATIONS *

W.C. Wallen[1], J.H. Dean[2], C. Gauntt[3], D.O. Lucas[3]

Introduction

Interferon (IF) inducers have been found to suppress the development of viral induced or transplanted tumors in vivo (1, 2). The mechanism of this inhibitory effect has not yet been determined. Administration of exogeneous interferon has also been shown to inhibit in vivo tumor development (3,4). In addition, several interferon containing preparations have been shown to inhibit the replication of cells in vitro including normal primary cells (5), transformed cell lines (6) and leukemia cells (7,8). In addition, crude exogeneous interferon has been found to inhibit the mitogenic response of mouse lymphocytes to phytohemagglutinin (PHA) and the immune response to allogeneic cells (9). In a preliminary report, we have confirmed the finding that interferon inhibits the blastogenic response to general mitogens by mouse lymphocytes (10). In this study we have examined the

[1] Department of Virology & Cell Biology, Litton Bionetics, Inc. 5510 Nicholson Lane, Kensington, Maryland 20795.

[2] Department of Immunology, Litton Bionetics, Inc., 5510 Nicholson Lane, Kensington, Maryland 20795.

[3] Department of Microbiology, University of Arizona Medical Center, Tucson, Arizona

*This work was supported in part by grants RR05675 and AI00372 Contract NIH-NCI-G-70-2320 from the U.S. N.I.H.

effect of pretreatment of mouse spleen cells with interferon on
the mitogenic response to concanavalin A as well as spontaneous
mitogenesis.We have also examined the effect of several partially purified interferon preparations on the blastogenic response
of mouse spleen cells to selected B- and T-cell mitogens.

Materials and Methods

Mice: CD-1 mice were obtained from the Animal Resource
Department, University of Arizona Medical Center and used as a
source of spleen cells for these experiments.

Interferon Preparations: Mouse interferon was prepared
from culture fluids of MM virus or Reovirus infected L-cells.
After 24 hours of infection the crude culture fluids were concentrated 100 fold by vacuum dialysis and then placed on a
Sepharose - 4B column. The eluate was monitored for absorbance
at 280nm interferon activity and for virus (Reo or MM virus) by
plaque assay. The eluate containing the interferon activity was
treated at pH - 2 for 24 hours at $4^{o}C$. The interferon activity
was titrated by a 50% vesicular stomatitis virus (VSV) plaque
reduction assay on mouse L-cells, as previously described (1).
Control culture fluids from non-viral infected L-cells in which
MM virus or Reovirus was added after harvest were collected and
treated in parallel with the interferon containing culture fluids.
A mouse serum interferon standard supplied by the National Institutes of Health was also utilized in some experiments. It was
determined by our plaque reduction assay that 8 interferon units
(IFU) were equivalent to one IFU of the mouse serum standard
interferon.

The L-cell culture fluid interferon was found to be resist-
and to treatment at pH-2 for 24 hours at $4^{o}C$, trypsin sensitive,
heat sensitive ($60^{o}C$ - 1 hour), DN'ase and RN'ase resistant, and

non-sedimentable at 100,000 x g.

Lymphocyte Stimulation: CD-1 mouse spleen lymphocytes were cultured with several doses of interferon for various time periods prior to the addition of the optimum blastogenic doses of the mitogens, phytohemagglutinin-P (PHA, Difco Lab, Detroit, Michigan), Concanavalin A (Con A, Calbiochemicals, San Diego, Calif.), Pokeweed mitogen (PWM, Grand Island Biological Company, Grand Island, N.Y.) and E. coli lipopolysaccharide (LPS, Difco). The spleen cells were cultured in triplicate at 5×10^6 cells/ml with or without interferon and/or mitogens. Each culture was pulse labeled for 18 hours prior to termination with tritiated thymidine (^{3}H-TdR)/(6.7 Ci/mM New England Nuclear, Boston, Mass). The incorporation of ^{3}H-TdR into acid insoluble material was assessed after 48 hours of culture by a filter pad technique as previously described (1).

Results

Effect of Interferon Pretreatment on Mitogenesis. Mouse spleen cells were cultured in the presence of the general mitogen Con A (10 mg/ml), to initiate a blastogenic response. This dose of Con A consistently induced an 8 to 15 fold increase in incorporation of ^{3}H-TdR into acid insoluble material when compared to spleen cell cultures without Con A. Some of the spleen cell cultures were pretreated for various time periods with partially purified mouse L-cell interferon at concentrations ranging from 0.1 to 250 IFU prior to the addition of Con A. The results of a typical experiment are presented in Table 1.

Presentation of interferon and Con A simultaneously to the spleen cell cultures resulted in minimal inhibition of DNA synthesis. Significant inhibition under these conditions was seen only with concentration of 10 IFU or greater. Pretreatment of the spleen cell cultures with IF for six hours resulted in a

slight increase in the inhibitory effect. The greatest inhibition
of DNA synthesis was found if the spleen cells were treated with
IF for 24 hours prior to the addition of Con A. Significant inhibition of the Con A - induced mitogenic response occurred with
doses of 1 to 250 units of IF. The suppression in this case,
ranged from 16% to 79% of Con A treated cultures which did not
receive any IF. Control L-cell culture fluids obtained from non-
virus infected cultures which had been treated in parallel with
the IF containing preparations was not found to suppress the
mitogenic response to Con A at a protein concentration equivalent
to the 100 IFU dose after 24 hours of pretreatment.

Suppression of spontaneous mitogenesis. While investigating the suppressive effect of IF on the mitogen-induced response,
we also found that IF reduced the normal background rate of DNA
synthesis by mouse spleen cells. The suppressive effect on spontaneous mitogenesis presented in Table 2. The suppression was
most apparent with 100 units of IF and appeared to be dose-depend-
ent. Pre-treatment of the spleen cells with IF for 6 and 24 hours
enchanced the suppressive effect at 10 IFU's when compared with
0 hr. There was little enhancing effect with 100 IFU's since the
suppression which occurred at 0 hr. (38%) was as great as that
which occurred at 24 hr. (42%).

Suppression of the response to B-cell or T-cell mitogens.
Mouse lymphocytes have been classified into 2 broad classes, bone
marrow dependent lymphocytes (B-cells) and thymus derived lymphocytes (T-cells). We have conducted several experiments in an attempt to determine if the suppressive effect of the IF-containing
preparations was specific for the response by mouse spleen cells
to purported B-cell mitogens, such as PWM (12) or LPS (13) and
T-cell mitogens, such as PHA or Con A (14). The results from a
typical experiment are summarized in Table 3.

TABLE 1

Suppression of Concanavalin A (10µg/ml) induced
lymphocyte stimulation in mouse spleen cell
cultures by Interferon preparations

| Treatment | Time of Interferon Pretreatment | | | | | |
| | 0 hr | | 6 hr | | 24 hr | |
	$\overline{x}$CPM ($\pm$S.D.)[1]	% supp.[2]	$\overline{x}$CPM ($\pm$S.D.)	% supp.	$\overline{x}$CPM ($\pm$S.D.)	% supp.
None	5238(192)	-	5338(171)	-	5412(52)	-
L-cell culture fluid[3]	-	-	-	-	5497(392)	+2
0.1 IFU[4]	5112(44)	2	5084(134)	5	4941(263)	9
1 IFU	4660(158)	11	4543(150)	15*	4526(182)	16*
10 IFU	4140(57)	21*	3497(85)	34*	2941(74)	46*
100 IFU	4137(123)	21*	3212(295)	40*	1260(198)	77*
250 IFU	3847(316)	23*	3143(197)	41*	1114(171)	79*

[1] $\overline{x}$CPM = mean counts per minute of ^{3}H-TdR incorporation obtained from 4 replicate cultures Standard Deviation. Values represent $\overline{x}$CPM of stimulated cultures minus the $\overline{x}$CPM of IF treated, but non-mitogen-stimulated, cultures.

[2] % supp. = percent suppression of ^{3}H-TdR incorporation in IF-treated cultures compared to untreated control. Values were compared for significant suppression (*) by the students "t" test at the 95% confidence interval.

[3] An IF negative equivalent L-cell culture fluid concentrated to a similar protein content.

[4] IFU = Interferon units per ml final concentration in each culture. Tissue culture prepared IF was derived from Reovirus type 3 infected L cells. Eight IFU of this preparation, as determined by our assay, was equivalent to one unit of the NIH mouse serum IF standard.

WALLEN, DEAN, GAUNTT & LUCAS

TABLE 2

Inhibition of spontaneous mitogenesis of mouse
spleen cells by an Interferon preparation

	Time of Interferon Pretreatment					
Treatment	0 hr		6 hr		24 hr	
	$\overline{x}$CPM ($\pm$S.D.)[1]	% supp.[2]	$\overline{x}$CPM ($\pm$S.D.)	% supp.	$\overline{x}$CPM ($\pm$S.D.)	% supp.
0 IFU[4]	525(+39)	–	645(35)	–	640(32)	–
1 IFU	552(38)	+7	545(35)	8	572(83)	14
10 IFU	438(122)	8	470(131)	28*	510(89)	21*
100 IFU	328(128)	38*	368(122)	44*	375(137)	42*

Legends are the same as those in Table 1.

TABLE 3

Effect of Interferon preparations
on selected B and T cell mitogens

Mitogen	% Suppression of Mitogenic Response[1]
PHA (2 μg)	82% (p<.01)
Con A (5 μg)	73% (p<.01)
PWM (1:50 dilution of stock)	87% (p<.01)
LPS (50 μg)	98% (p<.01)

[1] Spleen cells were pretreated for 24 hours
with 100 units of Interferon (MM virus)
prior to the addition of each mitogen.
These were compared to the mitogenic response in untreated spleen cell cultures.

PROLONGATION OF ALLOGRAFT SURVIVAL IN MICE BY INTERFERON INDUCERS AND INTERFERON PREPARATIONS[(x)]

Edward De Maeyer, Larry E. Mobraaten[(xx)]
and Jaqueline De Maeyer-Guignard

Institut du Radium,Université de Paris-Sud
Campus d'Orsay, Bât.110, 91405-ORSAY(France)

Introduction

Viral diseases can be accompanied by a temporary impairment of cellular immune responses. This phenomenon was first reported in 1908, by Von Pirquet, who noticed a decreased skin reactivity to tuberculin antigen in patients with measles (1).
Since this report, an impairment of delayed type hypersensitivi-
ty in patients with viral infections has been observed many
times. Another example of an alteration of a cell-mediated immune response during virus infection is the prolongation of skin
allograft survival in mice infected with lactic dehydrogenase
virus (2). Since the common denominator of many virus infections is the appearance of interferon in the host, we believe
that the effect of interferon on cellular immune reactions
should be investigated. Moreover, nonviral agents that have been
reported to prolong allograft survival in the mouse, such as

(x) This study was aided by a grant from the Fondation pour la
     Recherche Médicale Française.

(xx) Fellow of the Lady Tata Memorial Trust.

phytohemagglutinin and concanavalin A, are also interferon inducers (3, 4). Furthermore, interferon has been shown to inhibit
the proliferative phase of the mixed lymphocyte reaction (5) and
many people believe that this reaction represents an in vitro
correlate of allograft rejection (6).

We are currently studying the effect of interferon and
interferon inducers on two forms of cell-mediated immune reactions in the mouse: picryl chloride induced delayed type hyper-
sensitivity and skin allograft rejection. The presentation at
this symposium deals only with some results obtained in the skin
graft system; most of the results have been published in more
detail elsewhere (7, 8).

Materials and Methods

Interferon inducers: The effect of three totally different types of interferon inducers was examined: a paramyxovirus
(NDV), a double-stranded RNA mycophage (statolon) and a low molecular weight aromatic compound (tilorone).

a) Newcastle disease virus, Kumarov strain which had a titer of 5 x 10^7 median egg infective dose (EID$_{50}$) was inoculated
i.v. into the retro-orbital sinus (0.2 ml per mouse). Plain chick
allantoic fluid obtained from 12 day old embryos was used as control preparations.

b) Statolon, kindly provided by Dr. J.W. Kleinschmidt,Lilly
Research Laboratories, was injected i.p., 0.2 ml per mouse of a
suspension containing 15 mg of statolon per ml in a 1% bicarbonate solution; control animals received only an i.p. inoculation
of the bicarbonate solution.

c) Tilorone hydrochloride, (received from Dr. G.D. Mayer,
The Wm. Merrell Co.) was dissolved in the drinking water (0.3 mg

per ml).

Interferon preparations: Two different preparations of interferon were used. Brain interferon was produced by the intracerebral inoculation of West Nile Virus into mice according to the method described by Finter and modified by Gresser (9).Tissue culture interferon was produced in monolayers of Swiss mouse embryo fibroblasts induced by NDV. The preparation was kept at pH 2 for one week, centrifuged at 6000 rpm for 30', neutralized and centrifuged again at the same speed. Both interferon preparations were inoculated subcutaneously under the dorsal skin, as multiple 0.5 ml injections, beginning on the day of grafting and ending on the second day after grafting. Control preparations were processed in exactly the same manner as the interferon preparations, with the omission of the virus inducer.

Skin grafting: was performed by the method of Bailey and Usama (10). Briefly, this consisted of placing orthotopic tail-skin grafts about 2 x 5 mm on the dorsal side of the tail. In all experiments summarized here each recipient received two replicate allografts in addition to an isograft, and in all cases allografts included strong H-2 differences. Grafts were observed daily, the particular treatment of the graft recipient unknown to the observer, except in the case of tilorone treatment. The time of graft rejection was considered to be the day in which 50% or more of the graft appeared necrotic, and the mean of the two allograft rejection times on each host was taken as the time of response for that particular recipient: mice were between 5-12 weeks of age at the time of grafting.

Mouse strains: All mice came originally from the colony of D.W. Bailey at the Jackson Laboratory, in Bar Harbor. At the time of experimentation, the different strains had been maintained in Orsay for 4 to 6 generations. For some experiments mice belonging to Bailey's recombinant inbred lines were used (11).

Interferon titrations: All interferon titers are expressed in units as measured by the VSV plaque reduction assay in L
cells.

Results

A - Effect of inducers

The results of 3 experiments, each one with a different inducer, are summarized in table 1. Delay of rejection time as a
result of the various treatments was about 2 days except in the
case of tilorone, which caused a delay of about 5 days. All differences, while not large, were statistically significant as determined by the non-parametric Mann-Whitney U-Test. These differences are comparable to those recorded in the literature for
other agents that are potential interferon inducers, such as
Concanavalin A (4), PHA (3) and Lactic dehydrogenase virus (2).

B - Effect of interferon preparations

The results obtained with agents that induce interferon
suggested that the administration of interferon preparations
might also have a graft prolonging effect. Table 2 summarizes two
experiments, one carried out with a preparation of crude tissue
culture interferon, the other with a preparation of brain interferon. In both experiments, interferon preparations were administered subcutaneously, 0.5 ml for inoculation, starting the day
of grafting, continuing the first day after the grafting and ending the second day after grafting. This timing was adopted because a timing experiment with NDV had shown that an inoculation
the first day after grafting was most efficient to obtain graft
prolongation (7).

C - Differential effect of NDV inoculation into If-1^l and If-1^h
congenic mice

The levels of circulating interferon induced in mice after
intravenous inoculation of NDV are under the influence of the
If-1 locus; two alleles have been described for this locus:If-1^l
determining low interferon production as found in BALB/c mice,
and If-1^h, determining high interferon production as found in
C57BL/6 mice (12). It has been found that three congenic lines
of mice, all of which carry the H-28^c allele derived from the
BALB/c genome on a C57BL/6 genetic background, carry different
alleles for the If-1 locus. Thus, B6-C H-28^c (HW 110) was found
to have If-1^h while B6-C H-28^c (HW 81) and B6-C H-28^c (HW 97)
carry the If-1^l allele from the BALB/c genome (13). As far as is
known then, these three lines are identical except for the alleles at the If-1 locus. If allograft prolongation is determined
by interferon and not due to some other factors such as viral
particles, one would predict that inoculation of these congenic
lines with the same amount of NDV should produce differential
results in term of allograft prolongation; the line (HW 110) carrying the allele for high interferon production should show a
more pronounced effect on allograft prolongation than the other
line. As shown in Figure 1, this is what we found.

Discussion

Three different interferon inducers and two different interferon preparations were found capable of delaying allograft
rejection across an H-2 barrier in the mouse. The effect was not
dramatic - the average prolongation was of the order of two days
- but it was statistically significant and reproducible (8). It
was furthermore obtained with a relatively small amount of interferon units; the interferon amounts employed in this study,
having a total activity of 28,000 to 40,000 units, would have

very little antiviral effect if tested against an EMC virus challenge (14). Since interferon inducers may have multiple effects
in the mouse, for example all three inducers used did decrease
peripheral lymphocyte numbers (7), and moreover since only crude
interferon preparation were used in the present study, we cannot
at this stage be absolutely certain that the effect observed was
actually due to interferon itself, although the results obtained
with NDV in the congenic high and low producer lines are in favor
of interferon. Experiments with affinity chromatography purified
interferon (15) are in progress and should give the decisive
answer to this question.

The inhibitory effect of interferon on cell-mediated immune
mechanisms, as suggested by the present results, could explain
the tumor enhancing effect observed by Gazdar and co-workers
after administration of interferon preparations to mice, just before inoculation of Murine sarcoma virus or of tumor cells (16).
Such an effect is not necessarily in contradiction with the antitumor effect that has been so well documented by the work of
Gresser's group (17); continuous interferon treatment would have
an antiproliferative effect on division and growth of tumor
cells themselves, while pretreatment could have a predominant
anti-proliferative effect on the initial phase of an immune response against the tumor cells, allowing an enhanced tumor
growth. Thus, the action of interferon could very well have different consequences depending upon which cells are actively dividing at the time of administration and their response to the
particular dose given; the route of administration furthermore
may also influence the different cell types that will have optimum contact with the product administered.

Graft rejection is mainly a T-lymphocyte function, and
there are other indications that interferon affects T and also
B-lymphocyte functions. The report of Merigan and co-workers at

this symposium concerning the diminished number of antibody producing spleen cells as a result of interferon treatment of mice before immunization with sheep red blood cells indicates that other aspects of the immune response may also be affected (18). This is further borne out by the finding that antibody titers against a multitude of viral antigens were found to go down in patients that were treated for prolonged periods with concentrated preparations of human leukocyte interferon (19).

The depressive effect of interferon on cell-mediated immunity merits further attention, not only to clarify the mechanism of its action on the immune response, but also for its potential application in clinical transplantation. Interferon therapy, unlike other currently used immunosuppressive agents, could protect against viral infection and tumor growth, while at the same time helping to prevent graft rejection.

References

1. Von Pirquet, C. (1908). Deutsch Med. Wschr. 34:1295.
2. Howard, R.J., Mergenhagen, S.E., Notkins, A.L. and Doughertly, S.F. (1969). Transpl. Proc. 1:586.
3. Rosenau, W., Habler, J. and Goldberg, M. (1972). Transplant. 13:624.
4. Markowitz, H., Person, D.A., Gitnick, G.L. and Ritts Jr., R.E. (1969). Science 163:476.
5. Lindahl-Magnusson, P., Leary, P. and Gresser, I.(1972). Nature New Biol. 237:120.
6. Bach, G. and Hirschhorn, K. (1964). Science 143:183.
7. Mobraaten, L.E., De Maeyer, E. and De Maeyer-Guignard, J. (1973). Transplant. 16:415.

8. De Maeyer, E., Mobraaten, L.E. and De Maeyer-Guignard, J. (1973). C. R. Acad. Sc. (Paris) Série D, 277:2101.

9. Gresser, I. and Bourali, C. (1970). J. Nat. Cancer Inst. 45:365.

10. Bailey, D.W. and Usama, B. (1960). Transpl. Bulletin 7:424.

11. Bailey, D.W. (1971). Transplant. 11:325.

12. De Maeyer, E. and De Maeyer-Guignard, J. (1969). J. of Virology 3:506.

13. De Maeyer, E., De Maeyer-Guignard, J. and Bailey, D.W. (1973). Abstr. 73rd Ann. Meeting Amer. Soc. Microbiol., p. 261.

14. Gresser, I., Bourali, C., Thomas, M.T. and Falcoff, E. (1968). Proc. Soc. Expt. Biol. Med. 127:491.

15. Sipe, J.D., De Maeyer-Guignard, J., Fauconnier, B. and De Maeyer, E. (1973). Proc. Nat. Acad. Sci. (USA) 70: 1037.

16. Gazdar, A.F., Sims, H., Spahn, J.P. and Baron, S.(1973). Nature New Biol. 245:77.

17. Gresser, I. (1972). Adv. Canc. Res. 16:97.

18. Chester, T.J., Paucker, K. and Merigan, T.C. (1973). Nature 246:92.

19. Strander, H., Cantell, K., Carlström, G. and Jakobsson, P.A. (1973). J. Natl. Cancer Inst. 51:733.

TABLE 1

Effect of different inducers on graft survival

Treatment	Host strain	Number of mice	Donor strain	Mean survival time ± SD (in days)		P
Newcastle disease virus[x]	CXBH	8	CXBE	13.7	1.75	
Control allantoic fluid	"	9	"	12.0	1.54	≤ 0.05
STATOLON[xx]	C57BL/6	7	BALB/c	12.1	1.17	
Control bi-carbonate solution	"	6	"	10.2	1.44	≤ 0.05
TILORONE[xxx]	BALB/c	6	C57BL/6	13.6	1.46	
Control drinking water	"	7	"	8.9	0.54	≤0.001

[x] 0.2 ml of undiluted virus were inoculated i.v. 8 hours prior to grafting

[xx] 3 mg per mouse were given i.p. on the day of and on the 2nd and 5th day after grafting

[xxx] Tilorone hydrochloride was added to the drinking water starting one day before grafting and was then present throughout the experiment.

TABLE 2

Effect of different interferon
preparations on graft survival

Treatment	Host strain	Number of mice	Donor strain	Mean survival time ± SD (in days)			P
Control brain extract	BALB/c	5	C57BL/6	9.7	±	1.03	≤0.05
Brain inter-feron[x]		5		11.1	±	1.24	
Control tissue culture fluid	BALB/c	5	C57BL/6	8.8	±	0.57	≤0.001
Tissue culture inter-feron[xx]		5		10.9	±	0.89	

[x] Total dose received: 40,000 units

[xx] Total dose received: 28,000 units

All preparations were administered subcutaneously, 0.5 ml per inoculation.

An experiment in which 23,000 units of rat tissue culture inter-feron were administered did not show any prolongation of graft survival.

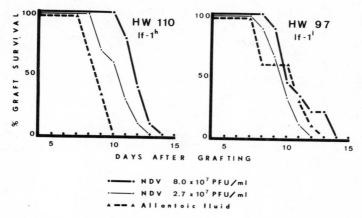

Fig. 1. Effect of NDV on allograft survival in high and low interferon producers. The figure shows the percent graft survival as a function of time in male If-1^l and If-1^h mice, after intravenous inoculation of NDV. One group received 0.2 ml of a preparation titering 8.0 x 10^7 PFU/ml, and a second group received one third of this amount. The control group was inoculated intravenously with 0.2 ml of plain allantoic fluid. All inoculations were carried out the day after grafting. The mice had received tailskin grafts from male BALB/c donors. Each group consisted of 5 mice, each mouse receiving two allografts and one isograft.

DISCUSSION

Epstein: Have you examined your interferon-treated grafts histologically at the time that the control grafts were being rejected and if so, what did you see?

De Maeyer: No, we have not examined them histologically, but it will be done.

Oxman: Was the number of circulating hymphocytes reduced in mice receiving the interferon preparations?

De Maeyer: It was, but only slightly.

Oxman: Was that also true in the one experiment in which the interferon preparation was ineffective?

De Maeyer: We didn't look there. We had two experiments where lymphocytes were down, but not so much down as with the inducers.

Levy: As you know, these compounds and poly I:C have had a reputation as being immune enhancers. Do you think that it is just a question of timing, that it is a biphasic thing?

De Maeyer: Well, I don't know. We did extensive timing experiments with NDV and we never saw enhancement of graft rejection. In other words, either it's prolongation or they reject at the same time as the controls. So I cannot say that we have ever seen enhancement of rejection. I know that it has been described for poly I:C and that's why we stayed away from it, because it seems more complicated than these compounds.

Grossberg: In the last experiment that you described where you had the low locus transfer in your back-cross mice, did you look at circulating lymphocytes? It seems to me that that would be the good experiment to do in order to differentiate the NDV suppressive, or lymphopenic, effect from the interferon effect on your allograft survival.

De Maeyer: I agree; I wonder why we didn't do it. We'll definitely do it.

FURTHER OBSERVATIONS ON THE MACROPHAGE-
ACTIVATING PROPERTY OF INTERFERON

Kun-Yen Huang and Robert M. Donahoe

The George Washington University Medical Center
Department of Microbiology
Washington, D.C. 20037

We have demonstrated previously, independently of Jahiel et al.(1), that interferon inducers suppress experimental mouse malaria (2). Attempts to elucidate the mechanism of suppression led to the finding that interferon-containing preparations are capable of enhancing the uptake of carbon particles by mouse peritoneal macrophages maintained in vitro (3). The enhancing factor exhibits characteristics that are indistinguishable from interferon (3, 4) and thus the authors concluded that the interferon molecule is capable of, among other things, enhancing the phagocytic activity of macrophages. This paper presents further observations made regarding such an effect of interferon preparations in vitro and in vivo.

Materials and Methods

Mice. Adult female NMRI Swiss mice weighing 20 to 22 g were used in in vivo experiments and to obtain peritoneal macrophages.

Interferon. Mouse interferons were induced either in vivo or in cultured cells. Serum interferons were induced by Newcastle disease virus (NDV). They were centrifuged for 90 min at 105,000 g, acid-treated for 5 days and stored at -70°C until used. The procedures for the induction of interferon in MSV-Ia cells have been described elsewhere (4). Controls for all these preparations consisted of serum or medium from animals or cell cultures which had undergone mock induction. All interferon preparations were assayed for antiviral activities as described previously (3).

Chemicals. Theophylline and cyclic adenosine 3', 5'-monophosphate (cyclic AMP) were purchased from P.L. Biochemicals Inc., Milwaukee, Wis.

Assay of phagocytic activities. Peritoneal macrophages were prepared and their phagocytic activities determined as described elsewhere (3). In experiments in which the effect of interferon on peritoneal macrophages in vivo was to be determined, interferon preparations were given either intraperitoneally or subcutaneously. At intervals, carbon (Günther Wagner, Germany) diluted in MEM was injected intraperitoneally into groups of mice. Thirty minutes later, peritoneal cells were harvested, maintained on coverslips in flat-bottom tubes for 2 hr to allow cells to attach firmly to the coverslips and then stained and evaluated for phagocytic activity (3).

Acid phosphatase determinations. Peritoneal macrophages were harvested as usual without prior stimulation. Cells were maintained in flat-bottom tubes with or without interferon for approximately 24 hr. They were washed with cacodylate buffer (pH 7.2) and then fixed at 4°C in 4% paraformaldehyde for 10 min. The cells were then incubated with the substrate(naphthol AS-MX phosphate, Sigma Chemical Co., St. Louis, Mo.) and fast blue for 20 min at 37°C and then counter-stained with methyl green.

Results

Demonstration of acid phosphatase. Acid phosphatase is an
enzyme considered to be mainly lysosomal in origin and thus
should be demonstrable in abundance in interferon-treated cells
if interferon is capable of activating macrophages. Peritoneal
macrophages incubated with either interferon prepared in MSV-Ia
cells or its control were therefore stained for acid phosphatase.
Interferon-treated cells contained a significantly larger amount
of acid phosphatase than did those treated with control specimens.
The enzyme response of macrophages was particularly conspicuous
after an overnight incubation of cells with 50 units/ml of interferon. In addition to the increased acid phosphatase reaction,
interferon-treated cells also showed a distinctive increase in
the number and size of vacuoles. Increased vacuolization was also
seen in peritoneal cells harvested from mice treated intraperitoneally with 160,000 units of interferon 65 hr before. These
cells also showed a greater tendency to attach and spread more
readily to glass surface than did cells from untreated mice.

In vivo effects of interferon on macrophages. Experiments
were also carried out to assess the effects of interferon or
interferon inducers on peritoneal macrophages in vivo. Peritoneal
macrophages were tested because in our original work the malarial
agent was introduced intraperitoneally. In one series of experiments, a total of 160,000 units of interferon which was prepared
in MSV-Ia cells and had been ultracentrifuged were given in two
intraperitoneal doses 30 min apart. In another series of experiments, a total of 240,000 units of the same interferon preparation was given in three equal doses, the first two intraperitoneally and the third subcutaneously at 30-min intervals. Seventy-
two hours after the last injection, 0.2 ml of carbon which was
diluted 1:2,000 in MEM was injected intraperitoneally and 30 min

later peritoneal cells were harvested and processed as described
in <u>Materials and Methods</u>. The results presented in Table 1 clearly show that, as in the <u>in vitro</u> experiments, the activity of
cells is significantly enhanced. Heating destroyed the enhancing
effects of interferon preparations while acid treatment and
ultracentrifugation had no effect.

When NDV was used in place of interferon preparations, the
results were quite different. Newcastle disease virus was injected intravenously into a group of mice. At intervals three mice
were sacrificed and peritoneal macrophages harvested, and the
phagocytic activity was evaluated as described. Control mice
received allantoic fluid instead of NDV. As shown in Fig. 1, the
phagocytic activity was clearly depressed in the first 20 hr.This
was followed by a secondary phase of enhancement which became
rather obvious only after 30 hr. Once the highest level was
reached, the level was more or less maintained for at least 66
hr. The peritoneal fluids harvested at intervals did contain measurable amounts of interferon. A short initial period of depression was also observed when an interferon preparation containing
residual NDV was used. However, ultracentrifuged interferon preparations induced no such depression.

<u>Preliminary</u> observations on the effect of cyclic AMP and
theophylline on the phagocytosis-enhancing effect of interferon.
The effects of cyclic AMP on both the antiviral activity of
interferon and phagocytes have been reported (5, 6). It is interesting therefore, to investigate the effect of this compound
on the phagocytosis-enhancing effect of interferon. Theophylline
was also used because it blocks the enzymatic degradation of
cyclic AMP by a phosphodiesterase and thus enhances an intracellular accumulation of cyclic AMP. In a series of preliminary experiments, macrophages were harvested as usual and then incubated
with culture medium, interferon, theophylline at 0.1 mM or cyclic

AMP at 0.1 mM or 0.001 mM, or a combination of any two of these, and then phagocytic activity was evaluated at 4 hr. The results are presented in Table 2. As has been shown previously (3),after a 4-hr incubation with interferon, no enhancement of phagocytosis was demonstrable. Both theophylline and cyclic AMP at 0.1 mM depressed phagocytic activity slightly. However, when either of these compounds was applied to cells in combination with interferon, significant enhancement was observed. Cyclic AMP at 0.0001 mM, either by itself or in combination with interferon, did not affect the phagocytic activity.

Discussion

The data concerning acid phosphatase and morphology provide histological evidence that supplement our previous observations that interferon enhances the phagocytic activity of mouse macrophages. Contradicting data still exist regarding the effect of interferon on the reticuloendothelial system in vivo (7, 8). The assessment of such an effect is difficult in vivo where factors affecting macrophage are far from being fully understood. The problem is further compounded when the determination of the interferon's effect is made with a pathogenic agent. Therefore, translation of in vitro data concerning interferon directly into an in vivo situation, as in any other biological phenomena, is difficult. Our present data clearly indicate that partially purified interferon preparations enhance the activity of mouse peritoneal macrophages in vivo. Newcastle disease virus or unprocessed interferon preparations are also capable of enhancing macrophages but only after an initial period of depression. The depression is clearly attributable to virus or components of virus because ultracentrifugation eliminates the depressive effect of unprocessed interferon. Such a depressive effect of NDV on macrophage activity may partly explain the enhancement of the mortality rate of certain experimental bacterial infections in mice (9) by NDV.

Some evidence is available which indicates that cyclic AMP may be a mediator of phagocytosis and the antiviral activity of interferon (5, 6). Our data obtained with cyclic AMP and theophylline are in line with these findings. Although our data are preliminary and no conclusion is possible at this stage, it is clear that studies in this direction are necessary to see if a unified explanation for all activities of interferon can be provided.

Acknowledgements

The excellent technical assistance of Mr. Ismail K. Al-Ghazzouli is gratefully acknowledged.

This study was supported in part by a grant from the Research Corporation, New York, N.Y., and by Public Health Service research grant USPHS 5-S01-RR-5359-12 from the Division of Research Facilities and Resources, National Institutes of Health.

References

1. Jahiel, R.I., Vilcek, J., Nussenzwig, R. and Vanderberg, J. (1968). Science $\underline{161}$:802-804.

2. Schultz, W.W., Huang, K. and Gordon, F.B. (1968). Nature (London) $\underline{220}$:709-710.

3. Huang, K., Donahoe, R.M., Gordon, F.B. and Dressler, H.R. (1971). Infect. Immun. $\underline{4}$:581-588.

4. Donahoe, R.M. and Huang, K. (1972). Infect. Immunity $\underline{7}$:501-503.

5. Friedman, R.M. and Pastan, I. (1969). Biochem. Biophys. Res. Comm. $\underline{36}$:735-740.

6. Weissman, G., Dukor, P. and Sessa, G. (1971). International Congress Series 229:107-120.

7. Remington, J.S. and Merigan, T.C. (1970). Nature (London) 226:361-363.

8. Herman, R. and Baron, S. (1970). Nature (London) 226: 168-170.

9. Hugh, R., Huang, K. and Elliott, T.B. (1971). Infect. Immunity 3:488-493.

TABLE 1

The effect of intraperitoneal interferon on phagocytic
activity of peritoneal macrophages

Exp. No.	Sample injected	Phagocytic activity[a] (%)			Mean (%)
1	interferon[b]	32,	48,		40
	control	13,	18,		16
2	Interferon[c]	37,	46,		42
	control	11,	6,	13,	10

[a] Determined 72 hr after injection of the last dose of interferon.

[b] 240,000 units in three equal doses delivered in 0.5 ml; the first two intraperitoneal and the third subcutaneous, 30 min apart.

[c] 160,000 units in two equal doses delivered in 0.5 ml; both intraperitoneal, 30 min apart.

TABLE 2

The effect of theophylline, cyclic AMP
and interferon on phagocytosis

Sample	Phagocytic activity[a] (%)	Mean (%)
EMEM	18, 23, 25	22
Theophylline (0.1 mM)	8, 6, 1	5
cAMP (0.1 mM)	12, 12, 9	11
cAMP (0.0001 mM)	17, 24, 22	21
Theophylline (0.1 mM) + interferon	46, 52, 55	51
cAMP (0.1 mM) + interferon	60, 54, 45	53
cAMP (0.0001 mM) + interferon	13, 22, 25	20
Interferon	25, 16, 19	20

[a] Activity determined after 4 hr of incubation.

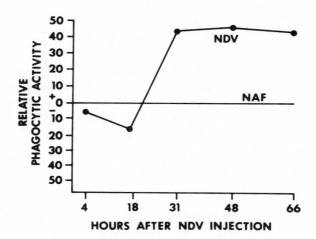

Fig. 1.   Kinetics of the phagocytic response <u>in vivo</u> after injection of NDV. NDV was given intravenously and the activity of peritoneal macrophages determined. Mice received normal allantoic fluid (NAF) served as the control.

their size and fluorescence (9,10). Thus, by virtue of the fact
that human B or bone marrow derived lymphocytes bear detectable
quantities of immunoglobulin on their surface, and that T or
thymic derived lymphocytes do not, the two populations of cells
can be separated by the FACS after their treatment with fluoresceinated anti-immunoglobulin reagents. Such fluoresceinated
reagents will label the B lymphocytes, and not the T.

Detailed description of the mechanical and electronic design of the FACS (9,10) and the tissue culture techniques employed in these studies have been described previously (7,8).
Briefly, however, human macrophage cultures were prepared from
leukocyte rich plasma by the growth and differentiation of monocytes in Leighton tubes. Several days later pure preparations of
lymphocytes from the same donor were obtained by their passage
through a nylon fiber column or from a Ficoll gradient. Erythrocytes which accompanied the lymphocytes off the nylon fiber column were lysed by an exposure to NH_4Cl. Monocytes which accompanied the lymphocytes from the Ficoll gradient were removed
by adsorption to glass. The lymphocytes were then sent to Stanford Medical School where they were treated with fluoresceinated
anti-Cohn fraction II, washed and passed through the FACS. The
cells were forced under pressure through a micronozzle into the
center of a stream of fluid which was illuminated by two lasers.
One, a helium neon laser, produces a signal which is proportional to the volume of the cell being illuminated, while the other,
an argon ion unit, produces a signal by the activation of the
fluorescent label on those cells which bear it. The cell stream
was vibrated to break it into 40,000 droplets per second. Those
droplets containing labelled cells of the proper size were giv-
en a positive electric charge and deflected into a collection
vessel. Those droplets containing no labelled cells were given
a negative charge and deflected into another collection vessel.

Empty droplets or those containing cells not of the proper size
remained unchanged and passed into the center container. Thus,
it was possible to adjust the instrument so that those cells
which contained $>10^5$ immunoglobulin molecules or B lymphocytes
would be collected in one container, and those containing <5 x
10^3 immunoglobulin molecules per cell or T lymphocytes would be
collected in another. Evidence that such immunoglobulin bearing
cells separate by the instrument were indeed B cells was provided
by previous experiments of Kreth and Herzenberg (11). They demonstrated that such cells developed into mature plasmacytes
with demonstrable intracytoplasmic immunoglobulin after prolonged
culture with PWM. Furthermore, in parallel studies, Bobrove et
al (12) demonstrated that such immunoglobulin-bearing cells
were unaffected by an anti-human T lymphocyte serum in the presence of complement. By contrast, those cells containing <5 x
10^3 immunoglobulin molecules were proven to be T cells, as they
were killed by the anti-human T lymphocyte serum in the presence
of complement.

The purity of T cell preparations was always greater than
99.9% and that of B cells 70-95% with a mean of 83%. The separated T and B cells were then returned to our laboratory in San
Francisco where they were placed on cultures either with or
without macrophages, PHA, or pokeweed mitogen (PWM). After an
incubation period of 3, 5, or 7 days, the cultures were pulse
labeled with ^{3}H-thymidine and harvested. The supernatants were
assayed for interferon by a viral plaque reduction method which
employs confluent monolayers of human foreskin fibroblasts and
bovine vesicular stomatitis virus. The cell pellet was studied
for the incorporation of ^{3}H-thymidine into DNA, as a measure of
lymphocyte proliferation.

The results were as follows: Figure 1 depicts the interferon response of T and B lymphocytes in the presence of macrophages in response to PWM after 3, 5, and 7 days of incubation. At 3 days there is a good T cell response, but no B response. The T cell response continues as the cultures are prolonged. Of interest was the observation that B cells can also produce interferon, but that the response is delayed as compared with T cells. The response observed at 5 and 7 days in the B cell-macrophage cultures was most definitely due to the B cells, and not due to the small contaminant of T cells which were present. Far too much interferon was produced than could be accounted for by that small number of T cells.

Similar observations were made when PHA was used as the mitogenic stimulus (Fig. 2). A good T cell interferon response was observed at 3 days and it reached its peak at 5 days.

Here again the B cell response was delayed to 5 and 7 days. In 7 additional experiments T cells in the presence of macrophages always produced interferon in response to either PHA or PWM at 3 days, whereas B cells did not. The same was true in most instances for the proliferative response, which followed the same pattern.

Then we performed a series of experiments to determine whether B cells could be induced to produce interferon at 3 days. First we tried increasing the concentration of B cells in combined B lymphocyte-macrophage cultures. Increasing the concentration of T cells in the presence of a fixed number of macrophages always resulted in increasing amounts of interferon, whereas increasing the concentration of B cells did not. Experiments were performed to determine if T cells or T cell products could stimulate interferon production by B cells in the presence of mitogens. In 3 experiments, varying amounts of T cells were added to cultures of B cells in the presence of macrophages and either PHA or PWM, and harvested 3 days later. The interferon titers observed in such cultures were never higher than would be expected from the number of T cells added to the cultures. Similarly, in 3 experiments in which 24-hour supernatants from cultures containing T lymphocytes, macrophages, and PHA or PWM or no stimulant were added to cultures of B cells with macrophages, no interferon was detected 3 days after the addition of the supernatants.

Finally, in some experiments most of the fluoresceinated anti-Cohn fraction II label was removed from the B cells by maintaining them in culture for 24 hours to induce capping and then by thorough washing of the cells. Subsequent stimulation of such thoroughly washed B cells with PHA or PWM in the presence of macrophages still did not result in the production of interferon after 3 days.

The proliferative response paralleled that of the interferon response at 3 days, i.e., a good proliferative response was noted in the combined T lymphocyte-macrophage cultures prepared with either PHA or PWM, but not in the B lymphocyte-macrophage cultures.

In summary, using highly purified T lymphocyte and enriched B lymphocyte preparations obtained by separation on the FACS, we demonstrated that both human T and B lymphocytes can respond to PHA and PWM in vitro in the presence of macrophages with proliferation and the production of interferon. However, selective T cell interferon production and proliferative response can be assessed at 3 days in culture; B cell interferon production and proliferative response is delayed to 5 and 7 days. T cells or T cell products are ineffective in inducing or accelerating B cell interferon or proliferative response at 3 days.

These studies are of importance for investigations of
patients with various immunological defects. Although T lymphocytes can be enumerated by several techniques, i.e. rosette-
forming ability (13), or lack of surface bound immunoglobulin,
the means by which their functional competence has been assessed
in vitro has been limited to their proliferative response to
various mitogens. The present studies demonstrate an additional,
new way by which T cell competence and effector function can be
evaluated - by the study of the 3 day interferon response to
PHA and PWM. Such studies could be of use in the detection, diagnosis, classification and further understanding of various
immunodeficiency states, and in other diseases in which abnormalities of T cell function are suspected.

It was for this reason, then, that we studied 11 patients
with various types of immunodeficiency in collaboration with
Dr. Arthur Ammann. We measured the amount of interferon produced
in three day cultures containing the patients' lymphocytes, macrophages, and either PHA or PWM, as an index of the competence
of T lymphocyte effector function (14). We found that 3 of 4
patients with selective IgA deficiency had depressed T cell interferon. In addition, another patient with selective IgA deficiency as well as thymic hypoplasia also showed a depressed
response. Similar studies were performed in collaboration with
Dr. Martin Cline on patients with chronic lymphocytic leukemia
and there also, T cell interferon measured at 3 days was depressed as compared with normals, and hence T cell effector
function was abnormal (15).

Thus, the ability of T lymphocytes to produce interferon
at 3 days was used as a measure of T lymphocyte competence, just
as antibody production is often studied to assess B lymphocyte
competence. The new technique does not require separation and

isolation of the T cells by the complex, unique and expensive
FACS, as highly purified preparations of human T cells can be
obtained by their passage through nylon fiber columns (8).

    Interferon is now well established as a mediator of cel-
lular immunity. It occurs after stimulation of lymphocytes with
mitogens (1,2,7,8,16-18), antilymphocyte sera (19), bacterial
(3,4,20,21) and viral antigens (5,6), and allogeneic lymphocytes (22). Such in vitro studies as we have reported herein
have particular relevance to events that occur in vivo, as, in
contradistinction to the other mediators of cellular immunity,
interferon has been demonstrated to occur in vivo in response
to the mitogen PHA (23) and to a specific bacterial antigen (24).
However, there are still numerous questions about interferon
produced in response to mitogen and antigen that remain to be
answered and pose quite a challenge for the future:

    1) What is the mechanism of induction of mitogen and/or
antigen stimulated interferon by lymphocytes?
    2) How does the macrophage or its membrane function to
augment production of mitogen or antigen stimulated interferon
by the lymphocyte?
    3) How broad is the spectrum of antiviral protection af-
forded by interferon produced in response to mitogen or antigen
- i.e. what cells are protected against which challenge viruses?
    4) Does interferon produced in response to mitogen or an-
tigen have effects on cell division, hematopoietic colony forming units, or the immune response, similar to that observed with
interferon induced by viruses and polynucleotides?

Acknowledgements

Many thanks to Virginia Hill and Miriam Debby for excellent technical assistance.

This work was supported by USPHS Grants CA11067 and by the Damon Runyon Memorial Fund, Grant DRG1205.

References

1. Epstein, L.B., Cline, M.J. and Merigan, T.C. (1970). In: Proc. 5th Leukocyte Culture Conference, J.E. Harris, editor. New York, Academic Press, p. 501.

2. Epstein, L.B., Cline, M.J. and Merigan, T.C. (1971). J. Clin. Invest. 50, 744.

3. Epstein, L.B., Cline, M.J. and Merigan, T.C. (1971). Cell. Immunol. 2, 602.

4. Epstein, L.B., Cline, M.J. and Merigan, T.C. (1971). In: Proc. 6th Leukocyte Culture Conference. R. Schwarz editor. New York, Academic Press, p. 265.

5. Epstein, L.B., Stevens, D.A. and Merigan, T.C. (1972). Proc.Nat.Acad.Sci.(USA) 69, 2632.

6. Merigan, T.C., Stevens, D.A., Rasmussen, L.E. and Epstein, L.B. (1973). In: A reexamination of non-specific resistance to infection. W. Braun and J. Ungar, editors. Basel, Karger, p. 41.

7. Epstein, L.B., Kreth, H.W. and Herzenberg, L.A. (1973) In: Proc. 8th Leukocyte Culture Conference. K. Lindall-Kiessling, editor, in press.

8. Epstein, L.B., Kreth, H.W. and Herzenberg, L.A.(1973). submitted for publication.

9. Bonner, W.A., Hulett, H.R., Sweet, R.G. and Herzenberg, L.A. (1972). Rev.Scient.Instr. 43, 404.

10. Hulett, H.R., Bonner, W.A.,Sweet, R.G. and Herzenberg, L.A. (1973). Clin.Chem. 19, 73.

11. Kreth, H.W. and Herzenberg, L.A. (1973).Submitted for publication.

12. Bobrove, A., Strober, S., Herzenberg, L.A. and De Pamphilis, J.D. (1973). J. Immunol. in press.

13. Wybran, J. and Fudenberg, H.H. (1973). New Engl.J.Med. 288, 1072.

14. Epstein, L.B. and Ammann, A.J. (1974). J.Immunol. in press.

15. Epstein, L.B. and Cline, M.J.(1974).Clin.Exp.Immunol. in press.

16. Wheelock, E.F.(1965). Science 149, 310.

17. Friedman, R.M. and Cooper, H.L.(1967).Proc.Soc.Exp. Biol.Med. 125, 901.

18. Wallen, W.C., Dean, J.H. and Lucas, D.O.(1973). Cell. Immunol. 6, 110.

19. Falcoff, R., Oriol, R. and Iscaki, S.(1972). Eur. J. Immunol. 2, 476.

20. Green, J.A., Cooperband, S.R. and Kibrick, S.(1969). Science 164, 1415.

21. Milstone, L.M. and Waksman, B.H.(1970).J.Immunol. 105, 1068.

22. Gifford, G.E., Tibor, A. and Peavy, D.L.(1971).Infect. Immunity 3, 164.

23. Epstein, L.B. and Merigan, T.C. unpublished results.

24. Stinebring, W.R. and Absher, P.M.(1970).Ann. N.Y.Acad. Sci. 173, 714.

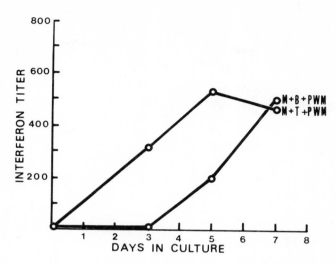

Fig. 1. Interferon production by human T or B lymphocytes in the presence of macrophages in response to PWM at 3,5 and 7 days in culture. L= lymphocytes; M= macrophages; PWM= pokeweed mitogen.

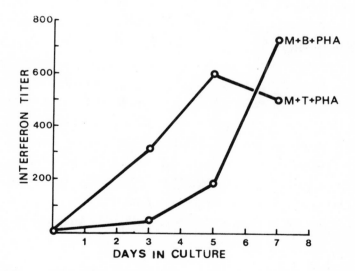

Fig. 2. Interferon production by human T or B lymphocytes in the presence of macrophages in response to PHA at 3,5 and 7 days in culture. L= lymphocytes; M= macrophages; PHA= phytohemagglutinin.

DISCUSSION

De Maeyer: I am very much impressed by these interesting
results, and also by the beautiful machine you used. But one
thing was not clear to me. Is the PHA and the pokeweed mitogen
there from the beginning of the culture, or do you add it on
days three, five, and seven?

Epstein: Both are added at the initiation of the culture.

De Maeyer: So, it is always there; thank you.

Merigan: With the cell sorter, is it possible that the
antiserum treatment that is required to detect the B cell in any
way influences the interferon response? So is it slower because
the cell has been damaged by antibody?

Epstein: We were very concerned about this and before we
even start the experiments with the machine we used mixed populations of T and B lymphocytes, exposed them to the antisera,
coated presumably only the B cells and studied the interferon
response. We could show no difference. To confirm this, after
we separated the B cells from the machine, we did experiments
which I mentioned briefly here. We tried to remove most of the
immuno-fluorescent complex by letting the B cells remain in culture for 24 hours and then thoroughly washing the cells. This
will remove most, but not completely all of the immuno-fluorescent complex. Even doing that and stimulating the cells with PHA
or poke weed mitogen, we did not get a B cell response at three
days.

Merigan: It will be very interesting to study: a patient
say with a pure T cell deficiency where you will be able to
study a population of pure B cells selected genetically to test

their response.

Epstein: Yes. Obviously chronic lymphocytic leukemics represent predomonantly B cell population, but they are abnormal
in other functional tests. There are now other means of isolat-
ing normal human B cells which do not involve the use of such a
complex machine as the FACS, and I hope to use those to study
just that kind of question.

Baron: Could you briefly compare the time of appearance
of the mitogenic response with the interferon response with both
the T and the B cells?

Epstein: Yes. For each experiment that we assayed interferon, we also assayed the proliferative response. 8 out of 9
experiments, after 3 days of culture B cells in the presence of
macrophages, showed no interferon or proliferative response to
either PHA or PWM. There was only one experiment in which we
saw a slight proliferative response of B cells to PHA at 3 days.
B cells in the presence of macrophages can produce interferon
and proliferate in response to PHA and PWM, but their response
is delayed to 5 and 7 days. The proliferative and interferon
responses of T cells to PHA peak at 3 days; their response to
PWM, both proliferative and interferon, peak about day 4.

Grossberg: It's very nice what you have described in the
human, but do the same kinetics pertain to the mouse?

Epstein: I guess I have a bias for studying human material! The situation is somewhat different in the mouse. Other investigators have used means other than the FACS for separating
T and B cells from the mouse. Greaves et al. (Greaves, M.F. and
Bariminger, S., Nature New Biol. 235, 67, 1972) have shown that
mouse T cells will repond to soluble PHA and poke weed with proliferation, but that B cells will only respond to poke weed

mitogen. However, if PHA is rendered insoluble by virtue of its
binding to Sepharose, then mouse B cells will show a proliferative response. We have shown that human B cells respond to both
of these two mitogens in the soluble form, and so the human response is different from the mouse. There is one other report in
the literature using human cells in which B cells have been
shown to respond to PHA. Phillips and Roitt (Nature New Biol.
1973, 241, 254) found that human B cells eluted from a Sepharose
anti-immunoglobulin column by dextranase did proliferate in response to PHA.

Grossberg: Do you have any observations on the production
of interferon in the patients that you studied with thymic dis-
plasia or hypoplasia?

Epstein: With regard to the IgA deficient patients we
were particularly intrigued. Several reports have indicated that
these patients have a normal T cell proliferative response to
PHA. We were pleased to find that we could pick up a defect of
T cell function which was separate from the proliferative response. This gives more credence to the fact that this test will
be of use in diagnosis and classification of patients with various immuno deficiency diseases. In fact, it was suspected in
the literature that there should be some kind of T cell defect
associated with deficiency of IgA. Percy et al. (Percy, D.Y.E.,
Frommel, D., Hong, R. and Good, R.A., 1970, Lab. Invest. 22,
212) demonstrated that rabbits which were thymectomized, irradiated, and reconstituted, all showed a selective depression of
plasma IgA. We also studied patients with thymic hypoplasia.
Some of them had received a thymic transplant and we were trying
to use this test of 3 day interferon levels to measure T cell
effector function to see whether it might also give us some indication of whether the thymic transplant had been successful.

By other criteria, namely by the proliferation of T cells to
PHA, one patient had not had a successful thymic transplant,
and no interferon was detectable. Another two, however, had successful transplants as evaluated by a good proliferative response to PHA. These two also had normal 3 day interferon levels. Now we are in the process of obtaining T lymphocytes both
before and after thymic transplants to follow the 3 day interferon response, to see if this would be an effective test to
monitor the success or failure of thymic transplants.

Grossberg: The only information I would like to add are
our observations made with Dr. Duquesnoy in anterior pituitary
dwarf mice which have thymic hypoplasia, and in which the circulating interferon response to the usual inducers is markedly
depressed. However, interferon nonetheless is produced to at
least a level of several hundred units. In the normal litter-
mates, the response is about ten-fold greater. We have only preliminary observations on the response of lymphocytes in vitro;
but since these are dwarfs we can get very few cells to study.

Epstein: It would be interesting to see whether these residual cells are indeed B cells and whether they are the ones
that are making the small amount of interferon that you see.

Baron: I can add a little bit of information towards an-
swering Dr. Grossberg's question about the differences between
the mouse and the human system. With Drs. Stobo and Green at
the N.I.H. we had a little experience with the mouse system and
the responses are substantially earlier in the mouse than you
describe here with the human system. Others have reported that
also. The interferon begins to appear between 12 and usually
reaches a maximum at 24 to 30 hours in mitogen stimulated spleen
cells while the proliferative response begins at 48 hours. So

there is about a 24 hour difference between the first interferon production and the increased thymidine uptake. Separation of the B cells from the T cells (using specific antisera for lysis of the appropriate B or T cell populations) indicates that mitogen will stimulate proliferation in the B cell population but no interferon was observed up to 3 days after stimulation of B cells. Splenic T cells produced interferon under these conditions.

Epstein: Did you have macrophages present in the culture?

Baron: Yes, they were present. I should also comment that the thymocytes free of macrophages did not produce interferon. The findings will be published in the Journal of Immunology.

Tan: Have you applied your system to study T and B lymphocytes from Down syndrome patients?

Epstein: No, it is something I would like to do. I would suspect that they might produce a large amount of interferon.

Tan: Is there any correlation between the interferon system and deficiency of the immune system in Down syndrome?

Epstein: To my knowledge, no one has yet studied mitogen or antigen stimulated interferon by the lymphocytes of these patients.

COMPLEMENT IN INTERFERON RELEASE IN THE INTACT ANIMAL

Juliana Larmie and Warren R. Stinebring

University of Vermont, Burlington, U.S.A.

Endotoxin and tuberculin in sensitized animals have long
been known to affect the complement system. Endotoxin injected
intravenously into non-immunized rabbits has been shown to reduce total complement levels significantly within one hour with
evidence of partial return to pre-injection levels by 3 hours
post-injection. These experiments by Gilbert and Braude (1) indicated most consistent results were obtained at doses approach-
ing the LD_{50} for this E. coli endotoxin. Immunized rabbits showed similar patterns of complement levels at these times. In 1954,
Rice, Boulanger, and Konst (2) demonstrated 18 hours after intraperitoneal injection of tuberculin into guinea pigs infected
with a moderately virulent strain of bovine tubercle bacillus
that survivors showed lowered total complement levels. Non-tu-
berculous animals showed no such effect on complement levels,
ruling out non-specific reactivity or endotoxin contamination
as problems. Furthermore, studies showed first, second, fourth,
but not third components of complement to be lowered in titre.
The third component of complement would also include C'5 and
C'6 and other later components according to newer nomenclature.
Füst and Föris (3) have presented interesting data which show
early deplection of C'3 and probably later components of the
complement cascade in the blood of rats treated with endotoxin
derived from Serratia marescens. They could find no such drop

in animals pretreated with increasing doses of endotoxin sufficient to render the animals tolerant to several minimal lethal
doses. Their conclusion was that in tolerant animals endotoxin
does not activate the full cascade and that formation of ana-
phylotoxin and chemotactic factor may be interfered with. Recently Borecky and his coworkers (4) have investigated effects of
various interferon inducers including Newcastle disease virus
(NDV) and endotoxin on the total complement in the circulation
of mice, or on guinea pig serum in vitro. Interferon titres in
vivo correlated in an inverse relationship with total complement, the late interferon system (NDV) showing slower depletion
of complement than the early (endotoxin) interferon system.

Our studies are concerned with the kinetics of interferon
response, and complement components C'1 and C'9. C'1 was chosen
because it is the first reactive component of the complement
cascade; C'9 because it is the last complement component in the
cascade and subsequent to activation of C'3 in the so called
by-pass known to be activated by endotoxin. We have also examined
the effects of lead acetate on interferon release and complement
because of the known effects of lead acetate in potentiating
interferon release as we have reported at an earlier International Interferon meeting (Lyon, 1970). The effect of pretreatment of mice with cobra venom factor which depletes C'3 and subsequent factors was also investigated. These experiments are
preliminary to a complete examination of hyporeactivity, effects
of poly I:C, the production of interferon by tuberculin, and
other interferon-cell related phenomena.

25 g. Taconic Farm female mice were injected intravenously with K235, E. coli endotoxin as indicated and were bled at
the times indicated. Serum was obtained in a manner to preserve
complement activity. Interferon was assayed in L cells using

the plaque reduction method with vesicular stomatitis virus as the indicator virus. Interferon titres are expressed as the reciprocal of the dilution reducing plaque numbers to half that of the controls. Complement component levels were determined using reaction mixtures for hemolytic assay as specified and supplied by Cordis Laboratories. Guinea pig serum reagents were used throughout and the spectrophotometric method was used to determine CH_{50} units. Results are expressed as the percentage activity of control sera from saline injected mice. Sera were from pools of ten or more mice.

Table 1 shows the characteristic time pattern of appearance of interferon with a peak at 2 hours and a subsequent drop. C'1 levels reach their low point at 2 hours but by 5 hours have returned to above normal. Table 2 illustrates that the C'9 level reaches its nadir at 2 hours, again at the interferon peak, and by 5 hours C'9 levels are normal. These patterns are reproducible. The results indicate that early and late components are depleted and that presumably the entire cascade has been activated , not just the C'3 by-pass. This is not unexpected in vivo because, as Gewurz (5) has pointed out, enzymatic action of trypsin can activate the cascade at C'1 and C'3 and that other proteases and lysosomal enzymes can activate the cascade at C'3 and C'5. Such enzymes circulate after endotoxin injection into the intact animal has injured especially the cells of the reticuloendothelial system.

Using lead acetate injection with small quantities of endotoxin causes enhancement of release of interferon. However, lead acetate alone releases no interferon and affects C'1 levels minimally if at all but probably reduces C'9 by 2 hours (Table 3). In combination lead acetate and endotoxin not only stimulate more interferon but seem to result in an additive ef-

fect on C'1 and C'9 levels. Admittedly, the data are not strong
and they should only be regarded as suggestive and preliminary.

Table 4 presents data from an experiment designed to test
the effect of lowering complement component levels on interferon
release. Cobra venom factor, a protein of molecular weight about
140,000 is non-toxic when separated from toxic components of raw
cobra venom. The presence of a normal serum beta-globulin, C'3
serum proinactivator, and CVF causes activation of the complement cascade at C'3 and beyond. Using doses of CVF known to reduce circulating C'3 to less than 10% of normal within 2 hours
in guinea pigs on a weight basis, we have attempted to study
effects of such depletion on interferon release in mice stimulated with endotoxin. Unfortunately, our mice are more resistant
to the effects of CVF than guinea pigs and the highest dose
tested , ten times that supposedly required, only causes a 22%
reduction in C'9 activity within 3 hours. Such a reduction does
not influence interferon production by endotoxin but the data
indicate CVF itself does not cause production of interferon although it does lower C'9 levels significantly. These experiments
failed to influence IF release but the 20% reduction still
leaves plenty of complement activity available for reaction upon
injection of endotoxin and indeed such an effect is found.

In conclusion, we have found, as has Borecky (4), that
complement levels change following endotoxin stimulation of mice
in an inverse relationship to interferon titres. Both C'1 and
C'9 levels are reduced indicating that in vivo the earlier parts
of the complement cascade are activated. Further experiments are
planned to determine if depletion of complement cascade past the
C'3 level will affect interferon production.

References

1. Gilbert, V.E. and Braude, A.I. (1962). J. Exp. Med. 116, 477.

2. Rice, C.E., Boulanger, P. and Konst, H. (1954). Canad. J. Comp. Med. and Veterinar. Sci. 18, 197.

3. Füst, F. and Föris, G. (1970). Experientia 26, 1362.

4. Rathova, V., Kociskova, D. and Borecky, L. (1972). Acta Virol. 16, 508.

5. Gewurz, H. (1971). In Biological Activities of Complement, ed. by Ingram, D.C., S. Karger, N.Y.

TABLE 1

Complement, interferon, and endotoxin in mice

Time (hr.)	IF Titre	C'l Titre (%)
0	<15	100
1	80	65
2	152	56
3	140	80
4	130	92
5	110	110

Endotoxin - E. coli, K235 - 250 µg i.v.

TABLE 2

Complement, Interferon, and Endotoxin in Mice

Time (hr.)	IF Titre	C'9 Titre (%)
0	<20	100
2	480	48
3	160	77
5	33	105

Endotoxin - E. coli, K235 - 250 µg

TABLE 3

Lead acetate, complement, interferon

	IF Titre	C'1 (%)	C'9 (%)
0 hr.	<20	100	100
ET* (2 hr.)	60	94	90
PbAC** (2 hr.)	<20	99	87
PbAC&ET (2 hr.)	400	89	77
ET (6 hr.)	50	95	94
PbAC&ET (6 hr.)	40	92	85

* ET - 1 µg
** PbAC - 5 mg

TABLE 4

Cobra venom factor, complement, interferon

	IF Titre	C'9 (%)
Endotoxin - 2 hr.	520	79
Cobra venom factor - 3 hr.	<30	78

Cobra venom factor
  - 3 hr., endotoxin
  - 2 hr.
	600	51

Endotoxin - 100 µg, Cobra venom factor - 50 units

DISCUSSION

Lebon: How are complement levels in mice treated with interferon?

Stinebring: The complement levels for these components
have been determined and they are quite well within the range
that Zarco has found at Cordis.

Chany: If I recall, Dr. Borecky showed that endotoxin-
induced interferon can be obtained at low temperatures using
leucocytes or macrophages from mice or from other animal cultures
in vitro. Did you ever try to see if complement has any effect
in such a system on interferon production?

Stinebring: No, but Dr. Borecky has reported that complement somehow interacts in reducing the amount of interferon produced in vitro in his system.

Paucker: How sensitive is your assay for C'1 and C'9 and is a reduction by 50% considered significant?

Stinebring: The reduction by 50% is certainly considered significant.

INTERFERON INDUCTION AND IMMUNOSUPPRESSION BY VIRUSES

I. Béládi, R. Pusztai, M. Bakay, K. Berencsi

Institute of Microbiology
University Medical School
Szeged, Hungary

Human adenoviruses are not pathogenic for a variety of common laboratory animals, however, marked antibody responses were noted in guinea pigs, cotton rats, rabbits and hamsters after single inoculation with different types. In contrast to these we found that types 6 and 12 were weak antigens in chickens. The primary immune response to a nonviral antigen, i.e., sheep blood cells (SRBC) was also suppressed. Chickens given SRBC stimulus within the first 48 hours of adenovirus infection or 16 to 20 days after virus injection responded with numbers of 19 S haemolytic plaque-forming cells in the spleen (HPFC) comparable to those obtained in uninfected birds. The response was slightly diminished when SRBC were injected 48 hours after adenovirus type 12 infection. Marked decrease was observed when antigen was given 4 to 6 days after type 6 injection (Fig. 1).

SRBC given together with type 12 adenovirus did not alter the production of 19 S HPFC in the spleen, rather a slight increase could be detected.

Spleen lymphocytes of adenovirus infected chickens were cultivated in vitro and their response to PHA was measured by
^{3}H-thymidine incorporation (Table 1).

The results showed that the stimulation ratio was much slower in the case of adenovirus infected chickens than in control birds. Spleen cells taken from adenovirus infected chickens at different times of incubation revealed a transient decreased response to PHA which could be detected from 1 to 14 days after virus infection.

Adenovirus infected chickens showed no gross pathological alterations. No marked change in the peripheral leukocyte counts was found rather a slight increase could be observed 2 to 4 days after infection. Chickens infected with adenoviruses had consistently similar total spleen cell counts as control animals. Cell viability studies showed no differences between infected and control birds. Interferon is formed in chickens infected with adenoviruses. A coincidence in time between the decreased response to antigenic stimulation and to a second interferon inducer could be observed. Spleen lymphocytes obtained from adenovirus type 12 infected chickens at different days of incubation were cultured in vitro in the presence and absence of adenovirus type 12 (Table 2).

Lymphocytes obtained 3 or more days after virus infection and rechallenged in vitro produced nothing or a very small amount of interferon. This is the time when the impaired immune response to SRBC could be demonstrated.

As the response to PHA of spleen lymphocytes from adenovirus infected chickens is impaired it is very likely that in virus infected birds the function of T cells is inhibited.

Similar results were observed in hamsters infected with NDV. After simultaneous administration of the virus and SRBC no immunosuppressive effect was evident, in fact a slight stimulation of the formation of 19 S HPFC in the spleen was found.

However, impairment in the HPFC was observed when SRBC were injected 1 to 14 days after NDV infection (Fig. 2).

The spleen weight and the total spleen cell number of NDV infected hamsters were similar to that of the control hamsters. NDV infected hamsters produced interferon very soon after virus infection. Maximum titer of interferon was observed at 8 hours after infection.

In hamsters injected with NDV and solubilized SRBC which do not need macrophages for the induction of antibody production, the formation of 19 S HPFC was also inhibited. Thus, in hamsters the impaired function of macrophages is not the reason for the decreased immune response.

We assume that in both virus-host systems the interferon formed was responsible for the transient inhibition of the immune response.

TABLE 1

Incorporation of ^{3}H-thymidine by PHA-stimulated spleen lymphocytes of adenovirus-infected and control chickens

Nº of animals	Stimulation ratio[a]	
	control	adenovirus-infected
1	33	16
2	150	7
3	35	13
4	85	6
5	18 52.6 ± 41.6[b]	9 9.3 ± 3.7[b]
6	47	12
7	17	8
8	45	4
9	44	9

[a] $\dfrac{\text{incorporation by PHA-treated cells (cpm)}}{\text{incorporation by untreated cells (cpm)}}$

[b] mean values $\pm$ SE

TABLE 2

Interferon titers in the spleen cells of chicks
infected with adenovirus type 12

Hours after infection	Titer of interferon			
	Virus infected		Control	
	-	Challenged in vitro	-	Challenged in vitro
3	8 , 32	32 , 64		
10	16 , 8	128 , 64		
24	4 , 4	32 , 64	<4 , <4	32 , 16
48	<4 , <4	4 , 4	<4 , <4	8 , 32
72	<4 , <4	8 , <4		
96	<4 , <4	<4 , <4		

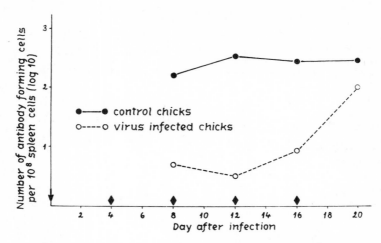

Fig. 1. The effect of adenovirus type 6 infection on the number of antibody forming cells (19 S IgM) in the spleens of chicks inoculated with sheep erythrocytes. ↓ virus inoculation; ♦ injection of sheep erythrocytes.

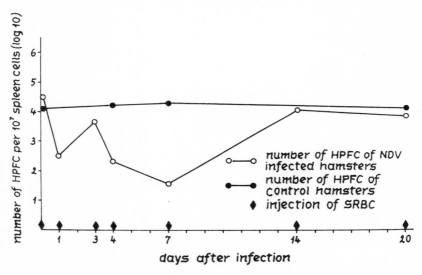

Fig. 2. The effect of NDV on the number of HPFC in the spleens of hamsters.

on, as we all know, for many days. So I think the two activities
of interferon are separable and we shouldn't confuse ourselves
by trying to explain the effects by too simplistic mechanisms.

Levy: I was just wondering whether you think this effect
on cells in tissue culture, or this lack of effect, bears any
relationship to the many times reported effect of interferon on
tumor growth in vivo. This is, I think, a pretty clear-cut phenomenon, the inhibition of tumor growth in vivo. Is that a different kind of phenomenon from that reported for inhibition of
normal cell growth?

Oxman: The growth of some tumors may depend upon the continued expression of tumor virus genes. If the expression of
these genes is sensitive to interferon, inhibition of tumor
growth could be accounted for by the antiviral action of interferon. This might even explain the inhibition of normal mouse L
cell multiplication by interferon, for normal mouse L cells contain RNA tumor virus genomes. If the rate of L cell division is
determined in part by the activity of endogenous tumor virus
genes, the antiviral action of interferon, by inhibiting the expression of these genes, would be expected to reduce the rate of
cell multiplication.

Some observations by Drs. Chany and Vignal may argue a-
gainst this hypothesis. If I remember correctly, a line of mouse
embryo cells transformed by the Moloney strain of mouse sarcoma
virus was carried in the constant presence of interferon. After
some 200 passages, the interferon treated cells showed no reduction in their content of infectious virus or virus-specific antigens. However, it is important to recognize that these are
really complicated experiments. Such cells may contain more than
one type of endogenous virus, and the virus genes whose expression you measure may not be those which determine the aspect of

the cells'behavior which you choose to study.

May I take a moment to propose a rather simplistic model for the origin of the interferon system which might also explain its effects on the multiplication of both normal and tumor cells?

Pereira: If it is brief I think it would be very nice to have something simplistic because I myself am pretty confused.

Oxman: The interferon system has evolved as a host defense mechanism in multicellular organisms in which, most of the time, most cells are nondividing. We may hypothesize that animal cells possess at least two distinct classes of genes: one class being active only during cell division, and the other being active in resting cells. If the division-associated genes are derepressed to initiate cell division, some natural regulatory mechanism must subsequently be brought into play to block their continued expression and thus return the cell to the nondividing state. Such a regulatory mechanism would have the capacity to distinguish between the two classes of genes, blocking the expression of only those associated with cell division. If the interferon system has evolved from such a regulatory mechanism, it may still retain some inhibitory activity for the division-associated genes.

Consistent with this hypothesis is the fact that most studies performed in confluent non-dividing cells have failed to document any effect of interferon on cellular synthetic functions.

Pereira: I wonder what would have happened if this explanation was not simplistic! I must confess it is still a little bit woolly to me and it will probably remain like that for a long time. I'm not even quite sure whether Dr. Oxman is defending the point that interferon has no action on cellular functions or whether it may under certain circumstances have some action on the cellular functions. I think this argument could go on for a long time, and I'm afraid we'll have to go on to the next speaker.

SUPPRESSION OF CELL GROWTH BY ELECTROPHORETIC
FRACTIONS OF L CELL INTERFERON

Y. Kawade and T. Matsuzawa

Institute for Virus Research,
Kyoto University, Kyoto, Japan

Interferon preparations have been found to suppress multiplication of cells in culture (1). Although interferon has not
been completely purified yet, various lines of indirect evidence
suggest strongly that interferon itself is responsible for the
"anticell" effects observed. In our laboratory, L cell interferon was purified to a maximum specific activity of 2×10^8 units/
mg protein, and to a higher degree after polyacrylamide gel e-
lectrophoresis (2) (interferon titers are expressed in this paper in international units), and such preparations were found to
suppress growth of various mouse cells in culture (3). However,
when the interferon was resolved electrophoretically into fast
and slow components, the cell growth inhibiting actvity of these
components was not parallel to the antiviral activity. That is,
the fast-moving component required a 10 - 100 times more antiviral dose than the slow component to effect the same degree of
inhibition of cell growth. An example is shown in Fig. 1, which
indicates the number of L cells after 4 days' cultivation in the
presence of various doses of the interferon components. It therefore appeared that either a non-interferon substance still contained in the purified preparation was responsible for the anticell effect, or the different interferon components had quantitatively different anticell activities. Lack of correlation be-

tween the antiviral and the anticell activities of electrophoretic fractions was also reported by Borecky et al. (4).

On the other hand, Gresser and his coworkers found no significant difference between the similar electrophoretic fractions
in their suppression of L 1210 cell colony formation (5).

In order to resolve this discrepancy, it was desirable to
improve both the antiviral and anticell assays. In our previous
study (3), the antiviral activity was assayed by the plaque reduction method using L cell and vesicular stomatitis virus (VSV),
and the anticell activity by counting the cell numbers after
several days' cultivation in the presence of interferon. Both
assays were tedious and suffered from considerable errors.

In the present study, the antiviral titer was determined
by a method based on the inhibition of VSV RNA synthesis measured by ^{3}H-uridine incorporation in the presence of actinomycin
D. It was originally developed by Drs. J. Suzuki and S. Kobayashi
of Basic Research Laboratory, Toray Industries, Inc., and found
to be much more rapid, simple and reliable than the plaque reduction method (Matsuzawa and Kawade, in preparation).

For the anticell assay, ^{3}H-thymidine incorporation into
DNA of L cells was measured. In preliminary experiments, it was
found necessary to have a relatively small number of cells per
culture for this assay to serve as a useful index of cell growth
inhibition. In practice, 3000 L cells were seeded in each well
of a microtiter plate, and after 3 or 4 days' incubation in the
presence or absence of interferon, ^{3}H-thymidine was pulsed for
1.5 - 2 h, and the acid-insoluble radioactivity in the cells was
counted (Matsuzawa and Kawade, in preparation). Fig. 2 shows the
interferon dose-response relationships determined in this way.

As can be seen in Fig. 2 (a), there was about a tenfold difference between the antiviral doses of the fast and slow components necessary for the same anticell effect, in agreement with our previous finding. This was true for the electrophoretic fractions obtained from a crude sample concentrated by zinc acetate, and from the ones purified by DEAE- and CM-Sephadex.

Peculiarly, in some preparations, the antiviral titer of the fast component dropped fairly rapidly on storage at -20°C (in 0.1% bovine plasma albumin in phosphate-buffered saline, pH 7.4), whereas the slow component was much more stable. For example, when the samples used in the experiment of Fig. 2 (a) were assayed again after 4 weeks of storage, the antiviral titer of the fast component was only 15% of the original value and that of the slow component was essentially unchanged. The thymidine incorporation-antiviral dose relationships for them at this time were indistinguishable from each other, as shown in Fig. 2 (b). Apparently, the anticell and the antiviral activities of the isolated components were not inactivated in parallel to each other.

Such a differential inactivation of the fast component was not always observed, and the reason for this variation among different preparations is not clear. When it did not occur, the quantitative difference in the anticell activity of the fast and slow components persisted after prolonged storage.

In conclusion. it was confirmed, using improved methods of the anticell and antiviral assays of interferon samples, that the fast- and the slow-migrating components of L cell interferon differ quantitatively in the anticell activity when compared at the same antiviral dose. However, in some preparations, the fast component lost its antiviral activity much faster than the slow component upon storage, and when this occurred, the anticell ac-

tivities of the two components became hardly distinguishable
from each other, indicating non-parallel inactivation of the anticell and antiviral activities.

This work was aided in part by grants from the Ministry of
Education and the Science and Technology Agency of Japan.

References

1. Gresser, I. (1972). Adv. Cancer Res. 16, 97.

2. Yamamoto, Y., Tsukui, K., Ohwaki, M. and Kawade, Y.
   (1974). J. Gen. Virol. , in press.

3. Ohwaki, M. and Kawade, Y. (1972). Acta Virol. 16, 477.

4. Borecky, L., Fuchsberger, N., Hajnicka, V., Stancek,
   D. and Zemla, J. (1972). Acta Virol. 16, 356.

5. Gresser, I., Bandu, M.-T., Tovey, M., Bodo, G., Paucker,
   K. and Stewart, W.E. II. (1973). Proc. Soc. Exp. Biol.
   Med. 142, 7.

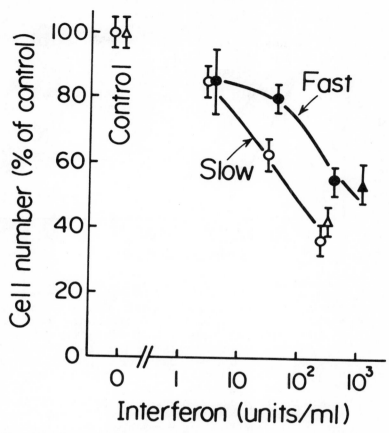

Fig. 1. Suppression of L cell growth by the fast and slow electrophoretic components of L cell interferon. Cells were cultured in 3 cm petri dishes in Eagle's medium plus 5% calf serum, starting with 4×10^4 cells in 2 ml, in the presence of the indicated concentration of interferon, and the cell numbers after 4 days' cultivation were counted in a hemocytometer (3). Five plates were used for each point, and each was counted twice. The vertical bars indicate the standard deviation of the mean. The circles and triangles represent independent experiments. The interferon preparation used in this experiment was purified by zinc acetate precipitation and chromatography on DEAE- and CM-Sephadex to a specific activity of 5×10^7 units/mg protein, then electrophoresed at pH 4.3 to separate the fast and slow components (2). Their antiviral titers were determined by the VSV plaque reduction method, using 3 - 5 plates for each interferon dilution, and average values from three assays were used.

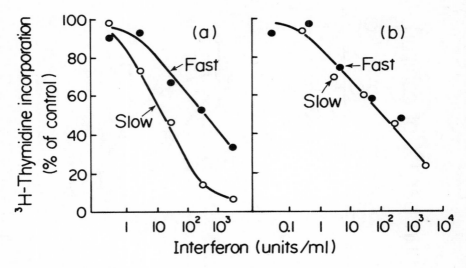

Fig. 2. Suppression of L cell growth by the slow and fast
interferon components as determined by ³H-thymidine incorporation. L cells in growth medium were seeded (3000 cells in 0.1
ml) in each well of a microtiter plate (6 mm diameter), containing the indicated antiviral doses of interferon, and after 3
days of cultivation, were pulsed with 0.5 μCi of ³H-thymidine
for 1.5 h. The acid-insoluble radioactivity is plotted against
the interferon dose, determined by the ³H-uridine incorporation
assay. The interferon preparation, column purified, had 2 x 10⁷
units/mg protein before electrophoresis. (a) Result obtained
using the fast and slow fractions 4 days after the electrophoretic separation (the ratio of their antiviral titers was confirmed by an independent plaque reduction assay). (b) The same
interferon fractions were re-assayed after 4 weeks' storage at
-20°C.

INTERFERON AND BONE MARROW COLONY-STIMULATING FACTOR

T.A. McNeill, M. Havredaki* and W.A. Fleming

Department of Microbiology
The Queen's University of Belfast
Belfast, BT12 6BN, N. Ireland

Introduction

During studies on the effect of antigens and infections on granulopoiesis we became interested in the inhibitory effects of interferon in a culture system which involves the multiplication and differentiation of granulocyte and macrophage cells from their primitive precursors. We feel that this is a suitable opportunity to summarise these observations and also to outline some recent studies which suggest a relationship between interferon and a stimulating factor which is necessary for cellular multiplication in this system.

The culture system

A system supporting the clonal proliferation of mouse granulocyte and macrophage cells in semi-solid agar was developed independently by Bradley and Metcalf (1) and Ichikawa, Pluznick

* Fellow of the International Atomic Energy Agency, Vienna.
Present address: Nuclear Research Center 'Democritos', Aghia Paraskevi Attikis, Greece.
This work was supported by grants from the Medical Research Council, London, and the International Atomic Energy Agency, Vienna.

and Sachs (4). In these cultures the primitive progenitor cells
of the myeloid series which are present in haemopoietic tissues
(approximately 1:500 of normal mouse bone marrow cells) give
rise to colonies of mature cell types. The progenitor cells (u-
sually termed in vitro colony-forming cells, CFC) are themselves
the progeny of the pluripotential stem cells which maintain the
production of all blood cell classes (19,3).

Colony formation in vitro is completely dependent upon the
presence of a glycoprotein termed colony-stimulating (CS) factor
the number and growth rate of colonies from any given cell suspension being dependent upon its concentration (13). Further details of the culture method, its applications and the biology of
CFC factor have been given by Metcalf and Moore (16).

Inhibition of colony growth by interferon

While studying the effects of several immunological adjuvants on granulopoiesis we found that serum taken from mice
three hours after an intraperitoneal inoculation of 100 microgram Poly rI:Poly rC inhibited colony growth in vitro (11). After fractionation on Sephadex the colony-inhibiting and interferon (antiviral) activities were closely associated in terms of
molecular size, active fractions showed that they had the same
sensitivity to heat, pH and trypsin and the colony-inhibiting
effect was more-or-less species specific (8,9).

It was interesting to observe that interferon not only inhibited colony growth in terms of the number of colonies per
culture and number of cells per colony but also interfered with
differentiation of cells within colonies (2). This may be of interest to those who find sympathy with the concept of protovi-
ruses and their possible role in cellular differentiation (17).

It will be remembered that colony formation requires the presence of CS factor and therefore the inhibitory effects of an interferon preparation must be measured against this background. Experiments in which the relative concentrations of interferon and CS factor were varied showed that the degree of inhibition by interferon was inversely related to the concentration of CS factor and could be overcome if a sufficiently high CS factor concentration was used (2). This effect was also encountered when, in collaboration with Dr. Gresser, we tested the colony-inhibiting effect of interferon preparations from different sources such as serum, brain and cell cultures. These experiments (10) showed that there was not necessarily a correlation between antiviral and anticellular activity in crude preparations, particularly those derived from cell cultures, and that this discrepancy was probably due to the high concentration of CS factor present in these preparations. Highly purified L-cell interferon free of CS factor, strongly inhibited colony development.

We believe that these experiments provide strong evidence that the colony inhibiting factor is interferon. They also raise the possibility that CS factor and interferon act as antagonistic regulators of cell division in this system.

Properties of CS factor relevant to interferon

The antagonistic effects of CS factor and interferon on colony growth in terms of their relative concentrations does not in itself mean that there is any fundamental relationship between the two factors. A similar type of relationship has been found with other colony-inhibiting agents as diverse as 5-iodo-2-deoxyuridine and methisazone (6) or chloroamphenicol (Table 1).

However, whenever we consider the general properties of

CS factor many similarities with interferon can be seen:

1. Glycoproteins of high specific activity.
2. Heterogeneity of molecular size and charge.
3. Stable within a wide range of pH and temperature.
4. Sensitive to alpha-chymotrypsin but resistant to most other proteolytic enzymes.
5. Produced by a wide variety of tissues in vivo and by cell cultures in vitro.

Much of the work on purification and biochemical properties of CS factor was carried out in Melbourne by Dr. E.R. Stanley and this, together with data relating to other biological properties, has been reviewed (15,16).

In vivo increases in CS factor levels can be induced by inoculation of many substances e.g., immunological adjuvants such as complete Freund's (5), bacterial products (14), and synthetic polyribonucleotides (11). Increases are also associated with both virus (12) and bacterial (18) infections of mice.

In vitro production of CS factor may also be modified by a variety of agents. Three examples which are relevant to a comparison with interferon are given.

(a) CS factor, like interferon, may be released during immunological reactions in spleen cell cultures (7).

(b) Interferon inducers such as rI : rC or Newcastle Disease virus (NDV) can alter the production of CS factor by L-cells. Figure 1 shows the results of experiments in which L-cell monolayers were washed and exposed to inducers (rI : rC 20 microgram per ml + DEAE-Dextran 100 microgram per ml, or 640 haemagglutinating units of NDV) for 1 hour at 37 C. Subsequently the monolayers were washed four times, refed with serum-free medium, incubated at 37 C and sample cultures removed at intervals for assay of the CS and interferon (antiviral, EMC virus in L-cells) activities in the medium. The reduction of CS activity after the appearance of interferon cannot be interpreted precisely since interferon affects the marrow assay system for CS factor, but it is interesting to note that during the first six hours, before interferon became detectable, there was a greater amount of CS activity released in induced cultures compared with controls.

Other experiments showed that this effect was also present in cultures treated with either rI : rC or DEAE-Dextran alone. Since these substances induce interferon in L-cells only when present together it must be concluded that the early increase in CS activity is not necessarily associated with interferon production.

(c) Preliminary experiments have indicated that, like interferon, CS factor may 'prime' cells for its own production. Table 2 gives results of experiments in which normal mouse marrow, spleen and thymus cells in agar culture were exposed to a low concentration of CS factor (0.07% mouse embryo conditioned medium). Cells at 10^6 per ml in an upper culture layer of Eagle's-0.3% agar were placed on an underlayer of Eagle's-1.2% agar which contained the CS factor. After 24 hours the upper layer of these primary cultures was removed and replaced with a fresh suspension of 5×10^4 marrow cells (secondary cultures) to measure the CS activity of the underlayers after conditioning by the primary cultures. Control primary cultures contained the same concentration of CS factor but no cells were present in the upper layers and the CS activity of the cell-conditioned underlayers was expressed as a percentage of the activity of these control cultures. These results can be compared with experiments in which underlayers were conditioned by cells not exposed to CS factor

during the primary culture period. It can be seen that in the
absence of CS factor in the primary cultures the cells had no
conditioning effect on the underlayers but in its presence marrow and thymus - but not spleen - cells gave an increase in
stimulating activity (Table 2).

Assuming that the increased CS activity of the culture
underlayers was due to CS factor and subject to confirmation
with more purified preparations of CS factor added to the primary cultures these results indicate a 'priming' effect of CS
factor on its own production. In addition, since thymus is virtually devoid of CFC they suggest that CS factor may act on cells
other than CFC - a necessary condition of any hypothesis propos-
ing relationships between interferon and CS factor as cell regulators.

Conclusion

We do not suggest that a relationship between interferon
and CS factor as cell regulators is proved by any of the various
studies outlined here. We do suggest that a hypothesis to this
effect has at least the right to exist and could stimulate many
investigations without respect for the confines of virology and
experimental haematology.

References

1.   Bradley, T.R. and Metcalf, D. (1966). Aust. J. exp.
     Biol. Med. Sci. 44, 287.

2.   Fleming, W.A., McNeill, T.A. and Killen, M. (1972).
     Immunology 23, 429.

3.   Haskill, J.S., McNeill, T.A. and Moore, M.A.S. (1970).

J. Cell. Physiol. 75, 167.

4. Ichikawa, Y., Pluznick, D.H. and Sachs, L. (1966).
    Proc. Nat. Acad. Sci. 56, 488.

5. McNeill, T.A. (1970). Immunology 18, 61.

6. McNeill, T.A. (1972). Antimicrob. Ag. Chemother. 1, 6.

7. McNeill, T.A. (1973). Nature New Biol. 244, 175.

8. McNeill,T.A. and Fleming, W.A. (1971). Immunology 21,
    761.

9. McNeill, T.A., Fleming, W.A. and McCance, D.J. (1972).
    Immunology 22, 711.

10. McNeill, T.A. and Gresser, I. (1973). Nature New Biol.
    244, 173.

11. McNeill, T.A. and Killen, M. (1971). Immunology 21,751.

12. McNeill, T.A. and Killen, M. (1971). Infec. Immun. 4,
    323.

13. Metcalf, D. (1970). J. Cell. Physiol. 76, 89.

14. Metcalf, D. (1971). Immunology 21, 427.

15. Metcalf, D. (1972). Aust. J. exp. Biol. med. Sci. 50,
    547.

16. Metcalf, D. and Moore, M.A.S. (1971). Haemopoietic
    Cells. North Holland, Amsterdam.

17. Temin, H. (1971). J.nat. Cancer Inst. 46, 111.

18. Trudgett, A., McNeill, T.A. and Killen, M. (1973).
    Infec. Immun. 8, 450.

19. Worton, R.G., McCulloch, E.A. and Till, J.E. (1969).
    J. Cell. Physiol. 74, 171.

TABLE 1

Bone marrow colony inhibition by 100 µg chloroamphenicol
Effect of CS factor

Relative CS factor concentration	Colonies per culture (mean of 4 $\pm$ 1 SD)		% inhibition
	Control	Drug	
1	69 $\pm$ 6	64 $\pm$ 3	7
1/2	67 $\pm$ 3	59 $\pm$ 4	12
1/4	59 $\pm$ 3	34 $\pm$ 3	42
1/8	40 $\pm$ 2	18 $\pm$ 1	55
1/16	22 $\pm$ 3	7 $\pm$ 2	68
1/32	13 $\pm$ 3	1 $\pm$ 1	92

TABLE 2

Conditioning effect of marrow and thymus cells
exposed to CS factor

Conditioning cells	Colony stimulating activity of culture underlayers % of unconditioned	
	CS factor not in primary cultures	CS factor present in primary cultures
Marrow	106 $\pm$ 5	158 $\pm$ 11
Spleen	99 $\pm$ 2	87 $\pm$ 12
Thymus	103 $\pm$ 2	149 $\pm$ 11

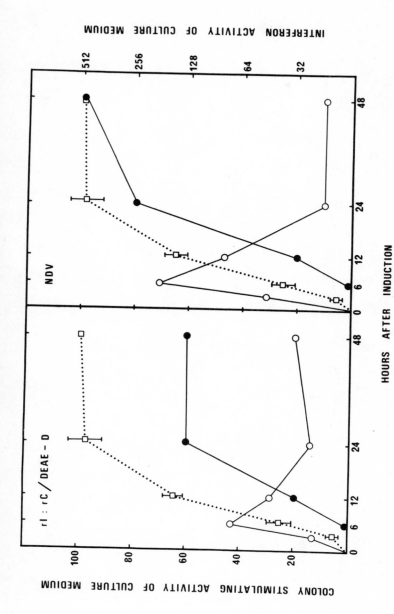

Fig. 1. Colony-stimulating and interferon activities of L-cell media after treatment of cultures with either rI : rC + DEAE-Dextran or NDV. O , colony-stimulating activity of treated cultures; ● , interferon activity of treated cultures; □ , colony- stimulating activity of control cultures.

MEMBRANE CHANGES IN L-CELLS TREATED WITH INTERFERON

L.J. Katz, S.H.S. Lee and K.R. Rozee

Department of Microbiology, Dalhousie University
Halifax, Nova Scotia, Canada

Introduction

Investigators in recent years have demonstrated that, in
addition to its well-documented antiviral effect, exposure of
cells to interferon results in a great variety of other cellular
changes (4,6,9,10).

Being interested in more rigorously investigating these
cellular effects, we recently turned our attention towards selecting a cell line that was unresponsive to some or all of the
actions of interferon. Such a cell would be an invaluable tool
for such studies. Gresser et al. (3), have already reported that
a cell line derived from murine leukemia cells (L1210) was resistant to some anticellular and antiviral actions of interferon.
These cells were obtained by culturing suspended L1210 cells in
the continuous presence of interferon. Chany and Vignal (1), also have similarly obtained a cell line (MSV-IF$^+$) which is resistant to the antiviral action of interferon.

We also attempted to select for interferon resistance by
continuously adding interferon to the growth medium at a low concentration and seeding the cells so that confluent monolayers
would be produced 5-6 days later. Specifically, we have found
that L-929 cells grown for over 6 months in the presence of in-

terferon can be shown to have a decreased responsiveness to both
the antiviral and growth depression actions of interferon. More
interesting, however, they have been found to be more susceptible
to the lytic properties of vesicular stomatitis virus (VSV) and
react differently than untreated L-929 cells when exposed to
certain membrane-active substances. The possible relevance of
these findings to the proposition that interferon affects the
cell membrane is discussed.

Methods

Mouse strain L929 cells were used throughout the investigation and grew as monolayer cultures in Eagle's minimal essential medium (MEM) supplemented with 10% inactivated fetal calf
serum (growth medium). They were used for the production of interferon, titration of interferon, and preparation of the different virus stocks.

The L-929 cell sub-strain referred to in the text as "L-
int" were grown in the same fashion as L-929 cells, but for more
than 6 months grew in the presence of 50 plaque reduction doses,
fifty percent (PRD$_{50}$) of mouse interferon. These L-int cells
were grown during this time as monolayer cultures in 8 oz. pre-
scription bottles and were seeded at each subculture at a cell
density so that confluent monolayers were just obtained after 5
days incubation. When cultures were required for experimentation,
cultivation was carried out in glass or plastic (Falcon) Petri
dishes, seeded at a cell concentration that produced confluent
monolayers after 3 days incubation in growth medium without interferon.

Stocks of VSV (Indiana), Reovirus (types 2 and 3), Vaccinia
virus (WR) and Mengo viruses were grown in mouse L-929 cells.
After growth they were stored in aliquots at -70°C. Newcastle

disease virus, California strain (NDV) was propagated in the allantoic cavity of 9 day old embryonated eggs.

Mouse interferon was prepared in 2.5-liter, cylindrical,
roller-bottle cultures of L-929 cells with ultraviolet-inacti-
vated NDV and interferon assays were performed by the plaque-reduction method in L-929 cells using VSV as a challenge virus as
previously described (8). Interferon induced and titrated by these
methods usually titered between 6,000 and 15,000 PRD_{50} units and
had a specific activity of 2-5 x 10^4 units/mg protein. "Spent"
media was produced by the same techniques except UV-NDV was o-
mitted in its preparation. This spent media was used as required,
for cultures carried as controls in interferon treatment experiments.

The antiviral and growth depression principles in these
interferon preparations were both non-dialyzable; did not sedi-
ment at 100,000 g within 3 hr; were not inactivated at pH 2.0;
were partially inactivated at 56°C for 1 hr at pH 7.4; were host
specific; contained no infectious NDV; were destroyed by trypsin;
and had molecular weights of about 38,000 daltons as estimated
by Sephadex G100 filtration techniques. Purified mouse L-cell
interferon, kindly donated by Dr. Kurt Paucker, had a specific
activity of 10^7 NIH reference units/mg protein.

Concanavalin A (2x crystallized) and Protamine Sulfate
(Salmine) were purchased from Nutritional Biochemicals Corp. and
DEAE-dextran (m.w. approximately 2 x 10^6) was purchased from
Pharmacia. Methylated albumin (bovine, B grade) was obtained
from Calbiochem. These reagents were sterilized by millipore filtration prior to use. Uridine-5-H^3 (S.A. 28 C/mM) and Thymidine-
methyl-H^3 (S.A. 6.7 C/mM) were purchased from New England Nuclear.

Results

When L-cells were cultivated in the continuous presence of
50 PRD_{50} units of mouse interferon cell yields were initially reduced by 40 to 60 percent as compared to those obtained with untreated L-929 cell cultures. However, when some 6 months had e-
lapsed it was observed that these treated cells had by this time
recovered their ability to grow in the presence of interferon
almost as well as L-929 cells did without interferon. We called
these cells L-int cells and proceeded to compare them in various
ways with their progenitor cell line L-929.

Differentiating L-int and L-929 cells by VSV plaque morphology. In the course of using VSV as a challenge virus for interferon assays it was found that the virus plaqued differently
in L-int cells as compared to L-929 cell cultures. A typical VSV
plaque-reduction assay for interferon activity using both L-int
and L-929 cultures was performed as follows. L-int cultures were
washed free of their interferon-containing growth medium, then
trypsinized and seeded at a cell concentration in growth medium
containing no interferon so that a usable monolayer culture was
formed in three days. L-929 cells were similarly washed and seeded in the same growth medium.

When monolayers of contiguous cells had formed, triplicate
cultures of these cells were washed and exposed for 16 hr to various dilutions of interferon. They were then challenged with VSV
at a dose calculated to produce about 100 plaques per control
culture. The virus was absorbed for 90 minutes then an overlay
of 0.6 percent agarose in medium placed over the culture. Two
days later 10% formalin in distilled water was introduced over
the agar. One hour later the overlay was removed. The fixed cells,
which remained attached to the surface of the Petri dish, were
then stained with 1% crystal violet. The results are given in

Table 1 and Figure 1.

Two observations are apparent from Table 1. First, L-int cells are more receptive to VSV, being able to detect by plaque formation, from 30 to 40% more virus from similar dilutions of the same virus pool as are L-929 cell cultures. Secondly, L-int cells are less responsive to the antiviral action of interferon than are L-929 cells. In interferon assays where comparable VSV challenge doses were used the number of antiviral units detected in L-int cultures was consistently about 25 percent less than that detected by L-929 cells. In separate observations it was found that this lack of responsiveness of L-int cells to the antiviral activity of interferon was paralleled by an unresponsiveness to growth depression by interferon. In clone size assays it required four times the amount of interferon to reduce L-int cell growth by 50 percent as that required for a similar activity in L-929 cell clone cultures.

A third observation is apparent in Figure 1. VSV plaques in L-int cultures are clear ,whereas the plaques in L-929 cultures are cloudy but both are of the same size. This is noteworthy because VSV has been used as a challenge virus in our laboratory for a number of years and we had never previously observed this virus to produce clear plaques in our L-929 cells.

In view of these findings, it was thought that the most plausible explanation for the variation in plaque morphology was not one directly related to the virus, but the L-int cells were more susceptible than L-929 cells to VSV lysis. We theorized that this might reflect a cellular membrane alteration occurring after prolonged growth in the presence of interferon.

We did experiments, however, to explore the possibility that the two cell cultures might yield different proportions of

incomplete virus during replication. It is well documented that
passage of VSV by high titer inocula results in a reduced amount
of infectious virus ("B") due to an increased percentage in the
virus yield of a competing, non-infectious, incomplete "T" virion
(5). The "T" component contains a smaller amount of viral RNA
and can be separated from the normal "B" component by density
gradient centrifugation.

We infected L-int and L-929 cells at an input multiplicity
of infection (moi) of 25 with VSV in maintenance medium containing 1 μc/ml of ^{3}H-uridine. The medium was collected 8 and 24 hr
post-infection, clarified by low speed centrifugation and re-
centrifuged for 1 1/2 hr at 30,000 rpm. The pellet was resuspended in 1 ml of 0.01 M Tris Buffer (pH7.4). This material was then
sonicated for 1 min prior to density gradient centrifugation on
10-50% (w/v) linear sucrose gradients for 90 min. at 30,000 rpm
in the SW 39 head of the Spinco Model L-2 Ultra-centrifuge. No
differences were found between the sedimentation pattern of the
L-int and L-929 cell VSV yields as revealed by ^{3}H-uridine incorporated into high molecular weight material by either 8 or 24
hr. Each culture products labelled with ^{3}H-uridine which when
processed and centrifuged, sedimented as a single peak identified by its position in the gradient and morphological appearance
in the electron microscope as being the B virion.

We reasoned that any other differences in VSV maturation
in L-int as compared to L-929 cells would be revealed by "one-
step" growth curve experiments at different moi.

We performed one-step growth curves using different moi
(0.25, 2.5, and 25) and both the exponential rate of virus replication and total yields of VSV were the same in L-int as compared to L-929 cells at each multiplicity as shown by Figure 2.

At this point we concluded that neither a difference in
degree of autointerference nor some other factor relating to virus maturation was responsible for the difference in plaque morphology.

The effect of interferon on membrane integrity. In order
to determine directly if L-int cells were more susceptible to
VSV initiated lysis than L-929 cells, a growth curve experiment
was carried out using cells which had been pre-labelled with ^{3}H-
thymidine. The release of isotope into the supernatant fluid at
various times after VSV infection and the amount of virus released by the cells were measured. The methods used for pre-la-
belling the cells and determining the proportion of label released were essentially those of Möller et al.(7).

L-int and L-929 cells were seeded in Petri dishes in growth
medium containing 0.25 µC of ^{3}H-thymidine per ml. After a 3 day
incubation at 37°C, the cultures were washed 6 times and VSV was
adsorbed at a moi of 25 for 1 hour. The cultures were then washed 3 times and incubated in medium containing 50 µg/ml of cold
thymidine. At 2 hr intervals, supernatant fluids were collected
to determine the amounts of virus and isotope released from the
labelled cells. Label was determined by adding 0.5 ml of culture supernatant to 15 ml of Aquasol scintillation fluid (New
England Nuclear) and reading activity directly in a scintillation
counter. The results of this experiment are presented in Figure
3.

A difference in the amount of labelled material released
was observed as early as 2 hrs post-infection when comparing culture supernatants from L-int and L-929 cells. As virus replication proceeded, the L-int cells proved to be significantly more
sensitive to lysis by VSV as determined by the release of label.
This data lends support to the proposition that L-int cells are

far more sensitive to lysis than are L-929 cells during the replication of VSV. L-int cells, however, do not yield appreciably
more virus than do L-929 cells (Figure 2).

    Another experiment which we performed to evaluate inter-
feron effects on cell membranes involved the use of neutral red
dye. Experiments were designed to discover if L-int cells had,
by their exposure to interferon, been compromised in their sensitivity to certain membrane active substances. We presumed that
if they had been, they would be unable to retain neutral red dye
after they had been exposed to concentrations of membrane active
substance which had no effect on the progenitor L-929 cell strain.
In this context then, the effect of DEAE-dextran, protamine sulphate and methylated albumin on L-int and L-929 cell cultures
was next examined.

    L-int and L-929 cells were subcultured in 60 mm Petri
dishes at a density so that confluent monolayers were obtained
in 3 days. The growth medium was then replaced with medium containing different concentrations of the respective substances
or, for controls, fresh growth medium alone. After a 24 hr incubation period the medium was removed and replaced with 2 ml of
a 0.01% solution of neutral red in Hank's balanced salt solution.
Cultures were then incubated at 37°C in the dark for one hour.
The neutral red solution was then removed, the plates washed 3
times with warm PBS, and 7 ml of phosphate buffered ethanol
(0.1 M NaH_2PO_4:ethanol, 1:1) was placed in each Petri dish. In
this way, the neutral red dye taken up by cells was eluted into
the ethanol solution. The optical densities of the eluates were
read at 540 nm and the effect of the polycations was expressed
as the percentage of inhibition of neutral red uptake in the
treated cultures as compared to the control cultures and the results are shown in Table 2.

It can be seen that L-int cells were significantly more susceptible than L-929 cells to the cytotoxic properties of DEAE-dextran, protamine sulphate and methylated albumin.

Of interest here are two experiments which also indicate that L-int cells do in fact have membranes with different functional activities than do L-929 cells.

Suspensions of L-int and L-929 cells were made and the amount of Concanavalin A required to cause agglutination was estimated. It was found that between 16 and 32 μg/ml was required to achieve an agglutination dose 50 percent, if the cell suspension was L-929. This figure was between 250 and 500 μg/ml if L-int cell suspension of the same density were used. This result despite the fact that if ^{3}H-labelled Concanavalin A was used it was found that, on a per cell basis, the same amount of Concanavalin A was bound by both L-int and L-929 cells.

In the other pertinent experiment L-int and L-929 cell cultures were evaluated for their ability to datect (plaque titrate) a selection of various viruses. In the cases of Sindbis, Mengo, EMC and vaccinia viruses, each cell strain served equally well. With reovirus types 2 and 3 it was observed that, as was the case with VSV, about 30 to 40 percent more virus was detectable by plaque assays on L-int cell cultures as compared to L-929 cells. In every example cited the data suggest that membrane alterations are indeed caused by interferon.

How stable are the purported membrane changes?   The experiments that have been described, were not designed to test if altered cellular characteristics were stable, but merely to show that the properties, found in cells after prolonged growth in interferon containing medium (L-int), were not lost after 2 - 3 cell generations in the absence of this interferon. To test the

stability of L-int cell characteristics, these cells were subcultured once in the absence of interferon and, as usual, clear
plaques were produced. If these L-int cultures were then trypsinized and subcultured a second time in the absence of interferon, it was found that VSV produced the cloudy plaques typical
of growth in progenitor L-929 cells. The production of clear
plaques with VSV was therefore not a stable characteristic and
was lost if L-int cells were cultured 4-6 cell generations in
the absence of interferon. The unresponsiveness of L-int cells
to the antiviral and growth depression action of interferon remained, however, unchanged.

The question that immediately occurred to us was whether
or not prolonged growth in the presence of interferon, hitherto
used, was necessary to procure membrane related interferon effects in L-929 cells. To answer this question we took normal L-
929 cultures and treated them overnight with interferon diluted
with MEM, trypsinized them, and after monolayers had formed they
were used to assay VSV. As can be seen from Table 3 in which the
results of three experiments are recorded, clear plaques were
produced. It can also be appreciated from Table 3 that such a
conversion of L-929 cells is a dose dependent phenomenon and the
cells are altered with less than 10 PRD_{50} units of interferon
per ml.

We soon found that a similar experiment to that described
in Figure 3 can be performed with almost identical results with
L-int cells replaced by L-929 after short-term growth in the
presence of interferon. These membrane related effects we now
consider to be rapidly induced phenotypic changes and amenable
to study in the context of other such changes caused by interferon.

In order to assure ourselves that the membrane changes we were observing were caused by interferon, and not some substance co-existing in our interferon preparations, we performed two experiments. We repeated the experiment which is described in Figure 3 with highly purified interferon obtained from Dr. K. Paucker. The response of L-929 cells treated overnight with 10 PRD_{50} units of this interferon having a specific activity of 10^7 NIH units per mg protein was in all essential respects the same as that detailed for L-int cells in Figure 3.

The second experiment involved fractionating our interferon on Sephadex G200 and testing the fractions individually for two different activities considered to be typical for interferon and for the ability to induce clear plaques with VSV. The antiviral activity and the property of inducing an increased sensitivity to the cytotoxicity of poly I:poly C and clear-plaque-induction activity were all found in the same fractions as illustrated by Figure 4. As illustrated, these fractions contain material with a molecular weight of from 35,000 to 40,000 daltons the correct figure for L-cell interferon which we employ.

Considering both experiments and the other biological properties stated earlier we can be reasonably sure that interferon is, in fact, causing these described membrane alterations in L-cells.

Discussion

We have presented evidence that changes, attributable to functional alterations of the cell membrane, occur when L-929 cells are exposed to preparations containing interferon. These changes are observable within 2-3 L-cell mean generation times after such treatment. Other evidence firmly suggests that the active principle causing these changes also has antiviral and

other anti-cell properties and can reasonably be identified as
interferon itself.

    The ability of interferon to affect cells in various ways
in addition to rendering them unresponsive to virus infection,
is now generally accepted. The list of actions of interferon has
grown so complex that a topical question that has arisen is
whether or not there is some underlying interdependency. Does
interferon ,in fact, trigger a cellular target which is capable
of initiating a cascade-like response causing alteration in a
variety of fundamental biological processes? For some time we,
as well as others, have considered it plausible to suppose that
such a mechanism or target exists that is the common initiator
of numerous biological responses. It has been our opinion that
a likely candidate for such a target is the cell membrane.

    In the past there has been little direct evidence to sup-
port this theory and our hypothesis was basically dependent on
two points. First, there is no convincing evidence that interferon actually passes beyond the cell membrane (2). Secondly, although the list of actions of interferon is complex, an assumption that is not contradicted by available data, is that all of
them could be initiated by cell membrane changes as a result of
a primary interaction with interferon.

    In our opinion, the recent publication of Stewart et al.
(11) showing that interferon treatment of cells quickly and
directly leads to an enhanced toxicity of double-stranded RNA
supports the view that interferon alters cell membranes. However,
these investigators found that all other membrane active materials tested except for vaccinia virus, failed to reveal any membrane alteration after interferon treatment. In this respect,
their findings differ from ours. However, it should be recognized
that unlike Stewart, we subcultured the cells after interferon

treatment. In fact, we have observed that cells treated overnight
with interferon alone without a subsequent period of incubation
in medium free of interferon does not produce cultures with an
increased susceptibility to DEAE-dextran.

More intensive investigation will hopefully clarify if induced membrane changes are of importance in the initial mechanism
of interferon action. In any event, studies on the changes caused
by interferon to the cell membranes will provide new insights
and bring us closer to resolving the question of how interferon
treatment alters cells. An answer to this question is of practical importance since interferon is considered by many to be a
potential agent for the therapeutic treatment of neoplasia.

Acknowledgements

The authors thank Lynne Johns and Paula Bird for their
fine technical assistance. This work was supported by a grant
(MT 1615) from the Medical Research Council of Canada.

References

1. Chany, C. and Vignal, M. (1970). J.gen. Virol. 7, 203.
2. Friedman, R.M. and Sonnabend, J.A. (1970).Arch. Int.
    Med. 120, 51.
3. Gresser,I., Brouty-Boyle, D., Thomas, M.T. and
    Macieira-Coelho, A.(1970 b). J.Nat.Cancer Inst.45,1145.
4. Gresser, I., Fontaine-Brouty-Boyle, D., Thomas, M.T.
    and Macieira-Coelho, A. (1970a).Proc.Nat.Acad.Sci.U.

S.A. 66, 1052.

5. Huang ,A.S. and Wagner, R.R. (1966). Virology 30, 173.

6. Lee, S.H.S., O'Shaughnessy, M.V. and Rozee, K.R. (1972) Proc.Soc.Exp.Biol.Med. 139, 1438.

7. Möller, G., Sjoberg ,O. and Andersson, J. (1972). Eur. J. Immunol. 27, 586.

8. O'Shaughnessy, M.V., Lee, S.H.S. and Rozee, K.R.(1972). Canad. J. Microbiol. 18, 145.

9. Paucker, K., Cantell, K. and Henle, W.(1962). Virology 16, 324.

10. Stewart, W.E., II, Gosser, L.B. and Lockart, R.Z. (1971). J. Virol. 7, 792.

11. Stewart, W.E., II, Le Clercq, E., Billiau, A., Desmyter, J. and De Somer, P. (1972).Proc.Nat.Acad.Sci. U.S.A. 69, 1851.

TABLE 1(a)*

Interferon preparation	Interferon titer[a] in different cultures		Ratio L-929/L-int
	L-int	L-929	
15-2	55	160	2.90
15-3	835	965	1.15
26-3	265	675	2.54
9-4	1660	1995	1.20
26-4	6000	9000	1.50
15-8	440	500	1.13
			Ave.1.74

[a]PRD_{50} per ml.

TABLE 1(b)*

VSV titration	The titer of challenge virus (VSV) in different cultures x 10^6 PFU/ml		Ratio L-929/L-int
	L-int	L-929	
15-2	55	44	0.86
15-3	72	64	0.88
26-3	111	74	0.66
9-4	230	211	0.91
26-4	47	21	0.44
15-8	44	39	0.88
27-9	55	29	0.52
1-10	123	62	0.50
			Ave.0.706

*Sensitivity of L-929 and L-int cell cultures to the antiviral effect of interferon (a) and to VSV (b) as indicated by plaque assay experiments. L-int cells are shown to be less responsive to interferon and more able to detect VSV in virus pools.

TABLE 2

The effect of various membrane-active substances on the a-
bility of L-929 and L-int cells to take up and retain neutral red dye following an 18 hour treatment

Membrane active substance	Dose reducing neutral red uptake by 50% μ/ml*	
	L-929 cells	L-int cells
DEAE-dextran	500-600	50-100
Protamine sulfate	300-400	100-200
Meth. Albumin	600-700	50-100

*Results are expressed as that amount of material required to
reduce the neutral red dye uptake of treated cells by 50 percent
as compared to the same cells, untreated.

TABLE 3

Clear plaque production on L-929 cells after overnight
interferon treatment and subculturing of cells to form
monolayers after three days growth*

Experiment 1		Experiment 2		Experiment 3	
Interferon (units/ml)	% clear plaques	Interferon (units/ml)	% clear plaques	Interferon (units/ml)	% clear plaques
90	100	75	100	360	100
45	100	37.5	100	120	100
22.5	100	18.8	100	40	100
11.3	100	9.4	99	13.3	100
5.6	93	4.7	60	4.4	59
2.8	32	2.4	43	1.5	5
1.4	0	1.2	0	0.5	0

*Monolayer cultures of L-929 cells were treated overnight with
interferon diluted in MEM. Two cultures from each dilution of
interferon as well as control plates were challenged with VSV
the next morning for a normal interferon plaque-reduction assay. A third culture from each group was trypsinized, the
cells washed twice, and plated so that confluent monolayers
were obtained after three days growth. These plates were then
challenged with approximately 100 pfu of VSV. After two days
incubation the plates were scored for clear plaque formation.

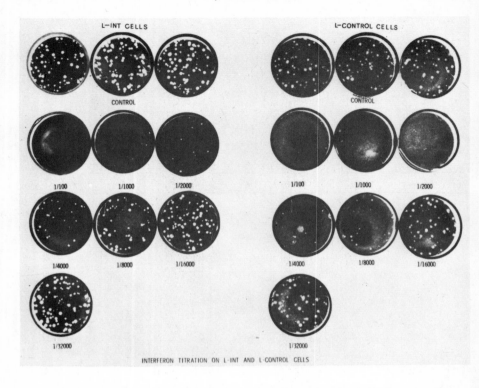

Fig. 1. Growth of VSV plaques in L-929 cell cultures and in interferon-treated L-int cell cultures. L-int cells, derived from the l-929 cell strain, show clear (a) while L-929 cells produce cloudy plaques with VSV (b).

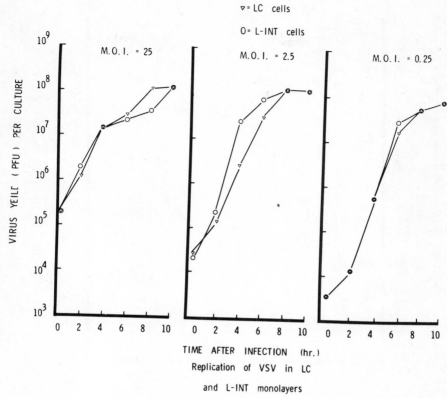

Fig. 2. One-step growth curves of VSV in L-929 cells (△) and L-int (○) cell cultures. The cultures were infected at zero time with different input m.o.i. and the figure demonstrates the essential similarity of replication of VSV in both cell cultures.

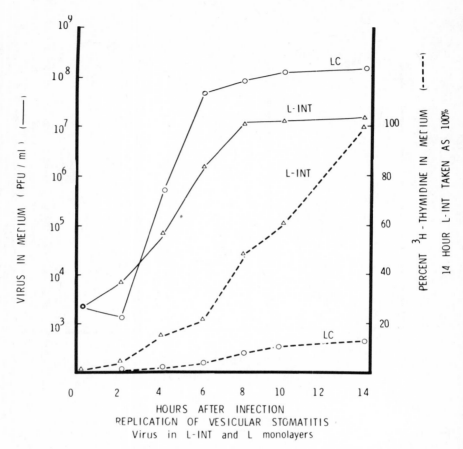

REPLICATION OF VESICULAR STOMATITIS
Virus in L-INT and L monolayers

Fig. 3. A one-step growth curve of VSV in L-929 and L-int cell cultures, pre-labelled with ^{3}H-thymidine. The figure illustrates the release into the medium of labelled material by both cell types during a single cycle of VSV replication.

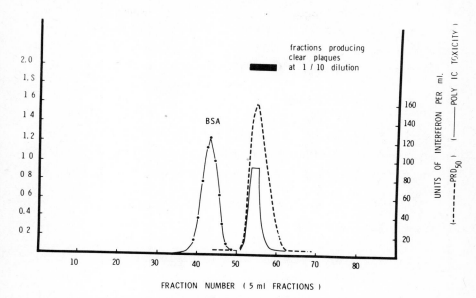

Fig. 4. Sephadex G200 fractionation of L-cell interferon with a bovine serum albumin (BSA) marker. The data reveals that fractions which are able to induce VSV clear-plaque changes, when diluted 1:10, are those fractions which have antiviral activity and are able to effect increased sensitivity to poly I:poly C.

DISCUSSION

Merigan: Your most recent findings of the effect would
make it seem to be not a genetic effect in the sense that true
genetic selection was not really operating to produce it.

Rozee: That's right.

Merigan: But on the other hand, it becomes then quite
reminiscent of the effects like priming and potentiation of poly
I:C toxicity that have been reported. How do you feel about this?

Rozee: I think that this is quite a valid comment. I think
it is a cellular membrane effect that is non-genetic in character.

Chany: A few years ago with Madeleine Vignal, we carried
out a series of MSV-transformed mouse cells and found that these
cells lost the capacity to produce colonies in gelified medium.
They recovered this capacity as soon as the interferon was removed from the medium. Another question concerning your observations is: have you ever looked at the capacity of the cells to
produce colonies? Are they morphologically modified?

Rozee: The L-int cells, the long term L-int cells, can
produce colonies. Cells of these colonies have acquired the a-
bility to grow with almost the same mean generation time as the
parental L-929 cells in the presence of concentrations of interferon that would, in fact, reduce the capacity of parental L-929
cells to grow. So I think that what we originally were looking
at was a modest selection and perhaps our L-int cells are consequently slightly more unresponsive to the antiviral and growth
depression effects of interferon. But at the same time I think
this response was complicated by phenotypic reactions which we
had originally naively assumed to be due to genetic selection.

Oxman: The marked phenotypic change following brief exposure to interferon could be explained by inhibition of some endogenous viral functions. L cells are known to contain endogenous
virus genomes, and thus I wonder if you have looked at primary
mouse or primary rabbit cells. This would certainly be worth
doing ,since the results might be easier to interpret.

Rozee: No, we haven't look at primary mouse cells. I hope
to, but we haven't yet. Our L cells, like everybody else's L
cells, are carrying a heavy load of latent viruses.

Oxman: Are they also carrying mycoplasmas?

Rozee: Well, I doubt it, but we have no evidence that they
do or don't. We do have evidence that they carry a heavy load of
C particles. We have other interesting data dealing with C particles, but I don't want to steal Ken Easterbrook's thunder.
Later on this year, he will present data with respect to C particles in L cells and interferon.

Pereira: Could I ask how uniform are L cells in this respect, although the question of genetic selection doesn't seem
to operate? If you pick many clones of these L cells, are they
uniform in these characters that you described? Do you get spontaneous variation or don't you know?

Rozee: I haven't done that. It wouldn't be surprising to
me if they were not uniform.

Pereira: Most cell lines vary quite a lot in that respect.
Have you compared your cells with the original ones in respect
with various interactions with the virus like the rate of adsorption ,penetration, growth cycle, etc.?

Rozee: Just with respect to the plaquing efficiency and

the yield. Just these two characteristics.

ENHANCEMENT BY INTERFERON OF THE EXPRESSION OF SURFACE ANTIGENS ON MURINE LEUKEMIA L 1210 CELLS

Pernilla Lindahl, Patricia Leary and Ion Gresser

Institut de Recherches Scientifiques sur le Cancer
94800 Villejuif, France

In addition to the well known antiviral action, interferon preparations have also been shown to exert a variety of biological effects on cells. The nature of some of these effects suggested the possibility that interferon treatment might engender modifications of the cell surface.

To test this hypothesis we have determined the effect of interferon on the surface antigen expression of mouse leukemia L 1210 cells by measuring their allo-antibody absorbing capacity.

Antibody absorbing capacity of L 1210 cells after interferon treatment.

Mouse lymphoid leukemia L 1210 cells (2 x 10^5 cells per ml) were cultivated for 24 hours with interferon, control preparation or left untreated. The antibody absorbing capacity of cells from each group was determined by incubating 1 x 10^7 cells with 0.25 ml of a dilution of a C57BL/6 anti-L 1210 serum and titering the residual antibody content by cytotoxicity for ^{51}Cr-labelled L 1210 cells in the presence of complement.

As illustrated in Fig.1A, interferon treated L 1210 cells

absorbed considerably more antibody than the same number of untreated or mock interferon treated cells. Similar results were
obtained when a C57BL/6-anti-Balb/c lymphocyte serum was used
instead of the C57BL/6-anti-L 1210 serum, that is interferon
treated cells again absorbed out more antibody than untreated
or mock interferon treated cells.

Fig. 2 illustrates the kinetics of the development of the
increased antibody absorbing capacity. Interferon treatment during 2 and 6 hr did not enhance the antibody absorbing capacity
of L 1210 cells, whereas an increase in antibody absorbing capacity was observed after 18 hr of treatment and was further
increased when cells were treated with interferon for 24 hours.

Fig. 3 illustrates the effect of varying amounts of interferon (after 24 hours of cultivation of L 1210 cells with interferon) on the antibody absorbing capacity of L 1210 cells.

Correlation between the antiviral activity of interferon preparations and their effect on the antibody absorbing capacity of
L 1210 cells.

All mouse interferon preparations tested were found to
enhance the antibody absorbing capacity of L 1210 cells. Purified mouse interferon preparations ($> 10^6$ units per mg protein)
were as effective as crude preparations of the same titer. Control preparations and heterologous interferon did not exert a
significant effect.

The factor·in the interferon preparations responsible for
the enhancement of antibody absorbing capacity displayed the
same physico-chemical characteristics as interferon and the activity could not be dissociated from interferon. Thus, procedures
used to inactivate interferon (i.e., trypsin, sodium periodate,

heating) inactivated the antiviral activity of interferon and the
factor that enhanced antibody absorbing capacity. Furthermore, as
illustrated in Fig. 1B, untreated interferon resistant L 1210-R
cells exhibited the same degree of absorbing capacity as interferon sensitive L 1210 cells (Fig. 1A) but interferon treatment
did not enhance their antibody absorbing capacity.

Specificity of the enhanced antibody absorbing capacity of L 1210 cells for anti-L 1210 sera.

The enhanced absorbing capacity of interferon treated L
1210 cells was immunologically specific. Thus interferon treated
L 1210 cells did not absorb an anti-EL4 tumor cell serum (anti-
C57BL). Likewise, interferon treated EL4 cells displayed an enhanced absorbing capacity for DBA/2-anti-EL4 serum but did not
absorb anti-L 1210 serum.

Effect of interferon on antibody absorbing capacity of L 1210 cells during logarithmic growth and at saturation density.

Fig. 4A shows the inhibitory effect of interferon on L 1210
cell multiplication. Both untreated and interferon treated cells
attained the plateau at 72 hours. As can be seen in Fig. 4B the
antibody absorbing capacity of control cells was slightly greater at saturation density at 72 hours and at 96 hours than in the
logarithmic growth phase. Interferon treated L 1210 cells (dashed lines) showed a marked increase in antibody absorbing capacity at 24 hours which was far greater than that observed for control cells at either 72 or 96 hours. The effect of interferon
was even greater at 72 and 96 hours.

L 1210 cells were seeded at a concentration of 2×10^6
cells/ml (saturation density) and at 2×10^5 cells/ml, and both
cultures were incubated with 2,500 units of interferon per ml

for 24 hours. Interferon treated cells seeded at saturation density displayed a greater antibody absorbing capacity than interferon treated cells in log phase growth (cells seeded at $2x10^5$
cells/ml) and both groups of interferon treated cells had a
greater antibody absorbing capacity than control cells at saturation density.

Relative concentration of surface antigen expression in inter-feron treated L 1210 cells.

To estimate the relative concentration of surface antigens
on the L 1210 cells a series of experiments was performed with
varying numbers of untreated and interferon treated cells for
absorption of a C57BL/6 anti-L 1210 serum.

As shown in Fig. 5 , there was no difference in the antibody absorbing capacity of control L 1210 cells after 24 and 48
hours of culture , and 4.8×10^5 cells were required to attain a
50% specific lysis at the antiserum dilution chosen. The number
of interferon treated L 1210 cells required for 50% lysis was
much less, 3.3×10^5 cells after cultivation with interferon for
48 hours. These figures indicate an increase of surface antigen
expression of 45% and 180% in interferon treated cells at 24 and
48 hours respectively.

Our data do not permit us to state which surface antigens
on L 1210 cells were increased by interferon treatment. The fact
that interferon treated L 1210 cells (H2-D) displayed an enhanced
antibody absorbing capacity for serum from C57BL/6 mice (H2-B)
immunized with L 1210 cells as well as for serum from C57BL/6
mice immunized with Balb/c (H2-D) splenic lymphocytes suggests
that we are measuring the expression of histocompatibility antigens on the surface of L 1210 cells.

Cikes and his coworkers found that the expression of surface antigens of a mouse leukemic cell line varied considerably during the growth cycle, but in general antigenic concentration increased as the growth rate declined. In agreement with their findings, antigen expression of L 1210 cells also increased as the cell population approached cell saturation density. Since interferon inhibits the multiplication of L 1210 cells (see Fig. 4A) it is possible that the effect of interferon on surface antigen expression is secondary to its effect on cell division. On the other hand we should point out that interferon treated cells displayed a far greater antibody absorbing capacity than untreated cells even when the former were tested in logarithmic growth phase (Fig. 4B). Furthermore, interferon enhanced the antibody absorbing capacity of L 1210 cells even when these were seeded at saturation density. Thus it is also possible that interferon may have a direct effect on the regulation of the expression of surface antigens.

In conclusion, the data presented show that interferon treatment of L 1210 cells is accompanied by modifications of the cell surface, measurable as an increased expression of surface allo-antigens. It would certainly be of interest to determine whether interferon might also modify the expression of other surface antigens and receptors. In particular, a possible effect of interferon on the expression of tumor specific antigens is relevant to the understanding of the mechanism behind the well documented antitumor effect of interferon in mice.

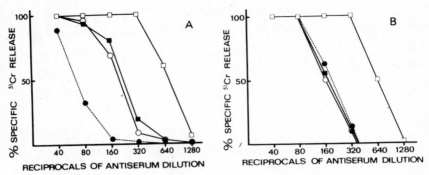

Fig. 1. Effect of interferon treatment (24hr) on the anti-body absorbing capacity of A. L 1210; B. interferon resistant L 1210-R cells. The symbols indicate the cytotoxic activity of C57BL/6-anti L 1210 serum on target L 1210 cells after: □ = no absorption; O = after absorption with 1x10^7 L 1210 cells; ■ = after absorption with 1x10^7 L 1210 cells treated with a control normal brain preparation; ● = after absorption with 1x 10^7 L 1210 cells treated with 2,500 units of C57BL/6 mouse brain interferon.

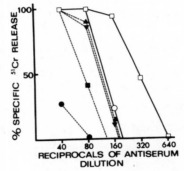

Fig. 2. Kinetics of the effect of interferon on the antibody absorbing capacity of L 1210 cells. The cytotoxicity of a C57BL/6-anti-L 1210 serum was determined on target L 1210 cells after: □ = no absorption; O = after absorption with 1x10^7 L 1210 cells; ▲ = after absorption with 1x10^7 L 1210 cells treated with 2,500 units of brain interferon for 2 hours; ▼ = after absorption with 1x10^7 cells treated with interferon for 6 hours; ■ = after absorption with 1x10^7 cells treated with interferon for 18 hours; ● = after absorption with 1x10^7 cells treated with interferon for 24 hours.

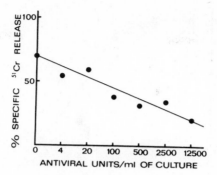

Fig. 3. Titration of the effect of interferon on the antibody absorbing capacity of L 1210 cells. A C57BL/6-anti-L 1210 serum dilution was assayed for specific cytotoxic activity on L 1210 cells after absorption with 1×10^7 L 1210 cells treated for 24 hours with varying doses of interferon.

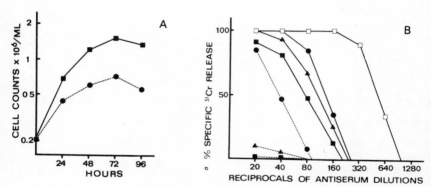

Fig. 4. Effect of interferon on multiplication and antibody absorbing capacity of L 1210 cells. A. Growth curve; ■ = untreated; ● = 2,500 units of mouse brain interferon per ml; B. Cytotoxic activity of a C57BL/6-anti-L 1210 serum on target L 1210 cells after: □ = no absorption; absorption with 1×10^7 control cells (solid lines): ● = at 24 hours; ▲ = at 72 hours; ■ = at 96 hours of culture; absorption with 1×10^7 interferon treated cells (dashed lines) at the same times, i.e., interferon treated cells at 24 hours, etc.

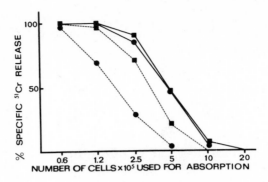

Fig. 5.   Quantitative absorption with interferon treated L
1210 cells. A C57BL/6-anti-L 1210 serum was absorbed with varying numbers of untreated L 1210 cells (continuous lines) and interferon treated L 1210 cells (dashed lines), after 24 (■) and
48 hours (●) of culture with 1,000 units of mouse brain interferon per ml.

DISCUSSION

Merigan: One question I have immediately is how do you
relate these findings to the prior observations in your laboratory in the past, that interferon will potentiate the toxicity
of sensitized lymphocytes for tumor cell monolayers?

Lindahl: The simplest answer is that it was those results
that prompted us to continue with surface antigens and I think
the first problem when trying to relate the two is that the kinetics are entirely different. For the enhanced cell mediated
cytotoxicity 2 or 3 hours of interferon action is enough to
reach a maximal effect. On the other hand you can't compare highly specialized lymphocytes that have just passed through the process of sensitization with the L 1210 cells that are transformed
cells that grow steadily in suspension. Furthermore, the kinetics

may mean nothing in terms of the effect of interferon , as it may
only be a matter of the property you're looking at. What is the
turnover rate for the different receptors you're looking at?
They may be entirely different for the specific receptors for
cell mediated cytotoxicity and for surface antigens like H 2.

Stewart: With Dr. Katz at Halifax I did some studies a-
long the same idea that interferon treatment might somehow expose surface antigens that aren't normally present and that this
might cause the cells to become sensitive to the toxicity of the
double-stranded RNA that we observe in interferon treated cells.
We thought that perhaps since in the cell cycle there are antigens exposed at times that aren't normally present, in a syn-
chronized culture we might be able to detect the toxicity at a
particular time without interferon pre-treatment. What we found
is that after a synchronization at all times in the cell cycle
the interferon treated cells were susceptible to the lytic activity with poly I:C but that at no time in the cell cycle were
normal cells susceptible to the lytic activity. So this did appear to explain one of our hypotheses.

Levy: In your experiments when you tried to relate to the
growth cycle did you try to synchronize the cells?

Lindahl: We have been thinking about that. I think the
possibilities you have to synchronize the cells would bother me
and in fact, what we are trying to do instead, is to utilize the
techniques that Caspersson has available in Stockholm, which
would involve measurement of quantitative immunofluorescence in
individual cells, at the same time determining the phase in the
growth cycle by cytochemical methods on individual cells, and
I hope that will give us a final answer.

Rozee: I just want to make a comment with respect to

cytotoxic antibody complement dependent lysis of cells. When we
use L-929 cells and L-int cells and did complement dependent
cytolytic antibody tests, we couldn't find any difference in the
levels of activity with the two cell types. In other words, they
were equally sensitive to the same levels of antibody. Perhaps
this type of test is not sensitive enough to pick up changes in
the surface of the cells.

Lindahl: First of all, we are not dealing with complement
lysis in these experiments. As you will appreciate, the adsorption
is done without complement. It is only the final assay for residual cytotoxicity that involves complement lysis. The other
problem is: I'm not sure what you would find if you do a titration of your antiserum on treated versus untreated cells. I don't
know how many sites you would need per cell in order to get a
100% lysis of the cells, but probably, if you have 50 versus
100 sites, you wouldn't see a difference in the titration of
your antiserum.

Rozee: This was my point, the fact that these membrane
changes are subtle enough that techniques like the complement
lysis probably do not pick them up.

Lindahl: No.

Oxman: Is it possible to do these experiments with primary cells?

Lindahl: We are doing this presently and the cells we've
chosen for obvious reasons are lymphocytes, as you would not
want to trypsinize the cells for these experiments. But it is
too early to give any details on the results.

De Clercq: I wanted to return to the immunolytic effect
of sensitized lymphocytes versus tumor target cells. As you have

published, this lytic effect of lymphocytes versus target cells
is enhanced by previous treatment of the lymphocytes with interferon. In this case, interferon causes an enhancement of the immune responsiveness of lymphocytes. How do you reconcile this
observation with the fact that interferon is immuno-suppressive
in many other conditions as reported during this meeting and
elsewhere (cfr. Lindahl-Magnusson, Leary, and Gresser, 1972,
Nature New Biology 137, 120; Chester, Paucker and Merigan 1973,
Nature 246, 92).

Lindahl: I think the important point is that the immune
response consists of several different phases; that is in order
for those lymphocytes to become sensitized they probably have to
undergo cell division. I think most people agree on that by now.
When they have undergone cell division, the cells gradually become able to express their specialized function. Thus, the examples described so far of immune depression with interferon
concern the early phase of cell division, whereas the enhancing
phenomena concerning lymphocytes are essentially a matter of the
terminal phase of the response. If I may go back to Michael
Oxman's suggestion this morning, which I liked very much, interferon may not only differ between cell division information and
resting cell information, it might even favor and enhance resting
cell information. Do you see my point? That is, if you look at
a lymphocyte when it is expressing cytotoxicity, for example,
it is certainly not at all the same cell as the one that in the
early phase of the response is supposed to undergo cell division.

Chany: Although that is not very much in agreement with
the findings that interferon depresses many of the cellular
functions in confluent resting cells, too; for instance, the
synthesis of ribosomal or messenger RNA.

Merigan: I asked my question in the beginning with a little different thrust. It was more to the question of what the
target cells are doing in the presence of interferon. If these
tumor cells are doing what you have been describing here, then
they provide a greater antigenic drive for the lymphocyte to be
reactive which could overcome any immunodepressent effect of
the interferon. An immunodepressent effect would most likely be
observed in the early phase of division of lymphocyte cell lines,
which might very well be important in the animal and not manifested in an in vitro assay. I think the effector limb is depressed in the in vitro assay and, if you're driving it with a
greater antigenic stimulus, it is reasonable that it will be
more brisk.

Lindahl: Yes. When you talk about the target cells, do
you mean in the in vivo situation?

Merigan: I meant specifically in your in vitro assay where
you've noted that interferon addition to sensitized lymphocytes
potentiates the action of sensitized lymphocytes on target cell
monolayers.

Lindahl: O.K. In those experiments first of all the whole
experiment is performed within a 6-hour period and during that
time there is absolutely no increase in the antigenic setup of
the target cell. We can also in that situation use interferon resistant L 1210 cells and that will not influence the results.
That is, in that situation the whole effect of interferon is on
the lymphocyte.

MODIFICATION OF THE RESPONSE OF DIPHTHERIA-TREATED HYBRID MONKEY-MOUSE CELLS BY HUMAN OR MOUSE INTERFERON

P. Boquet

Institut National de la Santé
et de la Recherche Médicale
U. 43 de Recherches sur
les Infections Virales
Hôpital St. Vincent de Paul
74, Avenue Denfert-Rochereau
75014 Paris, France

Diphtheria toxin inhibits protein synthesis in sensitive monkey or human cells by inactivating Transferase II (EF II) in the presence of nicotinamide adenine dinucleotide (1,2). Two steps are required for this inhibition process: firstly, the binding of the toxin proteins on specific cell membrane components, as shown by Gill et al. (3,4); and secondly, an active penetration of toxin in the cytoplasm. Immediately after, Transferase II is inhibited. Sensitive monkey or human cells have specific binding sites for toxin, whereas insensitive mouse cells have not.

It has been reported by Yabrov (5) that interferon-treated cells are protected against the cytopathic effect of diphtheria toxin. More recently, Moehring, Moehring and Stinebring (6) also have shown that homologous interferon decreases the toxic effect of diphtheria and suggest that protection involves a mechanism related to the cell membrane.

In our experiments, using somatic monkey-mouse hybrid cells, we were able to confirm this latter hypothesis, thus showing

mainly the involvement of cell membrane structures in this protective effect.

Material and methods.

Cell lines. Monkey-mouse cells, MKCV III clone 4, is a
somatic hybrid cell, sensitive to human and mouse interferon (7)
and also to diphtheria toxin.

BSC-1 cells were routinely propagated in the laboratory.
All cells were grown in Eagle's medium (MEM with 10% calf serum). Hybrid cells, MKCV III clone 4, were cultivated in the
presence of HATG (8).

Interferon. Mouse and human purified interferon were used
at the concentration of 500 units/ml.

Toxin. Pure diphtheria toxin was a gift of Dr. E.M.
Relyveld (Pasteur Institute). The titer was 115 floculation u-
nits/ml.

Toxicity assay procedure. Diphtheria toxin, at different
doses, and 0.1 mCi/ml of ^{14}C-leucine (CEA Saclay, France - 294
mCi/ml) were added to cells cultivated in 35 mm plastic Falcon
Petri dishes and maintained for 6 hr at 37°C. TCA (10%) was added
to the cells which were then chilled for 1 hr, scraped with a
rubber policeman, collected in glass tubes, and finally heated
at 90°C for 15 minutes. The precipitate was filtered on Watman
GF/C filters, washed 3 times with 5% TCA and once with ethanol,
dried and counted in a liquid scintillator counter.

Results.

Since monkey cells possess receptors and mouse cells do not,
it was of interest to investigate the response of monkey-mouse

hybrid cells in the presence of diphtheria toxin. It has been
shown that different hybrid clones are mostly mouse cells, carrying only 5-20% of the total monkey antigens (Wicker, unpublished
data). It is clear that the effect of either human or mouse interferon on such cells treated with toxin can be used to study
which species parts are involved in the protective action of interferon against toxin.

Somatic hybrid monkey-mouse MKCV III (clone 4, 57th passage) are used in these experiments. Firstly, the hybrid cells
are cultivated with either human interferon (500 units/ml) or
mouse interferon (500 units/ml) for 20 hours. Toxin is added at
different concentrations (10^{-7} M to 10^{-10} M). Untreated control
cells are simultaneously employed. The rate of protein synthesis
is expressed as the ratio of control minus toxin treated cells/
control. Homologous monkey interferon has a protective effect on
the intoxication process, while mouse interferon has very little.
The decrease of cellular protein synthesis in the presence of
either of the two interferons, but in the absence of toxin, is
comparable (about 20%). The protective effect decreases with increasing concentrations of toxin (Figure 1).

Effect of interferon treatment on the kinetics of inactivation of EF II by diphtheria toxin. Pappenheimer et al. (9) have
shown that inactivation of the EF II factor occurs after a lag
period which represents the time necessary to inactivate free
EF II. The decrease of protein synthesis is of a first order
process, depending on the time and the toxin dose used. The slope
of the curve is in relationship with the concentration of toxin
in the cell.

The effects of toxin on the rate of inactivation of the
EF II factor by diphtheria toxin on monkey BSC-1 cells are shown
in Figure 2. Different concentrations of toxin are added to cells

cultivated in Petri dishes. In the same experiment, two sets of preparation are used: one consists of cells pretreated with homologous interferon (human interferon 500 units/ml) for 20 hr; and the other without such a pretreatment. At 1, 2 and 5 hr after the addition of toxin, a pulse of ^{14}C-leucine is made for 1 hour. The amount of protein synthesis is estimated, as described in Material and methods. Pretreatment by homologous interferon for 20 hr changes the slope of the curve obtained with 10^{-7} M or 2.10^{-8} M. It may be assumed that under these conditions, less toxin penetrates into the cells (Figure 2).

Discussion and Conclusions.

We have shown, using monkey-mouse hybrid cells, that the protective effect of a pretreatment with interferon in the same hybrid cell is obtained only with primate interferon. Thus, in these cells the small amount of monkey components present in the membrane support both intoxication and interferon action. Interferon seems to decrease the number of inner cell toxin molecules which inactivate free EF II in the cell.

Two hypotheses may be proposed. Firstly, primate interferon produces a non-specific modification of the monkey cell components which interfere with the number (or the shape) of cellular toxin receptor sites. Secondly, primate interferon may compete with toxin for these binding sites. This latter hypothesis may be ruled out by the following arguments. A treatment by interferon for 20 hr is necessary (6), since before 17 hr, protection is almost non-existant. There is no direct effect of interferon on toxin when the two are mixed. In addition, a somatic monkey-mouse hybrid cell, resistant to toxin after several passages in the presence of low doses of diphtheria toxin, was recently isolated (unpublished data). This clone is fully sensitive to primate in-

terferon; thus the binding sites for toxin and interferon are
probably different. It could be postulated, therefore, that the
protective effect of homologous interferon against toxin in the
monkey cells is mainly due to modifications in the cell membrane,
resulting in a decrease of the ability of cells to bind diphtheria
toxin molecules.

References

1. Honjo, J., Nishizuka, Y., Hayaishi, O. and Kato, I.
    (1968). Biol. Chem. 243, 3553.
2. Gill, D.M., Pappenheimer, A.M.,Jr., Brown, R. and
    Kurnick, J.T. (1969). J.Exp.Med. 129, 1.
3. Gill, D.M., Pappenheimer, A.M., Jr. and Uchida, T.
    (1973). Fed. Proc. 32, 1508.
4. Ittelson, T.R. and Gill, D.M. (1973). Nature 242, 330.
5. Yabrov, A.A. (1966). Tsitologiya 8, 767.
6. Moehring, T.J., Moehring, J.M. and Stinebring, W.R.
    (1971). Infection and Immunity 4, 747.
7. Cassingena, R., Chany, C., Vignal, M., Suarez, H.,
    Estrade, S. and Lazar, P. (1971). Proc. Nat. Acad. Sci.
    USA 68, 580.
8. Littlefield, J.W. (1965). Biochem.Biophys.Acta 95, 14.
9. Uchida, T., Pappenheimer, A.M., Jr. and Harper, A.A.
    (1973). J. Biol. Chem. 248, 3845.

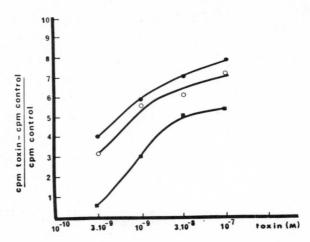

Fig. 1. Effect of primate or mouse interferon on the rate of protein synthesis in hybrid MKCV III clone 4 cells after 6 h of treatment with various doses of diphtheria toxin. ●——● control toxin; ○——○ mouse interferon + toxin; ■——■ primate interferon + toxin.

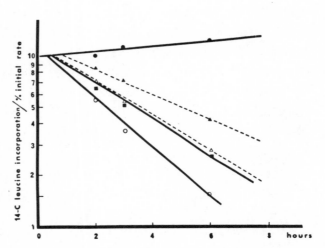

Fig. 2. Kinetic inactivation of EF II factor by diphtheria toxin in BSC-1 cells treated and untreated with primate interferon. Pulses of ^{14}C-leucine are made at 1, 2 and 5 hours after the addition of toxin. ●——● control; ▲--▲ 2.10^{-8} M toxin + primate interferon; △---△ 10^{-7} M toxin + primate interferon; ■——■ 2.10^{-8} M toxin; ○——○ 10^{-7} M toxin.

DISCUSSION

Tan: Have you looked at the antagonistic effect of interferon on cycloheximide and emetine in these hybrid cells?

Boquet: I have not looked at the effect of interferon on
such molecules, which are known to depress the translation. It is
well known that interferon acts at the level of translation and
probably only on elongation. Toxin acts on the Transferase II;
this enzyme is necessary for the step of translocation by binding GTP on ribosomes. When Transferase II is bound on ribosomes,
toxin is unable to inactivate Transferase II. The pool of free
Transferase II in cytoplasm is not very important; after each
translocation step, ribosomal-bound Transferase is released in
the cytoplasm. Thus, toxin activity may be in relationship with
the rate of elongation. If in interferon treated cells, elongation
is less important, it is possible that toxin has less effect on
Transferase II; but I think this is not very important.

Vilček: I have a question first and then perhaps a comment. You treated your cells with interferon for 20 hours. Does
it take 20 hours for this effect to get established or could you
treat for a shorter time?

Boquet: We have treated the cells for 4, 10 and 20 hours,
and like Moehring and Stinebring only at 20 hours we have the
protective effect. After 10 hours of treatment, the protective
effect is very low.

Vilček: Of treatment with interferon?

Boquet: Yes.

Vilček: Now, wouldn't that speak against an effect on the
receptor site? Since for the interferon to bind to the receptor

site, we know now, it takes around 30 minutes, perhaps even a
little less. Why would it then take so long for this effect to
take place if it is an effect on the receptor?

Boquet: I think this is not a direct competition on a same
receptor site, but a modification of the membrane induced by
interferon. Only after 18 hours the modification of the membrane
is able to modify the binding or the uptake of toxin.

Revel: Do you know if the penetration of diphtheria toxin
as an active process requires induction of protein synthesis
which itself may be blocked by interferon treatment?

Boquet: I think this is a very difficult question to answer. The target of diphtheria toxin is the translation at the
level of Transferase II. For this reason, it is not possible to
block protein synthesis by inhibitors. Actually the problem of
penetration of toxin has been fully studied by Pappenheimer et
al. Receptor sites are required for the uptake of toxin. Energy
is certainly necessary for the active process of uptake, but I
don't know if induction of protein synthesis is required. In
this case, toxin is able to block its own uptake.

Tan: A technical question. The amount of toxin you used
in these experiments was inhibiting about 30% of protein synthesis?

Boquet: No, for doses of 10^{-7} M of toxin, about 70%.

Tan: But that is not very much reversed by human interferon?

Boquet: No.

Tan: It is only when you went to about 10^{-8} where you get

30 to 40% inhibition. Only with lower percentage of inhibition did you see this effect with human interferon.

Boquet: No, human interferon is fully active from 10^{-8} M.

Tan: What happens in the case of mouse interferon? Would mouse interferon reverse it?

Boquet: Mouse interferon has just a little effect, but not comparable to human interferon on hybrid cells.

Tan: Could you see any reversal of this effect by mouse interferon at very low concentrations?

Boquet: We have with mouse interferon on hybrid cells a small effect as shown in Figure 1. This effect is the same for all concentrations of toxin. This data can be explained perhaps by an action at the level of translation.

Ankel: Do I remember correctly that the inactivation of Transferase II is a transfer of ADP-ribose to Transferase II from NAD? Is it possible that the effect of interferon could be a secondary effect on the concentration of NAD in the cell?

Boquet: No. I think not.

Ankel: There is precedence for that because if you grow cells in the presence of galactose as compared to the presence of glucose you have a change of morphology and of the ratio of NAD and NADH. So I mean, it is possible that morphological changes might also change the cell metabolism.

Boquet: Why in this case we have no modification on hybrid cells with mouse interferon.

Levy: Just to answer Dr. Ankel's question. If there were

an effect on NAD, did you expect it to be manifested in ways
other than just on this manifestation? There has been, as you
know, early reports that interferon affected lactic acid production and oxidative phosphorylation. All of these effects have
been eliminated and there appears to be no effect on respiratory
or glycolytic activity. If there were significant effects on NAD,
I think you would see this.

Merigan: We tried an experiment with NAD because of this
obvious possible interrelationship. Here, we grew and maintained
cells in very high concentrations of NAD, but couldn't alter the
interferon sensitivity of the cells by the exogenous NAD. We
didn't prove that our intracellular pool size went up. So this
experiment is not complete from that standpoint.

PRODUCTION OF INTERFERON-LIKE SUBSTANCE BY MOUSE SPLEEN CELLS THROUGH CONTACT WITH BHK CELLS CHRONICALLY INFECTED WITH HVJ

Yasuhiko Ito, Yoshinobu Kimura,
Akira Kunii and Ikuya Nagata

Germfree Life Research Institute (Y.I.,Y.K.,I.N.)
and 1st Department of Internal Medicine (A.K.)
Nagoya University School of Medicine
Showa-ku, Nagoya, Japan

This study is concerned with the production of an interferon-like substance in mixed cultures of mouse spleen cells and BHK-HVJ cells [baby hamster kidney cells chronically infected with HVJ (Sendai virus)] .

Spleen cells from C57BL/6 mice were used. The anti-HVJ HI titers of sera from the mice yielding these cells were less than 1:4.

The characteristics of BHK-HVJ cells were described previously (1). In brief, more than 80% of the cells in most passages exhibited a hemadsorbing capacity when tested after cells had been grown to confluence. The viral products released from the cells were noninfectious components.

Monolayer cultures of normal BHK cells and BHK-HVJ cells were washed once with fresh MEM and incubated at 35°C with 1 x 10^8 mouse spleen cells in 4 ml of the growth medium. Twenty-four hours later, the supernatant fluid was assayed for virus inhibitor, which I shall designate as "VI".

As shown in Table 1, the culture fluid from mouse spleen
cells co-cultivated with BHK-HVJ cells completely inhibited
plaque formation of VSV in mouse L cell monolayers, while no VI
activity was detected in the fluid from mouse spleen cells co-
cultivated with normal BHK cells. VI present in the culture fluid
inhibited plaque formation in mouse L cells infected with VSV
but not in hamster BHK cells. This finding indicates that VI is
produced by mouse spleen cells and not by BHK cells. The supernatant fluids of control cultures of spleen cells alone and BHK-
HVJ cells alone were shown to be free of VI.

In another experiment, BHK-HVJ cells suspended in the medium were sonicated in an ice bath for 30 seconds with an ultrasonic oscillator. The sonicated BHK-HVJ cells were added to mouse
spleen cell culture, and no VI production could be detected in
the fluid after 24 hours incubation at $35°C$.

Mouse L cells, mouse lymphnode cells, mouse thymocytes and
mouse liver cells were also tested for their capacity to produce
VI when they were co-cultivated with BHK-HVJ cells. The results
shown in Table 2, indicate that only lymphoid cells, i.e., the
cells of the spleen, lymphnode and thymus, are able to produce
VI in this system, while non-lymphoid somatic cells, i.e., fi-
broblastic L cells and liver cells appear to lack this competence.

In a similar experiment, mouse spleen cells were co-cultivated with normal HeLa cells or HeLa-HVJ cells (a cell line of
HeLa cells chronically infected with HVJ). Virus inhibitory activity could be detected in the culture fluid from spleen cells
co-cultivated with HeLa-HVJ, but not in that from cultures with
uninfected HeLa cells (Table 3).

Serial threefold dilutions of mouse spleen cell suspension, prepared in the growth medium, were co-cultivated with BHK-HVJ cells at 35°C for 24 hours, and VI in the culture fluid was assayed. In these experiments, VI production was proportional to the concentration of lymphoid cells present in the system (Fig. 1).

Certain properties of VI induced in the mouse spleen cell system were determined and compared with those of the interferons induced by NDV and E. coli endotoxin in mouse spleen cells in vitro (Table 4).

These inhibitors were all found to be nondializable, nonsedimentable, and relatively unstable at pH 2.0 for 24 hours. In contrast to the NDV-induced interferon, however, VI reported in this study is rather unstable at 56°C for 30 minutes. VI has no direct virus neutralizing properties and inhibits VSV plaque formation in mouse L cells but not in hamster BHK cells.

As shown in Figure 2, a linear relationship was observed between the concentration of VI and the degree of plaque reduction on L cells. In most experiments, the culture fluid of mouse spleen cells co-cultivated with BHK-HVJ cells for 24 hours exhibited 50% plaque reduction at dilutions of 1:100 to 1:200.

Whether or not an active metabolism, particularly DNA synthesis, of BHK-HVJ cells is required for VI induction was examined. As shown in Tables 5 and 6, the production of VI in ultraviolet irradiated and Mitomycin C treated BHK-HVJ cells was not inhibited. These results indicate that cells incapable of replication and probably non-viable, still induced VI in spleen cell cultures. Furthermore, taken with the demonstration that cells disrupted by sonication induced no VI (Table 1), this finding strongly suggests that organized structures, presumably located in the cell surface, play a role in the synthesis of this factor.

To explore further this possibility, an experiment was designed to test whether cell to cell contact was required for
production of VI in this system. A sterile type HA Millipore
filter was placed on BHK-HVJ cell monolayers, to which 1×10^7
mouse spleen cells suspended in the growth medium were added. In
control cultures, the same numbers of mouse spleen cells were
first added to BHK-HVJ cell monolayers and then a Millipore filter was placed over them. As shown in Table 7, intervention of
a Millipore filter between BHK-HVJ monolayers and mouse spleen
cells resulted in a marked reduction of VI production. This finding indicates that mouse spleen cells must be in contact with
BHK-HVJ cells in order to produce VI.

In the experiments to be described, the kinetics of VI production was studied. Spleen cells were co-cultivated with BHK-
HVJ cells in Petri dishes and after appropriate intervals culture fluid was harvested, cleared by centrifugation, and stored
at -20°C until assayed for VI activity. Figure 3A shows the time
course of VI production in the mixed cultures of mouse spleen
cells and BHK-HVJ cells. It appears that VI production begins
between 2 and 4 hours and reaches a maximal level by 8 to 24
hours of co-cultivation. Since VI release appears to start about
2 hours after the beginning of co-cultivation, this period of
incubation appears to be required for the mouse spleen cells to
release VI into the medium. Presumably during this period of 2
hours, cell to cell contact between mouse spleen cells and BHK-
HVJ cells, which has been shown essential for VI production must
take place.

In order to determine the period of cell contact necessary
for the initiation of VI production, the following experiment
was performed. A suspension of 1×10^8 mouse spleen cells in 4

ml was added to a BHK-HVJ monolayer in a Petri dish. At various
times of incubation, the culture fluid containing the mouse spleen
cells alone was transferred to another Petri dish and further
incubated. Twenty-four hours after beginning of co-cultivation,
the supernatant fluid was tested for VI activity. The results are
shown in Figure 3B. It is apparent that even one hour of co-cultivation results in production of an appreciable amount of VI.

In an attempt to study a possible cell-surface interaction
between mouse spleen cells and BHK-HVJ cells, the following experiments were performed. BHK-HVJ cell cultures in Petri dishes
were treated with anti-HVJ rabbit serum or normal rabbit serum
for 1 hour at 35 C. After washing once with Eagle's MEM, spleen
cells suspended in growth medium were added to each Petri dish.
After incubation at 35 C for 24 hours, the supernatant fluid was
assayed for VI activity. VI production by mouse spleen cells was
supressed almost completely when BHK-HVJ cells were pretreated
with anti-HVJ rabbit serum but unaffected by pretreatment of
BHK-HVJ cells with normal rabbit serum (Table 8).

This finding, together with the foregoing ones, indicates
that subsequent to the attachment of mouse spleen cells to BHK-
HVJ cells the next step required for VI production involves the
recognition, by mouse spleen cells of the virus antigen(s) present on the BHK-HVJ cell surface.

We have recently undertaken preliminary experiments to
clarify the mechanism of VI production in this system. Cell surface membrane, using the Warren's method (3) (Figure 4), were
prepared and tested to see whether such preparations were capable of inducing VI production by spleen cells. As shown in Table
9, these subcellular fractions (B, C, D, E, as indicated in Figure 4) which are considered to contain cell membranes, had the
capacity to induce VI. We are now trying to confirm this finding

by obtaining electron micrographs of these fractions. These observations confirmed our speculation that the surface membrane
of BHK-HVJ cells might initiate VI production in this system and
prompted us to perform the following experiments.

Induction of VI by HVJ or HVJ envelope material adsorbed
to erythrocytes was tested (Figure 5). We prepared envelope membrane from HVJ according to the method described by Hosaka (4).
The hemagglutinating subunits, which is considered to be envelope,
was adsorbed to formalin treated chicken erythrocytes after inactivation of neuraminidase activity by KIO_4. VI was detected in
the culture fluid of spleen cells co-cultivated with HVJ-erythrocyte (Table 10) and HVJ spike-erythrocyte complex (Table 11).
This result indicates that, although HVJ spike alone has no VI
inducing activity, its binding to erythrocyte surface results in
acquisition of VI inducing activity, thus stressing the importance of the surface-structural integrity of the inducers in the
present system.

Recent observations by Borecky et al.(5) and Gifford et al.
(6) have shown that there is a new type of interferon production
by lymphoid cells which requires a cell to cell interaction, and
specific immune recognition. On the basis of these observations,
we have following the production in vitro of VI by spleen cells
from mice previously immunized with HVJ when brought in contact
with BHK-HVJ cells. Adult mice were immunized by an intraperitoneal inoculation of 0.5 ml of HVJ (4096 HA), and 7 days later,
their spleen cells were tested and compared with those of non-
immunized control mice. Serum HI titers of immunized mice ranged
from 4096 to 8192, while those of non-immunized control mice
were less than 4. In this experiment, VI titers were expressed
as the reciprocals of dilutions causing 50% plaque count reduction. The results present in Table 12 suggest that VI production

by mouse spleen cells during co-cultivation with BHK-HVJ cells is
not related to the immune status of donor mice against HVJ.

The most significant of our findings may be summarized as
follows:

1.   Mouse lymphoid cells produce a virus inhibitor exhibiting the properties of interferon when cultivated in the presence
of hamster kidney cells chronically infected with HVJ. No inhibitor is produced by the lymphoid cells after exposure to culture
medium from the chronically infected cells or when co-cultivated
with normal BHK cells.

2.   For the production of the inhibitor in the system we
have studied, cell to cell contact between the lymphoid and the
BHK-HVJ cells is required under circumstances that permit recognition of the viral antigen(s) on the surface of the chronically
infected cell.

3.   VI production in this system might be initiated by
membrane-membrane interaction between mouse spleen cells and BHK-
HVJ cells.

4.   VI production by mouse spleen cells during co-cultivation with BHK-HVJ cells is not related to the immune status of
the donor mice against HVJ.

Acknowledgments

We wish to greatfully acknowledge Dr. John F. Enders
(Boston USA) for his kind help in preparing this paper.

We thank Dr. Hosaka (Osaka, Japan) for his kind supply of
some material to prepare viral components.

The study was partly supported by grant from the Department of Science and Technology, Japan.

References

1. Nagata, I., Kimura, Y., Ito, Y. and Tanaka, T. (1972).
    Virology 49, 453.

2. Maeno, K., Yoshii, S., Nagata, I. and Matsumoto, T.
    (1966). Virology 29, 255.

3. Warren, L., Glick, M.C., and Nass, M.K. (1966). J.Cell.
    Physiol. 68, 269.

4. Hosaka, Y. and Shimizu, Y.K. (1972).Virology 49, 627.

5. Borecky, L., Fuchsberger, N., Zelma, J. and Lackovic,
    V. (1971). Eur. J. Immunol. 1, 213.

6. Gifford, G.E., Tibor, A. and Peavy, D.L. (1971). Infec.
    Immun. 3, 164.

TABLE 1

Production of virus inhibitor by co-cultivation
of mouse spleen cells with BHK-HVJ cells

Culture fluid[a] harvested from:	Plaque counts[b]	Reduction rate(%)
BHK-HVJ cells + spleen cells	0	100
Normal BHK cells + spleen cells	90.5	2.9
Spleen cells	100.5	0
BHK-HVJ cells	100.5	0
Sonicated BHK-HVJ cells[c] + spleen cells	99.5	0
Culture fluid of BHK-HVJ cells[d] + spleen cells	·93.5	0
Control (MEM + 2% calf serum)	93.2	

[a]After twenty-four hours of cultivation, culture fluid was harvested from each culture dish, freed of cells by centrifugation, diluted threefold in MEM with 2% calf serum and assayed for virus inhibitory activity.

[b]An aliquot (3.0ml) of each specimen was placed on L cell culture in a Petri dish and, 24 hours later, the culture was challenged by VSV. On day 2 of virus challenge, the L cell monolayer was stained with neutral red and plaques were counted.

[c]BHK-HVJ cells suspended in the medium were sonicated in ice bath for 30 seconds with an ultrasonic oscillator.

[d]BHK-HVJ cells were grown to monolayers in Petri dishes for 2 days; the monolayers were then washed once with fresh MEM and incubated with 4 ml of fresh growth medium. Twenty-four hours later, supernatant fluids were harvested.

TABLE 2

Production of virus inhibitor by co-cultivation of mouse
various cells with BHK-HVJ cells

Experiment	Culture fluid[a] harvested from:	№ of dishes	Plaque counts[b]	Reduction rate(%)
	BHK-HVJ cells +	1	0	100
	spleen cells[c]	2	0	100
		3	0	100
	BHK-HVJ cells +	1	86	28.9
	liver cells[c]	2	70	42.1
1	BHK-HVJ cells +	1	2	98.4
	lymphnode cells[c]	2	5	95.9
		3	0	100
	BHK-HVJ cells +	1	10	91.7
	thymocytes[c]	2	15	87.6
	Control (MEM + 2% calf serum		121.3	
	BHK-HVJ cells +	1	0	100
	spleen cells[c]	2	0	100
		3	0	100
2	BHK-HVJ cells +	1	44.3	0
	L cells	2	39	9.3
	Control (MEM + 2% calf serum		43	

[a]After twenty-four hours of cultivation, culture fluid was
harvested from each culture dish, freed of cells by centrifugation, diluted threefold in MEM with 2% calf serum and assayed for virus inhibitory activity.

[b]An aliquot (3.0 ml) of each specimen was placed on L cell
culture in a Petri dish and, 24 hours later, the culture was
challenged by VSV. On day 2 of virus challenge, the L cell
monolayer was stained with neutral red and plaques were
counted.

TABLE 2 (continued)

[c]The spleen, liver, cervical lymphnode and thymus were aseptically removed from C57BL/6 mice and teased on steel mesh immersed in chilled TC-199 medium in a plastic dish.The cells passed through were then washed twice with medium and suspended in the growth medium.

TABLE 3

Production of virus inhibitor by co-cultivation
of mouse spleen cells with HeLa-HVJ cells

Culture fluid[a] harvested from:	№ of dishes	Plaque counts[b]	Reduction rate(%)
HeLa-HVJ cells + spleen cells	1	3	91.5
	2	0.5	98.5
HeLa cells + spleen cells	1	30	12.5
	2	44	0
Control (MEM + 2% calf serum)		34.3	

[a]After twenty-four hours of cultivation, culture fluid was harvested from each culture dish, freed of cells by centrifugation, diluted threefold in MEM with 2% calf serum and assayed for virus inhibitory activity.

[b]An aliquot (3.0 ml) of each specimen was placed on L cell culture in a Petri dish and, 24 hours later, the culture was challenged by VSV. On day 2 of virus challenge, the L cell monolayer was stained with neutral red and plaques were counted.

TABLE 4

Comparison of effects of various treatments on and properties
of virus inhibitors according to inducers

	Inducers		
Treatments and properties	BHK-HVJ cells	NDV	E. coli endotoxin
Centrifugation, 30,000 rpm 1 hour(supernatant assay)	$-^a$	-	-
56°C, 30 minutes	$\pm^b$	-	$+^c$
pH 2, 24 hours	±	+	+
Dialysis against Hanks' solution	-	-	-
Direct virus neutralizing activity	-	-	-
Species specificity	+	+	+

[a](-) indicates no reduction in titer of virus inhibitor after treatment or lack of a property.

[b](±) indicates about one half reduction in titer of inhibitor after treatment.

[c](+) indicates more than one forth reduction in titer of inhibitor after treatment or possession of property.

TABLE 5

VI production by spleen cells co-cultivated
with ultra-violet irradiated BHK-HVJ cells

UV treatment[a] (minutes)	VI titers[b]
3	88.5
1	97.7
0.5	108.5
0	93.5

[a]The monolayers of BHK-HVJ cells were throughly
washed once with fresh MEM, then completely
freed of the medium and ultraviolet-irradiated
at distance of 30 cm on ice box.

[b]Virus inhibitor was assayed by the plaque reduction method with L cells and VSV as challenge
virus. Titers of a virus inhibitor were expressed as the reciprocals of the dilutions causing
50% plaque count reduction.

TABLE 6

VI production by spleen cells co-cultivated
with Mitomycin C treated BHK-HVJ cells[a]

Dose of Mitomycin C	VI titers[b]	
	Exp. 1	Exp. 2
50.0 μg/ml	1050	1310
25.0 μg/ml	860	970
12.5 μg/ml	720	570
0	660	620

[a]BHK-HVJ cells were incubated with appropriate
doses of Mitomycin C for 20 minutes and washed
3 times with medium.

[b]As in Table 5.

TABLE 7

Blockade of VI production by interposing a Millipore filter
between mouse spleen cells and BHK-HVJ cell monolayers

Culture fluid[a] harvested from:	N⁰ of dishes	Plaque counts[b]	Reduction rate (%)
BHK-HVJ cells+MF+spleen cells[c]	1	67	30.3
	2	86	9.1
BHK-HVJ cells+spleen cells+MF[d]	1	0	100
	2	0	100
Control (MEM + 2% calf serum)		97	

[a]After twenty-four hours of cultivation, culture fluid was
harvested from each culture dish, freed of cells by centrifugation, diluted threefold in MEM with 2% calf serum and assayed for virus inhibitory activity.

[b]An aliquot (3.0 ml) of each specimen was placed on L cell
culture in a Petri dish and, 24 hours later, the culture was
challenged by VSV. On day 2 of virus challenge, the L cell
monolayer was stained with neutral red and plaques were
counted.

[c]A sterile type HA Millipore filter was placed on BHK-HVJ cell
monolayers, on which 1x10^7 mouse spleen cells in the growth
medium were added.

[d]The same numbers of mouse spleen cells were inoculated on
BHK-HVJ cell monolayers and then a Millipore filter was super-
imposed.

TABLE 8

Inhibition of VI production by pretreatment
of BHK-HVJ cells with anti-HVJ rabbit serum

Culture fluid[a] harvested from:	N.º of dishes	Plaque counts[b]	Reduction rate (%)
BHK-HVJ cells + spleen cells	1	0	100
	2	0	100
(BHK-HVJ cells + anti-HVJ rabbit serum)[c] + spleen cells	1	36	0
	2	21	38.7
(BHK-HVJ cells + normal rabbit serum)[c] + spleen cells	1	0	100
	2	0	100
Control (MEM + 2% calf serum)		34.3	

[a]After twenty-four hours of cultivation, culture fluid was harvested from each culture dish, freed of cells by centrifugation, diluted threefold in MEM with 2% calf serum and assayed for virus inhibitory activity.

[b]An aliquot (3.0 ml) of each specimen was placed on L cell culture in a Petri dish and, 24 hours later, the culture was challenged by VSV. On day 2 of virus challenge, the cell monolayer
was stained with neutral red and plaques were counted.

[c]BHK-HVJ cell cultures in Petri dishes were treated with anti-
HVJ rabbit serum (CF titer 256) or normal rabbit serum at 35°C
for 1 hour. After washing once Eagle's MEM, spleen cell suspension in the growth medium was added to each of the Petri
dishes.

TABLE 9

VI production by spleen cells incubated with
cell membrane fractions of BHK-HVJ cells

Fraction[a]	HA titers	VI titers[b]	
		Exp. 1	Exp. 2
A	16	NT	>1000
B	16	NT	>1000
C	4	11.7	131.0
D	6	41.0	320.9
E	6	18.6	301.6
F	6	5.3	178.7

[a]See Figure 1.

[b]Virus inhibitor was assayed by the plaque reduction
method with L cells and VSV as challenge virus. Titers of a virus inhibitor were expressed as the reciprocals of the dilutions causing 50% plaque count
reduction.

TABLE 10

VI production by spleen cells cultured
with HVJ-erythrocyte complex[a]

Culture fluid[b] harvested from:	VI Titers[c]		
	Exp. 1 (480)[d]	Exp. 2 (1,280)	Exp. 3 (2,560)
HVJ-erythrocyte complex+spleen cells	27.4	266.7	462.2
HVJ-erythrocyte complex + L cells	<3	<3	NT
Released HVJ[e] + spleen cells	<3	<3	<3
Erythrocyte + spleen cells	<3	<3	<3

[a]See Figure 2.

[b]Mouse spleen cells were cultured with the HVJ-erythrocyte complex for 24 hours and the culture fluid was assayed for VI activity.

[c]Titers of a virus inhibitor were expressed as the reciprocals of the dilutions causing 50% plaque count reduction.

[d]HA titer of periodate treated HVJ used for formation of HVJ-erythrocyte complex.

[e]means the culture fluid of complex after 12 hours incubation. HA could not be detected in the culture fluid.

TABLE 11

VI production by spleen cells cultured with
HVJ spike-erythrocyte complex[a]

Culture fluid[b] harvested from:	VI Titers[c]	
	Exp. 1 (640)[d]	Exp. 2 (640)
Spike-erythrocyte complex + spleen cells	10.1	10.3
Spike-erythrocyte complex + L cells	<3	<3
Released spike[e] + spleen cells	<3	<3
Erythrocyte + spleen cells	<3	<3
HVJ spike (10,000 HA) alone	<3	<3
HVJ spike (1,000 HA) alone	<3	<3

[a]See Figure 2.

[b]Mouse spleen cells were cultured with the HVJ spike-erythrocyte complex for 24 hours and the culture fluid was assayed for VI activity.

[c]Titers of a virus inhibitor were expressed as the reciprocals of the dilutions causing 50% plaque count reduction.

[d]HA titer of periodate treated HVJ spike used for formation of HVJ spike-erythrocyte complex.

[e]means the culture fluid of complex after 12 hours incubation. HA could not be detected in the culture fluid.

TABLE 12

Comparison of effects of immune-state against HVJ of spleen
cells donor mice on VI production[a]

Cell combination	Mouse Nº	VI titers[b]	Mean
BHK-HVJ cells + spleen cells	1	480	
from HVJ immunized mouse[c]	2	453.3	
	3	88.3	
	4	653.3	321.9
	5	130	
	6	126.7	
BHK-HVJ cells + spleen cells	1	560	
from non-immunized mouse[d]	2	146.7	
	3	120	
	4	413.3	310
	5	253.3	
	6	366.7	

[a]After twenty-four hours of co-cultivation, culture fluid from
each culture dish was assayed for virus inhibitory activity.

[b]Virus inhibitor was assayed by the plaque reduction method
with L cells and VSV as challenge virus. Titers of a virus
inhibitor were expressed as the reciprocals of the dilutions
causing 50% plaque count reduction.

[c]Adult mice were immunized by an intraperitoneal inoculation
of 0.5 ml of HVJ (4096 HA), and 7 days later, their spleen
cells were used. Serum HI titers of immunized mice ranged
from 4096 to 8192.

[d]Serum HI titers of non-immunized control mice were less than
4.

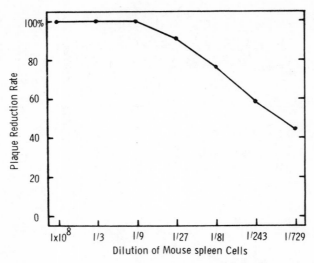

Fig. 1. Effects of mouse spleen cell numbers upon VI production. Serial threefold dilutions of spleen cells wer co- cultivated with BHK-HVJ cells for 24 hours. Culture fluid was harvested, and tested for virus inhibitory activity in L cells.

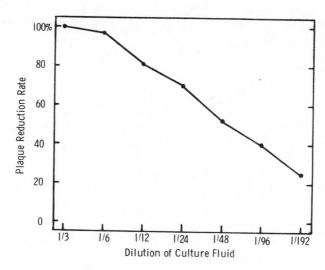

Fig. 2. Dose response of culture fluid. Serial twofold dilutions of culture fluid of mouse spleen cells co-cultivated with BHK-HVJ cells was placed on L cell culture in Petri dish and, 24 hours later, the culture was challenged by VSV. On day 2 after virus inoculation, the L cell monolayer was stained with neutral red and plaques were counted.

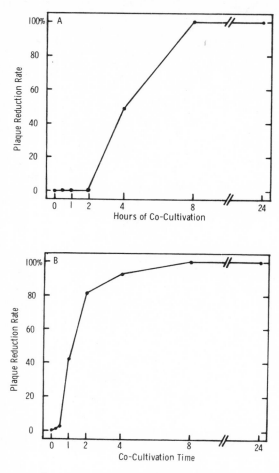

Fig. 3. A: kinetics of VI production. Spleen cells were co-
cultivated with BHK-HVJ cells in Petri dishes and after appropriate intervals culture fluid was harvested, cleared by centrifugation, and assayed for VI activity. B: the period of cell
contact necessary for the initiation of VI production. A suspension of mouse spleen cells was added to BHK-HVJ monolayer in a
Petri dish. At various times of incubation, the culture fluid
containing the mouse spleen cells alone was transferred to
another Petri dish and further incubated. At the end of incubation, 24 hours after the beginning of co-cultivation, the supernatant fluid was tested for VI activity.

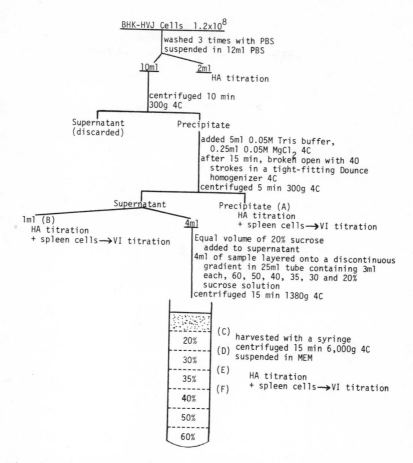

Fig. 4. Scheme of cell membrane fraction of BHK-HVJ cells.

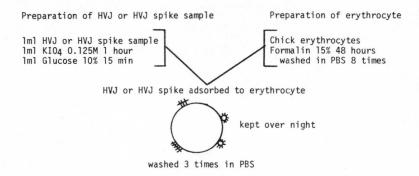

Fig. 5.   Method for formation of virus or spike-erythrocyte complex.

DISCUSSION

Friedman: Dr. Nagata has a very interesting paper but I'm not sure I followed exactly. How did you rule out that the phenomenon you see is not due to Sendai virus that's released by hamster cells, that it is not a direct virus stimulation of the spleen cells?

Nagata: In order to rule out such possibility, we cultured the spleen cells in the BHK-HVJ cell culture fluid that contained Sendai virus of about 1:64 HA titer. As was shown in the first slide, no VI activity was found in the spleen cell culture fluid.

Merigan: It might be helpful if you could tell us about the characteristics of the BHK cells that you're working with. Can you get virus out of those cells by any tricks?

Nagata: As far as we see it in hemagglutination titer, our cell line appears to release only a little virus particles into the medium which are not infectious to eggs, although about 50 to

80% of the cells contain viral antigens when tested after the cells have grown to confluence. We have tried to clean them from infectious virus, but failed.

Colby: In your cocultivation experiments, are the cells very close to each other? Are there two types of cells? Are they touching?

Nagata: I believe so, although I have no electronmicrographic evidence. You wonder if spleen cells contact with BHK-HVJ cells? As I have shown in the fourth slide we could not find any VI production when we put a Millipore filter between the BHK cells and the spleen cells. Therefore, we believe that they must be very close or touching each other.

Colby: Did you ever see any evidence of cell fusion that might be Sendai-mediated, indicating a direct transfer of the virus from one cell to the other?

Nagata: You mean Sendai virus mediated cell fusion could be related to the interferon production?

Colby: If you could visually see any fusion at all, that would be an indication that there was some Sendai at the surface that could be mediating that fusion and that there would be then a shared cytoplasm.

Nagata: You mean cell fusion between the BHK-HVJ cells and the spleen cells?

Colby: Yes. Have you ever seen any fusion?

Nagata: No, we haven't yet, as far as we tried.

De Maeyer: I'm interested in the origin of the spleen cells you're using. In other words, the strain of mouse involved in these experiments.

Nagata: We used C57BL.

De Maeyer: C57Black?

Nagata: Yes, C57Black mice, and we have got the same results using the other strain of albino mouse, DD mouse that have
been developed in Japan as inbred and are now widely used in Japan.

De Maeyer: What were the other strains?

Nagata: It's called DD strain.

De Maeyer: Did you use BALB/c mice? The reason I ask is
that we have recently shown in collaboration with Dr. Bailey of
Jackson Laboratory, that there are two genes in the mouse, expressed at the level of the lymphocyte and affecting interferon
levels induced by Sendai virus. So it would be very interesting
to use either high or low producer lymphocytes in your system
and see if the difference that is found in vivo is also found
in vitro. C57Black is a high producer.

Nagata: Thank you very much for your suggestion.

Morahan: Have you determined whether macrophages or lymphocytes in your spleen cell population are the interferon producing cells?

Nagata: I'm sorry, we haven't exactly done such experiments. However, I could tell you that the spleen cell suspension
we routinely use contains more than 90% nonadherent cell and
less than 10% adherent cell population and that, in a preliminary experiment, both populations seemed to be independently
involved in the VI production.

Planterose: Are you suggesting that the interferon production here is different from the well known fact that you get interferon if you take sensitized lymphoid cells and expose them to antigen? For instance, do you get any of the lymphokinins released at the same time, macrophage inhibition factor, for instance?

Nagata: Yes, I am. I think our experimental results are difficult to explain by the mechanism of so-called immuno-induction, I guess, you meant. The only reason why, we think, it is different from the immuno-induction of the donor mice and interferon producing ability of the spleen cells. As I have shown in the slide, interferon procuction was not enhanced by hyper-immunization of the donor mice against HVJ. I now realize that one objection to our interpretation may arise from the view that the observed dissociation might be just a reflection of that between cellular and humoral immunity.

Planterose: If in your system you have immuno-induction, do you get lymphokinins, such as macrophage inhibition factor?

Nagata: I think so, but the reverse may not be true.

Pereira: I would like a little clarification about the experiment in which you had red blood cells coated with virus spikes induce the virus inhibitor when in contact with lymphocytes, if I understood you correctly. Was this pure hemagglutinin? Would hemagglutinin itself non adsorbed to red cells do it or not?

Nagata: Yes, you understood me correctly. In control experiments we tried to induce VI with spike material alone which had 10,000 HA titer and failed. So we believe that our preparation of HVJ envelope itself does not have any capacity to induce interferon in the mouse spleen cells.

Pereira: Only when it is attached to red blood cells.

Nagata: Yes, that's right but I don't know why.

VI - MECHANISM OF ACTION AT THE MOLECULAR LEVEL

MECHANISM OF THE INTERFERON-INDUCED BLOCK OF mRNA TRANSLATION IN MOUSE L CELLS

M. Revel, J. Content, A. Zilberstein, H. Berissi,
B. Lebleu*, E. Falcoff*, and R. Falcoff*

Weizmann Institute of Science, Rehovot, Israel
and
*Institut du Radium, Paris, France

Addition of mouse interferon to L cells makes these cells unable to support the multiplication of viruses by blocking viral gene expression (1). Interferon is also known to reduce the rate of cell division(2) and the intracellular multiplication of various unicellular parasites (3). In an effort to determine what are the changes induced by interferon in the cell, studies of gene expression in cell-free systems have been undertaken in several laboratories. Recently, results indicating an effect of interferon on mRNA translation in vitro have started to accumulate (4,5,6,7). Our work (4) showed that cell-free extracts of interferon-treated mouse L cells have lost their ability to translate into protein exogenously added natural mRNA. This block in translation appears in uninfected L cells-extracts under conditions in which interferon induces the antiviral state (5). The translation of both the viral Mengo RNA and the cellular hemo - globin(Hb) mRNA can be inhibited almost completely in the ex - tracts. However, we have consistently observed that when the decrease produced by interferon treatment is only around 50-70 per cent, Mengo RNA translation is 2-3 times more inhibited than is Hb mRNA. Endogenous protein synthesis and poly U translation are

not significantly inhibited in interferon-treated cell-extracts.
Analysis of the mechanism of the translational block has indicated (5) the presence of an inhibitory factor, loosely associated
with the ribosomes. This inhibitor, which can be eluted from ribosomes by 0.5 M KCl, appears to be at least in part, a protein.
In addition, we now report that the translation activity of interferon-treated L cell-extracts can be almost quantitatively
recovered by the addition of a purified fraction of transfer
RNA, which can overcome the interferon-induced inhibition. The
nature of this tRNA and of its mechanism of action are described
here. The results suggest that interferon may alter a normal regulatory mechanism of protein synthesis in mammalian cells.

Materials and methods

Cell cultures and preparation of cell-free extracts. Mouse
L cells (strain CCL1), were grown in suspension cultures in Eagle Minimum Essential medium (MEM GIBCO) suplemented with 8% de-
complemented calf serum, 0.2% Bactotryptose, 0.1% methyl cellulose, glucose (5.5 g/l) and gentamycin (40 mg/liter), penicilin
(10^5 u/l) and streptomycin (0.1 g/l). Routinely 2 liters of culture to a density of 10^6 cells/ml were treated with 150-200 u-
nits/ml of mouse interferon. Interferon was prepared from NDV-
infected L cells and purified on CM-Sephadex as described previously (5). Specific activities ranged from 1-5x10^6 ref. units
per mg protein.

After 35 hours, cells were harvested, washed and a cell-
free extract S-10 was prepared as described before (5) except
that 0.02 M Hepes buffer, pH 7.5, was used instead of Tris-HCl
buffer. Preincubated S10 was used to translate Mengo RNA and
rabbit hemoglobin mRNA as before (5).Fractionation of S-10 into
ribosomes, ribosomal wash fraction and high speed supernatant

has been detailed before (5).

Cell-free extracts from Krebs ascites tumor cells were prepared as before (8). ^{14}C-radioactive protein-hydrolisate (50 µC/µAtC) or ^{35}S-methionine (>150 mC/µmole) from Radiochemical were used.

Preparation and purification of tRNA. Krebs ascites cells and L cells tRNA was prepared through phenol extraction, 1 M NaCl and isopropanol precipitation as outlined by Aviv et al. (9). Chromatography on benzoylated DEAE cellulose and DEAE Sephadex A50 was carried out according to Petrissant et al. (10). Purified rabbit liver tRNA$_{metF}$ was a gift from Dr. G. Petrissant. Total rabbit liver tRNA was a gift of Dr. D. Hatfield and rabbit reticulocyte tRNA was a gift from U. Nudel. E. coli B tRNA was purchased from Schwarz Co. Purified E. coli methionyl tRNA synthetase was a generous gift from Dr. J. Waller. RNA-free E. coli total supernatant enzymes was prepared to charge tRNA as described by Muench and Berg (11). For formylation, formylfolate reduced by hydrogen with a 5% rhodium-alumina catalyst was added. Over 60 per cent formylation was obtained as measured after alkali-hydrolysis and high voltage electrophoresis at pH 3.5 (12). MDMP was a generous personal gift from Dr. Baxter.

Results

1. Restoration by tRNA of translation activity in interferon treated extract. Cell-free cytoplasmic extracts are prepared from L cells, which have been treated in suspension cultures by 200 units of mouse interferon per ml, for 24 hours as described in detail previously (4). Such extracts, "S-10",translate very poorly Mengo virus RNA in comparison to S-10 from normal, untreated L cells. The correlation between this inhibition of in vitro mRNA translation and the antiviral effect induced

by interferon in L cells, has been well documented in a previous publication (5).

More recently we have observed that the ability of S-10 from interferon treated cells can be restored by adding transfer RNA. Fig. 1 shows that addition of rabbit reticulocyte tRNA and L cell high-speed supernatant (S-100) restores more than 80 per cent of its activity to the interferon extract. The S-10 from control L cells is not stimulated by tRNA. In this experiment only a small restoration is observed with tRNA alone, without S-100 supernatant. Both S-100 from normal and interferon treated L cells are active. Without tRNA, the addition of S-100 has no effect. The requirement of S-100 in addition to tRNA suggested that the active component is charged aminoacyl tRNA. Indeed, Table 1 shows that periodate treatment of tRNA, which oxydizes the terminal adenosine residue, completely abolishes its activity to restore the translation of Mengo RNA in S-10 from interferon treated L cells. E. coli tRNA has very little activity (Fig. 1B; Table 2) as compared to mammalian tRNA; when, however, E. coli tRNA was first charged with bacterial enzymes, some activity was observed. The restoration by tRNA was observed in many independently prepared extracts from interferon treated L cells, and the activity observed ranged from 75 to 120 per cent of that of the control S-10. The requirement for S-100 was on the other hand not observed in all the extracts used (e.g. Fig. 1B and Table 2). Preparations of tRNA from rabbit liver, Krebs ascites cells or L cells showed very similar activities in this system.

Restoration of mRNA translation was obtained with tRNA purified from both control and interferon treated L cells (Table 2).

2. Kinetic study of the tRNA effect in interferon treat-

ed extracts. A kinetic study of Mengo RNA translation at 30°C
(Fig. 2) shows that translation is initiated similarly in both
control and interferon-treated S-10, but stops in the interferon
treated S-10 after 20-30 minutes. In control S-10, with or without added tRNA, translation goes on linearly for more than 90
minutes. Strikingly, addition of tRNA to the interferon treated
S-10, allows translation of Mengo RNA to proceed linearly for
almost an hour, at a rate similar to that of the control S-10.
The difference between S-10 extracts from control and interferon
treated L cells is therefore even more clearly apparent if one
measures amino acid incorporation from 30 to 60 minutes after
starting the reaction. Table 3 shows that during this period the
interferon S-10 incorporates only 5 per cent of the methionine
incorporated by the control S-10. Moreover, if the tRNA is added
30 minutes after starting the reaction with Mengo RNA, the following incorporation is restored to a value similar to that of
the control. This clearly demonstrates that incubation of the
messenger RNA in the interferon S-10, under conditions where
little translation is observed, does not lead to any loss of
template activity. In line with this conclusion, the addition
of new Mengo RNA did not reactivate the interferon treated S-10
in the absence of added tRNA.

What reaction is affected by the addition of tRNA? Using
inhibitors of protein synthesis initiation (such as MDMP) (13)
we determined that under our conditions new initiations still
occur in control S-10 as late as 30-40 min after the beginning
of incubation at 30°C. The abrupt drop in the rate of translation which occurs in the interferon treated extract could therefore result from a lack of reinitiations.

To determine what reaction is affected by the addition of
tRNA, we used two different inhibitors of initiation, MDMP and
ATA, and studied their effect on the stimulation of the inter-

feron treated S-10 by tRNA. Fig. 3 shows the results obtained
using ATA. The translation of Mengo RNA is allowed to proceed 15
minutes at 30°C and then ATA is added. This addition produces
almost no inhibition (compare curve 3 to 1), although ATA added
at 0 minutes (compare curve 0 to 1) or added at 15 min to the
reaction containing tRNA from time 0 (compare curve 5 to 6) produced the expected inhibitions. This suggests by itself that after 15 minutes, no reinitiations are observed in the interferon
treated S-10. Addition of tRNA at 15 minutes, stimulates markedly Mengo RNA translation (curve 4) as mentioned above. However,
if ATA is added together with tRNA, no stimulation is observed
(curve 2) which strongly suggest that addition of tRNA stimulates
reinitiation of Mengo RNA translation. Identical results were
obtained when MDMP was used as inhibitor of initiation instead
of ATA. Therefore, tRNA does not stimulate elongation only, but
requires new initiation to exhibit its effect.

3.   Nature of the active tRNA. We investigated if the active tRNA species was the initiator met $tRNA_F$. Purified $tRNA_{metF}$
was obtained from rabbit liver (a generous gift from Dr. G. Petrissant) (10) or from Krebs II ascites tumor cells. Addition
of this purified tRNA to S-10 from interferon treated L cells
did not restore Mengo RNA translation (Table 4). Addition of
tRNA Met_F sometimes stimulated methionine incorporation in the
control S-10, indicating that the initiator tRNA may be limiting.
However, the ratio between interferon and control activities remained unchanged. Precharged ^{35}S-met $tRNA_{met\ F}$ also had no effect. Addition of total tRNA almost fully restored the transfer
of methionine from purified precharged ^{35}S-met $tRNA_{met\ F}$ to protein in the interferon S-10 (Table 4).

We have prepared N-formyl-(^{35}S)met-$tRNA_{met\ F}^{rabbit\ liver}$, using a tRNA-free E. coli enzyme and formyl donor. This species
did not reactivate Mengo RNA directed free ^{35}S-methionine incor-

poration in the interferon treated S-10; (Table 5) a small increase was observed, essentially as a result of inhibition of
the control S-10. On the other hand, addition of a similar amount
of restoring tRNA (purified as described below) had a very marked stimulatory effect on the interferon treated extract. (Studies on the direct transfer of methionine from fmet-tRNA are
presented in a following paragraph).

The nature of the tRNA active in the restoration reaction
was investigated after chromatography on BD cellulose according
to Petrissant et al. (10). Fig. 4 shows the elution of the ac -
tive species. It is clear that the activity is separated from
the bulk of the tRNAs. As mentioned above, $tRNA_{met\ F}$ which e-
lutes early from BD cellulose is not active in the restoration
reaction; moreover, $tRNA_{met\ M}$ is also inactive. The active fractions, devoid of methionine accepting activity, stimulated the
Mengo RNA dependent incorporation of ^{35}S-methionine by the interferon treated S-10. The species which restore activity to the
interferon S-10, did not stimulate the control S-10. The same
fractions of the BD-cellulose chromatogram of Fig. 4, reactivat-
ed two different, independently prepared, interferon treated extracts. Reactivation was observed for both Mengo RNA and hemo -
globin mRNA. The active species were further purified on DEAE-
Sephadex A-50 (10) and rechromatography on BD-cellulose. The
most active fractions restored activity at a dose of 0.03 µg
tRNA under the conditions of Fig. 1A. A 100 fold purification
was therefore obtained. By filtration on Sephadex G-75 and polyacrylamide gel electrophoresis in sodium dodecyl sulfate, only
4S RNA was seen in the active material. The precise nature of
the active tRNA species is as yet unknown.

4. Translation inhibitory activity from ribosomes of interferon treated cells. In previous experiments we showed (5)

that the fraction washed-off ribosomes from interferon-treated
cells contained an inhibitor of protein synthesis. This inhibitor can be assayed in cell-free extracts S-10 from untreated L
cells or even from Krebs ascites tumor cells (cells which by
themselves are resistant to interferon). The inhibitor is precipitated by ammonium sulfate at 70-85 percent saturation and
blocks completely translation of Mengo RNA (Fig. 5). In some cases, ribosomal wash proteins from control cells also inhibit,
but the concentration of inhibitory activity is usually about 5
times higher in fractions obtained from interferon-treated L
cells than in control cells. It is not clear if the inhibitor
present in control extract is the same as that which appears in
interferon-treated cell extracts.(It remains possible that the
inhibitory activity exists in normal ribosomal wash, but is masked by a stimulatory factor. Mixing experiments do not, however,
support this interpretation). Heating for 7 minutes at 50 C destroys the inhibitor activity. The inhibitor is adsorbed on DEAE
cellulose from which it can be eluted by washing with 0.3 M KCl.
These characteristics suggest that the inhibitor is a protein or
contains a protein moiety.

The inhibitory factor of interferon-treated extract does
not inhibit the translation of poly U. It has no effect also on
endogenous protein-synthesis in L cells extracts (Fig. 6 and
Table 6). Since this synthesis represents mainly completion of
in vivo initiated chains it cannot be easily compared to the
translation of exogeneous mRNA. Table 6 also shows that the inhibition of Mengo RNA translation by adding ribosomal wash proteins from interferon-treated ribosomes to the control S-10, can
be overcome by the addition of tRNA and supernatant enzymes. Actually the inhibitory factor makes the control S-10 stimulable
by tRNA, normally a characteristic of the interferon treated S-
10. This observation would suggest that the interferon induced

inhibitor is the cause of both the block in mRNA translation and of the dependence on tRNA.

One possible inhibitor was clearly separated from this inhibitory activity, namely, the enzyme deacylase (14); this enzyme as assayed by hydrolysis of ^{35}S-met tRNA was not increased after interferon treatment and was separated from the present inhibitor on DEAE cellulose.

Discussion

The main new result is that the block in exogenous natural mRNA translation observed in extracts of interferon-treated L cells is overcome by the addition of tRNA. There does not seem to be permanent damage to the protein synthesis machinery but a rather specific requirement for this tRNA species.

We do not know what reaction is blocked in these interferon extracts. The simplest possibility would be that some tRNA species are limiting. However, since endogenous mRNA translation is almost unaffected, a general effect on polypeptide chain elongation is unlikely. In non-preincubated extracts in which endogenous mRNA activity is measured, the translation of Mengo RNA is inhibited to the same extent as in extracts preincubated without mRNA for 30-60 minutes. The detailed kinetic studies presented here show that translation of Mengo RNA starts normally in interferon-treated extracts but stops after a few minutes. Addition of tRNA restores activity even after translation has stopped. There may be either a depletion of some essential component (a tRNA ?) or accumulation of an inhibitory material (whose activity is blocked by tRNA). This arrest does not occur in the absence of mRNA. However, mRNA is not degraded during this first incubation period, since delayed tRNA addition re - stores translation. Binding of mRNA to ribosomes (15) is still

normal even when translation is blocked. Since polysome degradation is observed (15) the block may be in some initiation step
or early elongation, and further work is needed to determine the
precise reaction(s) blocked.

Does interferon treatment affect the tRNA population di -
rectly or indirectly? Although a decreased acceptance of methionine and other amino acids was observed in the interferon
treated S-10, it should be recalled that tRNA from these treated cells appear to have normal restoring activity. The possible
accumulation of an inhibitor, which may be the ribosome-associ-
ate inhibitory activity, remains a likely possibility.

Inhibition of initiation has been reported in eukaryotic
cell extracts starved for amino acids (16). Furthermore, amino
acid starvation during interferon treatment was shown by Kerr
et al. (17) to potentiate the in vitro translation inhibition
produced by interferon. Further work on the mechanism of the
interferon-induced block and on the nature of the restoring
tRNA is still needed, but our observations, already, focus the
attention on the possible function of a particular tRNA in the
regulation of mammalian protein synthesis and in the mode of
action of interferon.

Acknowledgment

The technical assistance of Mr. Shulman and Mrs. Federman
is very gratefully acknowledged. A grant from the Israel Acad-
emy of Science and Humanities partly supported this research.
E.F. and B.L. were recipient of EMBO fellowships.

References

1. Vilček, J. (1969). "Interferon", in Virology Mono - graphs, vol. 6, Springer-Verlag, Wien and New York.

2. Gresser, I., Bandu, M.T., Tovey, M., Bodo, G., Paucker, K., and Stewart, W.E. (1973). Proc. Soc. Expt. Biol. Med. 142, 7.

3. Hanna, L., Merigan, T.C., and Jawetz, E. (1966). Proc. Soc. Expt. Biol. Med. 122, 417.

4. Falcoff, E., Falcoff, R., Lebleu, B., and Revel, M. (1972). Nature New Biol. 240, 145.

5. Falcoff, B., Falcoff, R., Lebleu, B., and Revel, M. (1973). J. Virol. 12, 421.

6. Friedman, R.M., Metz, D.H., Esteban, R.M., Tovel,D.R., Ball, L.A., and Kerr, I.M. (1973). J.Virol. 10, 1184.

7. Gupta, S.L., Sopori, M.L., and Lengyel, P. (1973). Biochem. Biophys. Res. Comm. 54, 777.

8. Nudel, U., Lebleu, B., and Revel, M. (1973). Proc. Natl. Acad. Sci. US 70, 2139.

9. Aviv, H., Boime, I., and Leder, P. (1971). Proc. Natl. Acad. Sci. US 68, 2303.

10. Petrissant, G., Boisnard, M., and Puissant, C. (1971). Biochimie 53, 1105.

11. Muench, K., and Berg, P. (1966). in Proced. In Nucl. Acid Res., Cantoni and Davis Ed., Harper and Row, p. 375.

12. Groner, Y., and Revel, M. (1971). Eur. J. Biochem. 22, 144.

13. Baxter, R., Knell, V.C., Sommerville, H.J., Swain, H. M., and Weeks, D.P. (1973). Nature N.B. 243, 139.

14. Gupta, N.K., and Aerni, R.J. (1973). Biochem. Biophys.

Res. Comm. 51, 907.

15. Lebleu, B., Content, J., and Revel, M. unpublished re-
     sults.

16. Vaughan, M.H., and Hansen, B.S. (1973). J. Biol. Chem.
     248, 7087.

17. Kerr, I.M., Friedman, R.M., Esteban, M., Brown, R.E.,
     Ball, L.A., Metz, D.H., Risby, D., Tovel, D.R., and
     Sonnabend, J.A. (1973). Advances in the Biosciences
     Nº 11, in press.

18. Tal, J., Deutscher, M., and Littauer (1973). Eur. J.
     Biochem. 28, 478.

TABLE 1

Effect of periodate treatment on the ability of tRNA
to restore translation in interferon-treated S10

Additions	^{14}C-amino acid incorporation in interferon - treated S10	
	c.p.m.	Δ
None	1645	–
Stripped tRNA, 5µg	4695	3050
Periodate treated tRNA,6.5µg	2195	550

Assay as in Fig. 1A. Rabbit reticulocyte tRNA was stripped by
incubation in 0.5 M tris-HCl pH 8.9 for 30 min at 37°C and
subsequently oxydized with periodate as detailed by Tal et al.
(18). Incorporation in the absence of Mengo RNA was 550 cpm.

TABLE 2

Effect of tRNA from various sources

^{14}C-aa incorporation

Additions		Control S10	Interferon	S10
		c.p.m.	c.p.m.	per cent
Exp.1	None	11,950	1,250	(11)
	+tRNA$^{\text{rabbit liver}}$, 3µg	12,755	7,602	(60)
	+tRNA$^{\text{rabbit liver}}$, 6µg	10,925	8,133	(75)
	+tRNA$^{\underline{\text{E. coli}}}$, 4µg	9,579	2,211	(23)
Exp.2	None	14,380	1,615	(11)
	+tRNA$^{\text{rabbit liver}}$, 6µg	7,330	4,510	(61)
	+tRNA$^{\text{L cells}}$, 2.9µg	8,410	5,435	(65)
	+tRNA$^{\text{L cells}}$ interferon treated, 2.9µg	9,750	6,250	(64)

Conditions as in Fig. 1B. Incorporation without Mengo was 330 cpm. tRNA was extracted from suspension culture of control and interferon treated L cells as described in Methods.

TABLE 3

Effect of the delayed addition of tRNA

	Extract	Addition at 30 min	^{35}S methionine incorporation from 30 - 60 min at 30°C
			cpm
Exp.1	Control-S10	none	73,170
	Interferon-S10	none	2,310
	Interferon-S10	+tRNA,6μg	62,920
Exp.2	Control-S10	none	60,000
	"	+tRNA,6μg	101,150
	"	+Mengo RNA,1μg	80,000
	Interferon-S10	none	3,750
	"	+tRNA,6μg	62,810
	"	+Mengo RNA,1μg	3,660

Conditions as in Fig. 1B, except that reaction mixture contained from 0-30 min cold methionine, 1 μM. At 30', 2.3 uC of ^{35}S-
methionine (195 mC/μmole) were added. Mengo RNA 1 μg was present
from zero time and an additional 1 μg was added at 30 min where
indicated. Rabbit liver tRNA was added at 30 min where indicated.

TABLE 4

Effect of tRNA$_{met\ F}$ on translation of Mengo RNA
in extracts of interferon-treated cells

Additions	^{35}S methionine incorporation		
	Control-S10	Interferon-S10	
	cpm	cpm	per cent
Exp.1 None	103,150	8,480	(8)
tRNA$_{met\ F}$,1µg	62,500	7,480	(12)
" ,5µg *	55,110	5,120	(10)
tRNA$_{met\ F}$,1µg +tRNA total,9µg	75,962	61,215	(81)
Exp.2 None	133,350	31,550	(23)
tRNA$_{met\ F}$,1µg	280,375	41,240	(15)
tRNA$_{met\ F}$,1µg+S100	374,700	47,300	(13)
tRNA total,9µg	247,600	234,300	(95)
Exp.3 ^{35}S-met-tRNA$_{met\ F}$ (0.2ug-6x10^5 cpm)	91,800	5,950	(7)
idem+tRNA total,9µg	87,100	73,750	(85)
idem, no Mengo RNA	4,750	3,450	

Conditions as in Fig. 1B. Purified tRNA$_{met\ F}$ was from rabbit liver (10). Total tRNA from rabbit liver. In experiments 1 and 2,
free ^{35}S-methionine (5 µc; 195 mc/µmole) were added. In Exp. 3,
the transfer of met from charged ^{35}S-met tRNA$_{met\ F}$ was measured
and no free methionine was added. Incorporation from 0-60 min at
30° C was measured.
* from separate experiment.

TABLE 5

Absence of restoration by N-formyl-^{35}S-met tRNA$_{met}$ F

Additions	Control-S10	Interferon - S10	
	cpm	cpm	percent
None	33,600	7,000	(21)
fmet tRNA$_{met}$ F,0.3µg	33,100	8,200	(25)
" ,0.6µg	23,100	8,750	(38)
fmet tRNA,0.15 ug +restoring tRNA,0.5 µg	35,800	29,600	(83)

Conditions as in Fig. 1B. ^{35}S-fmet tRNA$_{met}$ F was prepared as in Methods. Free ^{35}S-methionine (1µc and 55 pmoles for 0.05 ml) was added. Without Mengo RNA, 600 cpm was incorporated from 20-60 min at 30°C.

TABLE 6

Effect of ribosomal wash fraction on L cell translation

Additions	L cell endogenous protein synthesis	Mengo RNA translation
	percent	percent
None	100	100
tRNA$_{retic}$,5µg + S100	–	85
Control ribos. wash,20µg	72	74
Interf. ribos. wash,25µg	63	27
Idem + tRNA$_{retic}$, 5 µg+S100	–	83

Conditions as in Fig. 1A. ^{14}C-amino acid incorporation was measured in control L cell - S10; non preincubated for endogen-ous protein synthesis (100 percent = 8,950 cpm in 60 min at 30°C) or after preincubation and addition of 1 µg Mengo RNA (100 percent = 2330 cpm).

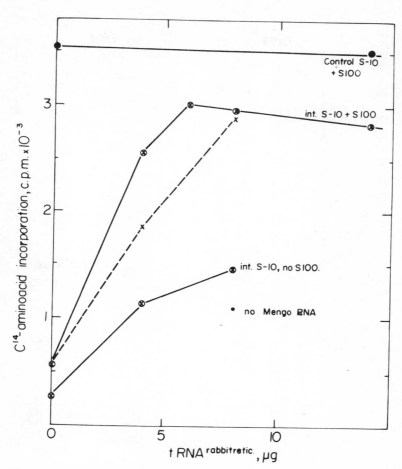

Fig. 1A. Restoration by tRNA of Mengo RNA translation in Interferon-treated L cell S-10. Conditions of assay as in Methods with 0.3 A_{260} units of S10 from control or interferon treated L cells and 1 μg Mengo RNA in 0.05 ml. Incubation for 60 min at 30°C. Ammonium sulfate (90%) precipitated-high speed supernatant (S100) was added (0.15 A_{280} units) where indicated. Hot TCA insoluble radioactivity of a 0.04 ml aliquot determined.

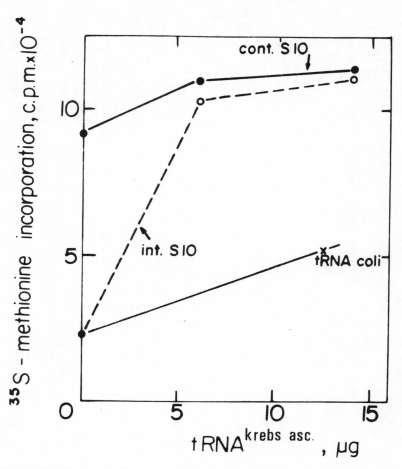

Fig. 1B.   Restoration by tRNA of Mengo RNA translation in interferon-treated L cell S-10. Conditions as in Fig. 1A with different S10 extracts (0.2 A_{260} units) and ^{35}S-methionine. No supernatant added.

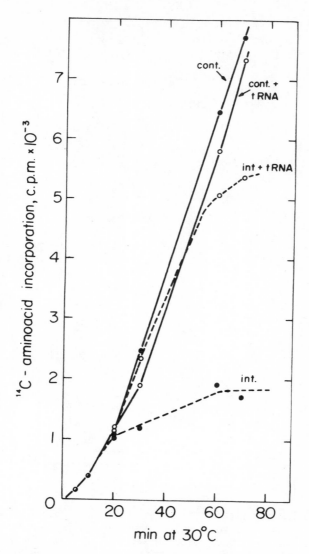

Fig. 2.   Kinetic study of the tRNA effect. Conditions were as in Fig. 1A. L cell extracts used were either treated with 150 units mouse interferon per ml culture for 18 hours, or untreated. Rabbit liver tRNA (15 µg) was used.

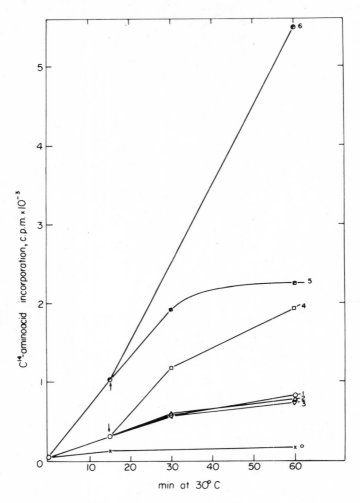

Fig. 3. Effect of Aurintricarboxylic acid (ATA) on restoration by tRNA. Conditions were as in Fig. 1A, but radioactivity incorporated in a 0.02 ml aliquot was determined. Only reaction mixtures containing interferon-treated S10 and 1 μg Mengo RNA are shown. Curve 1: interferon-treated S10; curve 6: same plus rabbit liver tRNA, 9 μg at time 0 min; curve 0: same as 6 but with ATA, at 15 min; curve 4: interferon-treated S10 plus 9 μg tRNA at 15 min; curve 3: interferon-treated S10 plus ATA at 15 min; curve 2: interferon-treated S10 plus tRNA and ATA at 15 min. Control S10 gave 6500 cpm at 60 min.

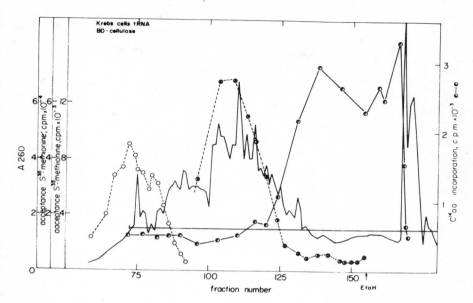

Fig. 4. Chromatography of restoring tRNA on a BD-cellulose column. A 0.9 x 12.5 cm column of BD-cellulose (Schwartz) was loaded with 12.5 mg tRNA extracted (9) by phenol and 1M NaCl from Krebs ascites tumor cells. The column was washed with 0.35 M NaCl, 0.01 M MgCl₂, 0.01 M Na acetate buffer pH 4.5 and eluted with a 100 ml gradient of 0.35-1.0 M NaCl in the same buffer. Fractions of 0.5 ml were collected, dialyzed against Hepes buffer pH 7.5 0.02 M, KCl 0.12 M, MgCl₂ 0.005 M, β mercaptoethanol 0.007 M, glycerol 10 p.cent and assayed for their ability to restore Mengo RNA translation in S10 extracts from interferon treated L cells as in Fig. 1. (without S100). (●———●). Fractions were also assayed for acceptance of ³⁵S-methionine with purified E. coli methionyl tRNA synthetase (0----0) or L cell S-100 (◐-----◐).

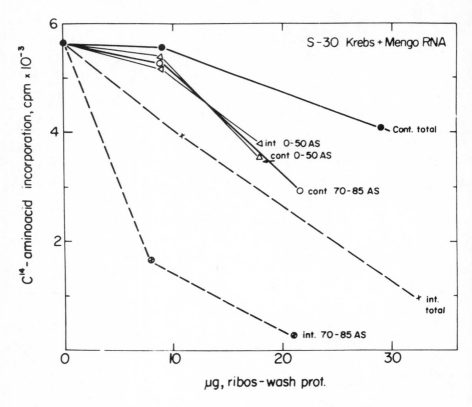

Fig. 5.   Protein synthesis inhibitory activity from ribosomes of interferon-treated L cells. Ribosomes from L cells (5),
normal or treated by 200 units/ml interferon for 38 hours, were
treated for 4 hours at 0°C by 0.5 M KCl in Hepes buffer pH 7.5,
0.02 M $MgCl_2$, 0.005 M β mercaptoethanol 0.007 M, glycerol 20
p.cent. After centrifugation, 3.5 hours at 50,000 rpm in Spinco
R65, the ribosomal wash fraction was dialyzed against the same
buffer but with 0.12 M KCl. Fractionation by ammonium sulfate at
4°C, was followed by dialysis with the same buffer. Fractions
were assayed at the indicated protein concentration for their
effect on the translation of Mengo RNA in Krebs ascites tumor
cell S-30 (5).

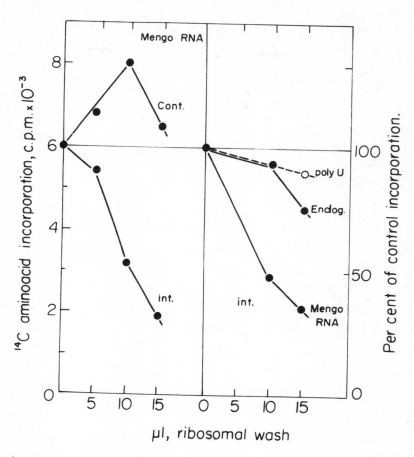

Fig. 6. Effect of ribosomal wash fraction on the translation of different mRNAs in Krebs ascites tumor cells S-30. Total ribosomal wash fraction prepared as in Fig. 5 was assayed. The 100 p.cent value for Poly U translation was 7,800 cpm ^{14}C-phenylalanine incorporated. For endogenous activity, a non preincubated Krebs S-30 was used (3350 cpm ^{14}C-aminoacid incorporated). The two panels represent different experiments. In the right panel, only interferon-ribosomal wash was used.

DISCUSSION

Chany: It may be a little difficult, but is there a possibility to get the protein which accumulates on the ribosome
into a fresh cell and to find out if it affects or not the normal messengers of the cell?

Revel: You would like to introduce it in the cell?

Chany: If this is possible.

Revel: I think it would be an interesting experiment, but
we would like to try it on the purified factor and not on the
crude material we have for the moment. The fact that it seems
to be able to cross some species specific barrier may be interesting. I didn't mention that in some preliminary experiments
this material seems to affect also rabbit reticulocyte ribosomes so that it may be nonspecies specific.

Chany: The experiments which we have performed on somatic
monkey-mouse hybrid cells (Chany et al. Proc. Nat. Acad. Sci.
USA 70, 557-561, 1973) seem to indicate as I mentioned earlier,
that the antiviral protein should not be species specific.

Ankel: I was just wondering, do you require the intact
transfer RNA to reverse the effect or have you tried to treat
it with CCA enzyme or periodate?

Revel: We have tried to treat it with periodate; after
periodate treatment, there is no more activity for restoration.
So it requires the intact adenine residue.

Oxman: Dr. Revel, your proposal that the "antiviral protein" itself is not specifically antiviral, but that it exerts
its effect by altering the ribosomes in such a way that the concentration of certain transfer RNAs becomes a limiting factor
in translation is extremely interesting. I wonder how it fits

with the observation that when two viruses with very different sensitivities to interferon infect the same cell, the difference in their sensitivities is maintained?

Revel: You may be right. Making hypotheses is attractive, but the best way is to try and get the answer by experiments.

INTERFERON INHIBITS THE TRANSLATION OF VIRAL
mRNA IN ANIMAL CELL-FREE SYSTEMS

Mariano Esteban

National Institute for Medical Research,
Mill Hill, London NW7 1AA

The interferon effect in virus infected cells

Pretreatment of animal cells with interferon prevents viral replication and this phenomenon is thought to be due to the
induction by interferon of a factor(s) which acts directly upon
an early stage(s) in virus replication. There have been several
conflicting reports suggesting that the interferon-mediated inhibition acts at the level of transcription (1,2,3,4) or translation (5,6,7,8,9,10,11) of viral messenger RNA. A priori it
may be that both of these events can be affected by a common
factor or perhaps that interferon has indeed more than a single
locus of action. It is fairly well established, however, that
in cells pretreated with interferon and infected with vaccinia
virus, viral protein synthesis is inhibited while viral mRNA
synthesis is stimulated (12,13). The inhibition of viral protein
synthesis in intact L-cells appears to be mainly due to the
failure of the small ribosomal subunit (40S) to bind with the
viral messenger. There is as well an additional effect on the
rate of elongation of viral protein synthesis (14). It is important for a fuller understanding of the mechanism of action
of interferon to use cell-free systems which can reproduce the
same basic conditions as occur in the intact cell. Thus, when

crude post-mitochondrial extracts (S10) were prepared from interferon-treated, vaccinia-infected cells and assayed for their
ability to translate added viral mRNA, a marked inhibition (50
to 90%) of viral translation was observed (9). No such clear-
cut inhibition was seen with similar minimally treated extracts
from cells subjected to interferon treatment alone in the absence of infection, although a small inhibition ($\leqslant$ 20%) of
polypeptide chain elongation was frequently observed (9). From
this it was concluded that infection may be required to trigger
the full development of this inhibitory response.

     a) The interferon effect in EMC virus infected-L cells and
cell-free systems. There has been some question as to what extent it is possible to discriminate between the role played by
the viral infection and that due to interferon. One approach to
this problem is to consider another virus system and study the
interferon effect under conditions where there is no apparent
effect of viral infection on host protein synthesis. We have selected EMC virus infection of L-cells for a number of reasons.
EMC virus multiplies in the cytoplasm of infected cells, so is
similar in this respect to vaccinia, but the inhibition of host
protein synthesis does not develop under our conditions of infection with 10-20 pfu/cell before 2 hr of viral infection (Fig.
1). Using pulse-labelling of EMC virus-infected L-cells at different times post-infection with ^{35}S-methionine as a precursor,
followed by polyacrylamide-SDS gel electrophoresis and autoradiography it has been possible to detect 17 different virus
specific polypeptides by 3 hr after infection. Their synthesis
is inhibited in cells pre-treated with interferon. This does
not, however, prevent the inhibition of host protein synthesis
from occurring later in infection. No effect on host protein
synthesis is observed at or before 2 hr of virus infection. Accordingly, we have prepared cell-free systems from EMC virus-

infected L-cells and interferon-treated, virus-infected L-cells
at different times after infection and assayed them for their
ability to translate exogeneous EMC RNA (Fig. 2). With a crude
post-mitochondrial supernatant (S10) it is possible to observe
a marked inhibition of viral RNA translation in cell extracts
prepared from cells pretreated with interferon and then infected
with EMC virus. Inhibition of viral RNA translation in these
extracts can be clearly observed by two hours after infection
and even earlier and it is fully expressed by 4 hr after infection. In the absence of infection we can detect only a very small
inhibition (≤ 20%) of translation of EMC RNA in these crude
extracts. Thus we are able to observe an inhibition of viral
RNA translation in cell-extracts from interferon-treated EMC virus-infected cells at times where there is no obvious effect on
host protein synthesis in the intact cell. This result would
suggest that the inhibitions of host and viral protein synthesis are developing independently after infection and may be different. If this is so, one would predict that these extracts
will discriminate viral messenger RNA from host mRNA in vitro.

    b) The translation of EMC RNA and mouse globin mRNA. We
have used mouse globin mRNA (the kind gift of Dr. R. Williamson)
as a model for host mRNA and EMC RNA for viral mRNA. The translation of EMC RNA and mouse globin mRNA has been compared in
cell-free systems using cell-sap from interferon-treated, EMC
infected cells at times where there is no apparent effect of virus infection on host protein synthesis in vivo. With systems
showing a 50% inhibition of viral RNA translation, no effect on
the synthesis of authentic mouse globin polypeptide in response
to mouse globin mRNA was observed (Fig. 3). There is, as well,
no effect on poly U translation. With cell-extracts showing a
greater inhibition (≥ 70%) of translation of EMC RNA about
(≤ 30%) inhibition of mouse globin mRNA was observed. These re-

sults would suggest that there is some specificity of the inhibitor(s) for viral mRNA as opposed to host messenger RNAs.

   c) Site of action of the inhibitor(s). We have further characterised the site of action of the inhibitor(s) by analysis of the products synthesised in response to EMC RNA using poly-acrylamide-SDS gel electrophoresis.

   Fig. 4 represents a time-course study of the EMC RNA directed protein synthesis in cell extracts prepared at 2 hr after infection from interferon treated and untreated virus infected cells. It is quite clear that under these conditions the ratio of some of the viral polypeptides synthesised in response to EMC RNA in interferon-treated, infected cell extracts appears to be different from untreated infected cell extracts. Thus, for example, polypeptide 130 which is completed in the cell-free system by 60 min of incubation at 30°C is not in interferon extracts and takes about 120 min for it to be synthesised. This result probably reflects an inhibition on the rate of elongation of viral polypeptide synthesis as one would predict if this rate is slower than in control. We have furthermore fractionated by centrifugation at 100,000 g/2 hr the post-mitochondrial supernatant fraction (S10) into ribosomes and cell-sap and located the interferon effect in this fraction. Assaying L-cell ribosomes from interferon-treated, EMC virus infected cells in the cell-free system with cell-sap (post-microsomal   supernatant) from untreated, virus infected L-cells and the products synthesised in response to EMC RNA analysed by polyacrylamide-SDS gel electrophoresis, the major inhibitory effect (mediated by the ribosomes) appeared to be on the rate of elongation of viral polypeptide chains (not shown). Assaying cell-sap from interferon-treated, EMC virus infected cells with L-cell ribosomes or with preincubated normal Krebs microsomes (see Fig. 3) where a 50% inhibition of viral translation was observed, the polypepti-

des synthesised in response to EMC RNA appears to be equal in
size, but less in amount in interferon-treated, virus infected
cells. This result would indicate that the inhibitory effect
mediated by interferon and associated with the cell-sap is primarily on initiation. Thus, the interferon-mediated inhibitor(s)
can be found both in the cell-sap and ribosomes. Whether the cell
sap associated inhibitor factor(s) is the same, or different
from that ribosome associated inhibitory factor(s) remains to be
seen.

The interferon effect on uninfected cells

In the absence of virus infection we can detect only a ve-
ry small inhibition ($\leqslant$ 20%) of translation of EMC RNA in a crude post-mitochondrial supernatant fraction (S10). The interferon
effect is expressed only following virus infection in these extracts. These results imply some role of the virus, such as a
very early function, in triggering the interferon-mediated in-
hibitor(s) of viral RNA translation in the cell-free system.
However when cell extracts either from interferon-treated, uninfected cells or interferon-treated, EMC virus infected cells,
were preincubated under an amino acid incorporating system conditions then, the interferon-mediated inhibitor(s) is fully expressed. The extent of this inhibition depends on the dose of
interferon used (not shown). Fig. 5 shows a time-course of pre-
incubation at 37°C under cell-free system conditions using post-
mitochondrial supernatant (S10) from untreated or interferon -
treated, uninfected cells. The interferon effect develops with
time and is triggered during preincubation. The fact that treatment other than infection can induce in interferon-treated L-
cells an inhibition of viral translation in the cell-free system
indicates that the triggering effect is important for the full
activation of the inhibitor(s) mediated by interferon.

References

1. Bialby, H.S., and Colby, C. (1972). J. Virol 9, 286.
2. Manders, E.K., Tilles, J.G., and Huang, A.S. (1972).
   Virology 49, 573.
3. Marcus, P.I., Engelhardt, D.L., Hunt, J.M., and Sekellick, M.J. (1971). Science 174, 593.
4. Oxman, M.N., and Levin, M.J. (1971). Proc. Nat. Acad.
   Sci. 68, 299.
5. Falcoff, E., Lebleu, B., Falcoff, R., and Revel, M.
   (1972). Nature New Biology, 240, 145.
6. Falcoff, E., Falcoff, R., Lebleu, B., and Revel, M.
   (1973). J. Virol. 12, 421.
7. Friedman, R.M. (1968). J. Virol. 2, 1081.
8. Friedman, R.M., Esteban, M., Metz, D.H., Tovell, D.R.,
   Kerr, I.M., and Williamson, R. (1972). Febs. Letters
   24, 273.
9. Friedman, R.M., Metz, D.H., Esteban, M., Tovell, D.R.,
   Ball, L.A., and Kerr, I.M. (1972). J. Virol. 10, 1184.
10. Joklik, W.K., and Merigan, T.S. (1966). Proc. Nat.
    Acad. Sci. US 56, 558.
11. Kerr, I.M. (1971). J. Virol. 7, 448.
12. Metz, D.H., and Esteban, M. (1972). Nature 238, 385.
13. Esteban, M. and Metz, D.H. (1973). J. gen. Virol. 20,
    111.
14. Metz, D.H. and Esteban, M. (1974). (submitted)
15. Esteban, M. and Metz, D.H. (1973). J. gen. Virol. 19,
    201.

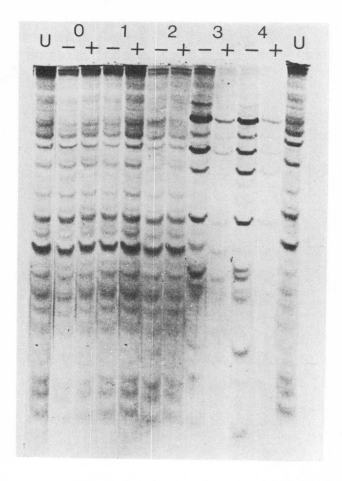

Fig. 1. Electrophoretic analysis of polypeptides synthesised in control and interferon treated EMC virus-infected L - cells. Cells were treated for 22 hr at 37°C with 50 units/ml of purified mouse interferon (specific activity 10^7 units/mg protein), infected with 10 pfu/ml of purified EMC virus and labelled for 20 min periods at 37°C with ^{35}S-methionine (120 Ci/mmol) as described (12,15). Electrophoresis of the reduced proteins in SDS polyacrylamide gels in the presence of 8 M urea has already been described (12,15). U denotes uninfected cells (interferon alone has no effect on the pattern seen with uninfected cells). Gels plus (+) and minus (-) pretreatment with interferon are shown for time points 0, 1, 2, 3 and 4 hr post-infection. The times indicated are for the start of each 20 min pulse.

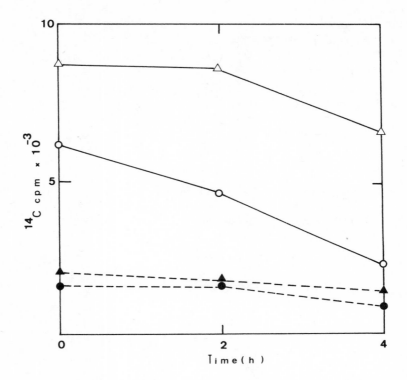

Fig. 2. Development of the interferon-mediated inhibition of
EMC RNA translation with time post-EMC virus infection. L-cells
(1.5 x 10⁶ cells/ml) were treated for 4 hr at 37°C with 50 u-
nits/ml of interferon, diluted with an equal volume of medium
and incubated for a further 18 hr. The cells were washed and
infected with purified EMC virus (10 pfu/cell). Infection was
as Fig. 1 for 30 min at 37°C at 10⁷ cells/ml prior to dilution
to 10⁶ cells/ml for further incubation. The time of dilution
was taken as zero time. After 0, 2 and 4 hr post-infection the
cells were washed and cell extracts prepared and assayed in the
cell-free system as previously described (9). With EMC RNA (20-
40 μg/ml) incubations were in the presence of a ¹⁴C-amino acid
mixture (57 mCi/mA) for 2 hr at 30°C. Untreated, infected plus
(△) and minus (▲) EMC RNA; interferon-treated, infected plus
(○) and minus (●) EMC RNA.

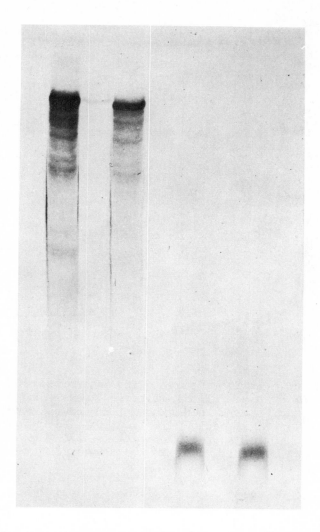

Fig. 3a. Autoradiography of the ^{14}C-labelled polypeptides synthesised in response to EMC RNA and mouse globin mRNA employing preincubated Krebs cell ribosomes and L-cell sap preparations. L-cell sap (100,000 g/2 hr) was obtained from untreated or interferon-treated, EMC virus infected cells at 2 hr after infection. Pretreatment of the cells, preparation of the cell-free system and their assay were as described in Fig. 2. The stimulation by mouse globin mRNA was optimal at 3.5 mM Mg^{++} and 50 mM K^+.

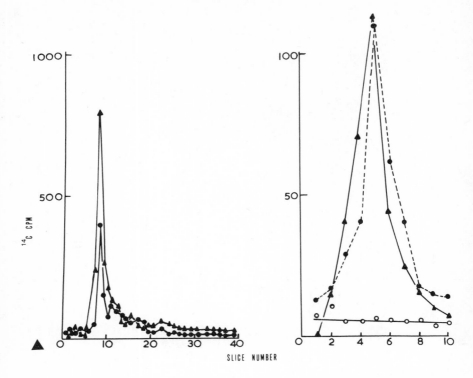

Fig. 3b. Direct quantitation of the interferon effect. The corresponding gels were sliced, dissolved in H_2O_2 and counted. Polypeptides synthesised in response to EMC RNA in untreated, infected cells (▲) and interferon-treated, infected cells (●). On the right, globin polypeptide synthesised in response to globin mRNA in untreated, infected cells (▲), interferon-treated, infected cells (●), and in the absence of globin mRNA (O).

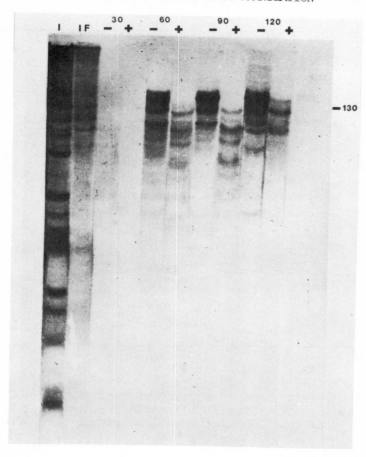

Fig. 4. Characterization of the polypeptides synthesised by EMC RNA with time in cell-free systems from untreated or interferon-treated, EMC virus infected cells. Pretreatment of the cells with interferon, conditions for infection and preparation of the cell extracts were as in Fig. 2. Unfractionated post - mitochondrial supernatant (S10) prepared at 2 hr post-infection were preincubated and passed through Sephadex G-25 (9). Incubation at 30 C in the cell-free system with added EMC RNA was followed at 30, 60, 90 and 120 min. Numbers on top of the gels indicates the times of incubation in the cell-free system, without (-) interferon treatment or with (+) interferon treatment. No polypeptides can be seen in the absence of EMC RNA. Gel (I) shows the ^{35}S-methionine labelled polypeptides for 20 min from EMC virus infected intact cells at 4 hr after infection and gel (IF) denotes the labelled polypeptides from the same cells but pretreated with interferon.

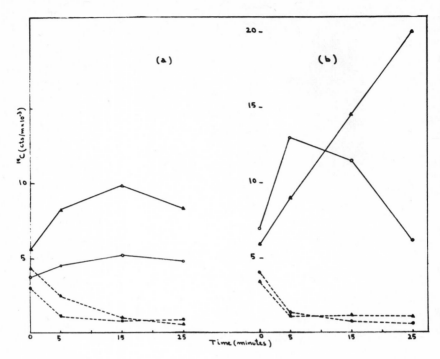

Fig. 5. Development of the interferon-mediated inhibition of EMC RNA translation with time during preincubation at 37 C. Post mitochondrial supernatant (S10) prepared as described in Fig. 2 from untreated or interferon-treated, uninfected cells was pre-incubated at different times at 37 C in the standard 50 μl assay (9) under amino acid incorporating conditions. At the end of the incubation at 37 C, EMC RNA and ^{14}C-amino acid mixture were ad-ded to the systems and further incubation was continued at 30 C for 2 hr. (a) denotes total protein synthesised in response to EMC RNA from untreated (△) or interferon-treated, uninfected cells (O). Dotted lines indicate total protein synthesised in the absence of EMC RNA from untreated (▲) or interferon-treated uninfected cells (●). (b) same as (a) but cells were incubated in buffered salt for 30 min at 37 C prior to the preparation of cell-extracts.

DISCUSSION

Levy: Just a couple of points I want to clarify. In these last experiments where you showed there was a specific effect on EMC translation, were these done with preparations made from uninfected cells?

Esteban: Yes.

Levy: I'm not quite sure what the situation is. Do uninfected cells show the interferon effect or not?

Esteban: Yes, they clearly show it, but in order to have the expression of the interferon-mediated inhibitor(s) of viral RNA translation in the cell-free system, you need some tricks such as virus infection to the cells or preincubation of the cell-extracts under cell-free system conditions.

Levy: The other thing, where you show that extracts from interferon treated cells translated globin messenger RNA normally. Were those from uninfected or infected cells?

Esteban: Those were done from EMC virus infected cells.

De Maeyer: There was no effect on translation of mouse globin messenger RNA in extracts from interferon treated cells. Now would it be possible in your system to try translation of rabbit globin messenger RNA, which in a way is a foreign messenger for the mouse system?

Esteban: Yes.

De Maeyer: Have you tried it?

Esteban: No. I have not tried it but I would expect rabbit globin mRNA to be translated similarly as mouse globin mRNA in extracts from interferon-treated cells.

THE INHIBITION OF PROTEIN SYNTHESIS IN CELL-FREE SYSTEMS FROM INTERFERON-TREATED, INFECTED CELLS*

Robert M. Friedman

National Institute for Medical Research,
Mill Hill, London NW7 1AA, England

After several years in which very little new work had appeared on the mechanism of interferon action, several reports have been recently published on this phenomenon (1,2,3). The conclusions reached by these studies however, appear to be quite contradictory, and, as a result there is some confusion on this subject. We propose in the present report to summarize some of the results of work on interferon action that our group has obtained.

Numerous studies on intact cells in tissue culture have suggested that interferon acts by inhibiting virus directed protein synthesis (4). Other studies which attempted to confirm this hypothesis in cell-free systems proved either inconclusive or, while uncovering some inhibition of viral messenger RNA translation, in cell-free systems, failed to demonstrate clearly that this inhibition was related to the antiviral action of interferon and was not due to a relatively non-specific toxic

---

* This work was carried out while the author was a visitor at the Biochemistry Department of the National Institute for Medical Research, London. Collaborators on the project were L.A. Ball, D.H. Metz, R.M. Esteban, D.R. Tovell, J.A. Sonnabend, D. Risby, R.E. Brown, and I.M. Kerr.

effect of the interferon preparation employed (5,6). On the other hand, reports from this laboratory have presented evidence
for the inhibition of the translation of viral RNA in a cell -
free protein synthesizing system from interferon-treated, virus-
infected cells. This effect seemed quantitatively sufficient to
account for the inhibitory action of interferon pretreatment on
virus replication and was seen on treatment with small doses (5
to 50 NIH reference units of mouse interferon per ml) of highly
purified (> 10^7 units/mg protein) interferon (1,7).

   With cell-free systems from interferon-treated, vaccinia
or EMC virus-infected L-cells, the response to EMC RNA was inhibited, and in some systems the polypeptides which were formed were of somewhat lower molecular weight while in others, they
were normal. The inhibition affected the rate as well as in some
systems the size of the product formed in response to the added
RNA and was not reversed by the addition of excess EMC RNA. In
addition, the results of a number of control experiments have
indicated that this effect is interferon mediated. It was seen
with highly-purified mouse interferon from two sources. In other
studies, chick interferon was without effect; inactivation of
the antiviral activity of interferon by heat or trypsin treatment abolished the inhibition of translation in the cell-free
system; and a 60% inhibition was seen after exposure of the
cells to as little as 5 units/ml of interferon. No such effect
was seen with polyuridylic acid as a messenger RNA. These results indicate that a marked inhibition in viral mRNA translation is demonstrable in extracts from interferon-treated, virus-infected L-cells and that this inhibition has many of the
characteristics one would expect if it were indeed interferon
mediated.

   In our hands virus infection of cells is required to demonstrate regularly marked inhibition of translation in the cell-free system. This develops rapidly after vaccinia or EMC virus infection since there was a 72% inhibition of EMC RNA translation in such systems with extracts from cells which had been exposed to vaccinia virus for only 15 min at 37°C. Because of this rapid development of inhibitory activity in interferon-treated cells after virus infection activation of a precursor may be taking place. It is also possible that a virus function may be required for the inhibition to develop.

Mixing experiments were carried out in order to test whether there was a factor in the extracts from interferon-treated, virus-infected cells which would inhibit EMC RNA directed protein synthesis in extracts from untreated, virus-infected cells. In two experiments the mixture of equal volumes of both extracts responded considerably less well to added EMC RNA than did the extracts from untreated, virus-infected cells. In this respect, the mixtures resembled the extracts from interferon-treated, virus-infected cells, although in neither experiment was the inhibition of EMC RNA-directed protein synthesis as profound as was seen in the extracts from interferon-treated, virus-infected cells. The results of these experiments therefore suggested the presence of an inhibitory, rather than the absence of a required factor in interferon-treated, virus-infected cells.

Preliminary results indicated that the inhibitory activity in the cell-free system was associated with both the cell sap and the ribosome fractions (7). In most preparations from interferon-treated, vaccinia virus infected cells, the bulk of the inhibitory activity is present in the cell sap fraction. In fact, the addition of cell sap from vaccinia virus-infected, interferon-treated L-cells to ribosomes from interferon insensitive Krebs ascites cells also results in an inhibition of the trans-

lation of EMC RNA. In a few experiments inhibitory activity was
present in the ribosome fraction from interferon-treated, virus-
infected cells but, since in most experiments the ribosome fraction does not inhibit translation, while the cell sap does, our
results taken together suggest that the inhibitory activity may
be primarily associated with a cell sap factor which becomes
under some conditions ribosome associated.

Studies in intact cells with inhibitions of RNA or protein
synthesis have suggested that interferon action requires the
production of an "antiviral protein". It may be, therefore, that
the inhibitory factor we are studying is this postulated "antiviral protein". Inhibition of initiation of protein synthesis
has proved an attractive hypothesis to explain the action of interferon and our results are in accord with an inhibition of
initiation in cell-free systems. In these systems the incorporation of ^{14}C amino acids was inhibited in extracts from interferon-treated, virus-infected cells, as compared to extracts
from virus-infected cells. We intended to study whether initiation of protein synthesis was also inhibited. This was accom -
plished by assaying EMC RNA stimulated polypeptide synthesis by
extracts in the presence of formyl ^{35}S methionyl tRNA$_F^{MET}$ which
is incorporated into polypeptides only at the N-terminal site.
In this system no difference in ^{35}S incorporation was observed
despite marked inhibition of ^{14}C amino acid incorporation. The
major polypeptide product from extracts of interferon-treated
cells which had incorporated the formyl ^{35}S methionine was approximately the same molecular weight (about 130,000) as the
normal product of these cell-free systems. The results suggest
that in the presence of the formyl methionyl tRNA the translation inhibiting activity induced by interferon treatment is cir-
cumvented. While we are still uncertain of the exact site that
this inhibition takes place,the latter finding makes it like-

ly that the initiation of protein synthesis is involved.

Previously reported work together with our current results
have suggested to us the following explanation for interferon
action. When cells are treated with an appropriate interferon
for a sufficient period of time an inactive protein is formed.
Interferon treatment may have a specific inhibitory effect on
the growth of some cells (8); however, such effects are small
and no gross inhibition of any cell function so far studied can
be detected. On the other hand when the interferon-treated cell
is virus infected, rapid activation of the protein induced by
interferon treatment takes place. Virus growth is markedly inhibited in intact cells and translation of viral messenger RNA
is reduced in extracts from the interferon-treated, virus-infected cells. Our experiments have not progressed to the point
where we can pinpoint the locus of inhibition during the translation process but the results so far suggest that a factor is
present in the cell sap of interferon treated, virus infected
cells which inhibits a normal function necessary for translation. This inhibited function seems necessary for chain initiation of viral polypeptides, but we have some evidence that it
may also be involved in chain elongation. Other laboratories
have recently reported inhibition in translation of virus messenger RNA directed protein synthesis in extracts from interferon treated cells (2,3). Although the results reported from various laboratories differ in some details, these may involve
matters of technique and not be fundamental differences. In
another set of recent reports, however, it seemed that pretreatment of cells with interferon inhibited the intracellular accumulation of viral messenger RNA produced by the parental infecting virion polymerases of vesicular stomatitis and vaccinia viruses (9,10). These findings together with those of Oxman et al.
on early SV-40 messenger RNA synthesis (in this case involving

a cell polymerase) have led to the suggestion that the primary action of interferon is on transcription (11). It is certainly possible that interferon does indeed possess two basic mechanisms of action, the one on translation, the other on transcription. At present, studies in cell-free protein systems may be helping to clarify the mechanism of action of interferon, but, as yet, no satisfactory system has been found to study the possible effect of interferon treatment on virus directed transcription.

References

1. Friedman, R.M., Metz, D.H., Esteban, R.M., Tovell, D. R., Ball, L.A., and Kerr, I.M. (1972). J. Virol. 10, 1184.

2. Falcoff, E., Falcoff, R., Lebleu, B., and Revel, M. (1973). J. Virol. 12, 421.

3. Gupta, S.L., Sopori, M.L., and Lengyel, P. (1973). Biochem. Biophys. Res. Commun. 54, 777.

4. Friedman, R.M., and Sonnabend, J.A. (1970). Arch. Int. Med. 126, 51.

5. Carter, W.A., and Levy, H.B. (1968). Biochim. Biophys. Acta 155, 437.

6. Kerr, I.M. (1971). J. Virol. 7, 448.

7. Friedman, R.M., Esteban, R.M., Metz, D.H., Tovell, D. R., Kerr, I.M., and Williamson, R. (1972). FEBS Letters 24, 273.

8. Paucker, K.B., Berman, B.J., Golger, R.R., and Stancek, D. (1970). J. Virol. 5, 145.

9. Marcus, P.I., Engelhardt, D.L., Hunt, J.M., and Sekellick, M.J. (1972). Science 174, 593.

10. Bialy, H.S., and Colby, C. (1972). J. Virol. 9, 286.

11. Oxman, M.N., and Levin, M.J. (1971). Proc. Nat. Acad.
     Sci. USA <u>68</u>, 299.

DISCUSSION

<u>Levy</u>: In view of our finding of differences in tRNA frac-
tions in control and interferon-treated cells, would you think
it worthwhile to try to see whether or not you can reverse the
interferon effect if you use tRNAs from interferon-treated cells?
I would predict that you would not be able to reverse the interferon effect.

<u>Friedman</u>: I'm not sure I follow. Do you mean using tRNAs
from interferon-treated cells?

<u>Levy</u>: Yes. It may be that there is a modification in the
tRNAs from interferon-treated cells which prevents those tRNAs
from forming an initiation complex with viral RNA.

<u>Friedman</u>: I have to think about that. Maybe I'll follow
this suggestion.

<u>Revel</u>: I would like to mention, maybe to solve some of
the confusion mentioned in Dr. Friedman's lecture, the experiments done by Peter Lengyel at Yale University. He has worked
with a very purified mouse interferon (I think he has now an interferon which has two bands on electrophoresis polyacrylamide
gel) and finds in noninfected L cells the same type of inactivation of translation that we have observed. I think it may depend on the type of cell one is using, but at least two laboratories on both sides of Atlantic have seen it.

<u>Colby</u>: On your 45 minute at 37°C reversal, was that a
warming of the total extract or was that a warming of your cell
sap? Was that just a standard sort of pre-incubation in which

the effect disappeared or was it the cell sap?

Friedman: This was a standard sort of pre-incubation, but as I said, this does not happen with every extract. The first few we made were inactivated without exception. We would see in-activation just incubating for 40 minutes at 37°C - that was just taking the whole extract and incubating it, not just the cell sap. I don't remember if we have ever tried the cell sap alone. Since then, we've had some extracts to which we could do that. I don't know really what the explanation is.

Oxman: A question for both Dr. Friedman and Dr. Revel. Have you compared the level of RNAase activity in preparations from interferon-treated and control cells? Dr. Revel, have you tested the inhibitory material which you can elute from inter-feron-treated ribosomes for RNAase activity?

Friedman: We have, by looking at the integrity of the EMC RNA after it has been incubated with the extract for a while. It is really surprising but Andrew Ball found that EMC RNA holds together quite well, even after 2 hours.

Kerr: There is no difference in the stability of the EMC RNA in interferon and control extracts that we can test. This is Andrew Ball's work. Moreover, you can re-extract the RNA and put it back into another cell-free system and it's not modified by pre-incubation in the interferon system compared with the appro-priate control.

Revel: We have not seen any evidence for degradation of the RNA in the interferon-treated extract. One of the experiments we have been able to do recently since we have the possibility to reverse the effect by adding tRNA, is to preincubate for 15 minutes the interferon-treated extract (which is completely inactive) with the messenger RNA and then add the tRNA: the reaction starts at the same rate as in the control. So the messenger RNA does not get degraded in the interferon extract during this preincubation time. With radioactive mRNA we find, as I said, binding to the ribosomes as in normal extracts.

Colby: Most research groups studying the mode of interferon action in in vitro protein synthesis systems have found that the effectiveness of both viral and host mRNA's in directing the incorporation of amino acids could be equally inhibited with extracts prepared from interferon-treated cells. It has recently been determined that mammalian messenger RNA's are functionally stable for periods ranging from one to several days. These two results suggest the possibility that the mechanism of action of the interferon-mediated antiviral activity may be to block the initiation of translation of all new mRNA's for the period that the block is present. Friedman and his coworkers have reported that aryl hydrocarbon hydroxylase induction is stimulated in interferon-pretreated cells. Dr. Gordon Tompkins and I have studied effect of interferon pretreatment on the induction of tyrosine aminotransferase in rat hepatoma cells. We obtained rat interferon from the NIH group. We used a concentration of interferon that resulted in a 1.5 $\log_{10}$ reduction of vesicular stomatitis virus growth in these cells. We found no difference in the inducibility of tyrosine aminotransferase whether or not the cells had been pretreated with interferon.

Kerr: I wonder if that would still be true if you used either infected cells or cells using one of the tricks for mimicking infection. If you starve the cells, for example, although I am quite sure you can see an effect in uninfected cells, I am equally certain, and I think Dr. Revel agrees, that it is en - hanced on infection. I think it would now, with hindsight, be

very intriguing to do exactly that same test with interferon-
treated starved or infected cells.

   Friedman: I just had one other comment I wanted to make
on that since some work I've done bears on it. That was carried
out with Dan Nebert on aryl hydrocarbon hydroxylase "induction".
There have been some recent surprises with the system. While it
had all the earmarks of an inducible system, recently Dan has
found a quantitative method of studying the ion atoms in the
molecule of the enzyme. He has found that the process is not a
true induction but is an activation of the enzyme. That which
appeared to be an induction was really an increase in the activity of the enzyme which was there all the time and there is no
true increase in the level of the enzyme, only of the enzyme activity. So it isn't a true induced system and it isn't really a
good test of Bud's idea. Why interferon has the effect it has,
I don't know, but it all goes to show that you never know about
these things in animal cells. It's a pretty complicated business.

   Colby: I think that your results could be explained in
the light of other work that has been presented here at this
Symposium. That is, concomitant with the establishment of the
antiviral state by interferon treatment are a variety of cellular changes including some changes in the surface membrane such
that a more efficient interaction of the aryl hydrocarbon with
the membrane could result in a higher level of activation in
this case. To answer Dr. Kerr's question, we did the experiment
exactly as I described in the hepatoma cells that were not viral infected nor were they amino acid starved. We could go back
and do that. In answer to your comment, Bob, I don't know of
anyone who has looked for and found any sort of metal ions associated wiyh tyrosine aminotransferase and I think that some of

the studies involving incorporation of radioactive amino acids into purifiable tyrosine aminotransferase indicate that that system really is truly inducible.

EFFECT OF INTERFERON TREATMENT ON CELL mRNA SIZE

Hilton B. Levy and Freddie Riley

Laboratory of Viral Diseases
National Institute of Allergy and Infectious Diseases
National Institutes of Health
Bethesda, Maryland 20014

After a number of disagreements among different laboratories, I think that today everyone has come around to agree with the idea that at least one effect of interferon treatment is to modify the cell's translation machinery so that there is a relatively selective inhibition of translation of viral RNA and perhaps of other heterologous RNAs, with only a minimum effect on the translation of normal host cell messenger RNA. Whether this is the only effect of interferon is another story. How the cell makes the distinction between viral messenger RNA and host messenger RNA has not been understood. While levels of interferon that can strongly inhibit virus growth have no immediate effect on total cellular RNA, protein or DNA synthesis, it is self-evident that interferon treatment of a cell must initiate a change, probably biochemical, that is ultimately responsible for this ability to recognize differences between virus and host RNAs. Because of the fact that new RNA and protein synthesis is needed in order for interferon treatment to lead to a virus resistant state, it has been suggested that there is a newly synthesized protein or proteins that is the active mediator of the virus resistant state. This protein has never been demonstrated, however. We'd like to report some interferon induced changes in certain cellular RNA species that may bear on the mechanism by which cells can distinguish between virus and cell RNA.

Cells were treated either with interferon or control fluid overnight. The interferon was removed and then the cells were exposed to radioactive RNA precursors such as labelled uridine. Polysomes were prepared from these cells as follows: The cells were washed, broken by exposure to hypotonic salt solution with douncing and the polysomes precipitated from the postmitochondrial supernatant by the addition of magnesium. The polysome of course consists basicaly of ribosomes held together by magnesium and messenger RNA or rather messenger ribonucleoprotein, with some transfer RNA in the structure as well. By lowering the magnesium concentration we separated the polysome into messenger ribonucleoprotein, transfer RNA and ribosome subunits. We then spun out the ribosome subunits and left the messenger RNP and tRNA in solution. This messenger RNP and tRNA therefore represents material that was in the state of being translated at the time the experiment was terminated. The RNPs from control and interferon treated cultures were analyzed by electrophoresis on 7% polyacrylamide gels. After the run the gels were scanned at 260 nm, sliced into 80 1mm slices, the slices digested and counted. In order to facilitate comparison between interferon and control gels, the data are presented in the following way. The numbers representing the disintegrations per minute from each of the slices were fed into a computer which determined the percentage of the total counts present in each slice. The computer then plotted the log to the base ten of this percentage in order to accomodate the large range in percentage distribution in the slices. Fig. 1 presents in this way the data from an experiment where L cells were treated with 50 units of interferon, labelled messenger RNPs were prepared and compared on gels with comparable messenger RNPs from control cells.

The two curves are very similar to each other, point by point, except that the curve representing the interferon preparation is displaced just a bit to the left of the control curve. That is, each interferon component moves a bit slower than the corresponding control component. The small peaks and dips are so parallel that I believe in their reality. Just for substantiation , Fig. 2 shows another identical experiment. You can see that the same phenomenon, point by point, exists as was seen in Fig. 1. The lines represent the places where 4S, 5S and 7S peaks showed up in a separate gel run with whole cell RNA for optical density markers. This optical density tracing marker gel is shown in Fig. 3. There were big radioactive peaks seen in Figs. 1 and 2 in the messenger RNP preparations which correspond in position to the 4S peaks, but no radioactive peaks at 5S and 7S. There are two radioactive peaks corresponding in position to the optical density peak marked x and y in this graph. Roughly they correspond to 11 to 12S and 15S.

Differences in migration rates in a RNP could be due ei - ther to differences in RNA or protein or conceivably to both. RNA was prepared from the ribonucleoprotein by phenol extraction and analyzed in the same way. Fig. 4 shows the results. Again the interferon components moved more slowly than did the control components.

Differences in RNA migration speed in a polyacrylamide gel might be due to differences in size or in charge. It is generally considered that running the RNA in a gel containing sodium dodecyl sulfate minimizes the effect of charge differences. Fig. 5 shows that when the messenger RNAs are run in the presence of SDS the RNA components from the interferon treated culture still move more slowly. It appears then that the tRNAs and messenger RNA components from interferon treated cells are slightly larger

than the control components. Structural alterations conceivably
might play a role in determining this effect but two things tend
to make this unlikely. (1) The gels were run under low salt conditions and (2) the same findings were observed when urea was
present in the gel.

7% gels exclude 18S RNA and larger species. Figure 6 shows
data obtained with L cells using 2% gels which allowed larger
components to enter the gel. The same phenomenon is present. The
arrows indicate where 18 and 28S ribosomal RNA appears in control
marker gels. There was no evidence of the presence of ribosomal
RNA in our so-called messenger RNP fraction. On rare occasions we
did have some evidence of ribosomal subunit disintegration. We
did not use these experiments.

Comparable experiments were done with primary mouse embry-
o cells with typical results shown in Fig. 7. Two things can be
seen here. (1) The characteristic profile of distribution of
messenger RNP in the gel is somewhat different for primary mouse
embryo than for L cells and (2) the slower movement of the interferon components is present also in experiments with primary
mouse embryo cells. In both primary mouse embryo and L cells
both mouse serum interferon and mouse tissue culture interferon
are equally effective but rabbit interferon is not. However, in
rabbit cells both rabbit serum interferon and rabbit tissue
culture interferon kindly supplied by Jan Vilček are effective
while mouse interferon is not (Fig. 8).

Treatment of L cells with interferon for 4 hours or more
brings on the virus resistant state and the biochemical changes.
Treatment for 2 hours brought on neither.

Levels of interferon of 5 units/ml or more bring on the
biochemical changes but less than 1 unit do not.

The effect is restricted to the fraction of cell RNA that we have described, in that ribosomal RNA is not altered nor is total nuclear RNA. The ribosomal RNA and nuclear RNA of course constitute the great bulk of the cell RNA.

The RNA that remains in the supernatant after removing the ribosomes consists of tRNA and unbound messenger RNA. This supernatant fraction sometimes showed the effect and sometimes not.

There are some thoughts I have about what this may mean and I'll briefly describe three things. (a) What indeed are the RNA species that are altered here (b) what is the molecular nature of the alteration and (c) what does all this have to do with the antiviral action of interferon.

Polysomes are generally recognized as having in them three types of RNA, ribosomal 28S and 18S, transfer (4S) and messenger species. That the RNA's whose differences we note here are not ribosomal is shown by a)- ribosomal RNA does not enter a 7% gel b)- there were no ribosomal subunits, or 28S and 18S RNA species detectable in sucrose gradients, or on 2% gels and c)- ribosomal RNA's do not show the differences. There is transfer RNA in the preparations; added carrier tRNA migrates to the point where the big, fastest moving component moves. This fast moving component does not bind to poly dt cellulose column, therefore it doesn't contain poly A, and is probably not mRNA. The remainder of the RNA must be mRNA. Preliminary data on the radioactivity that does adhere to a poly dt cellulose column are consistent with this. It would appear therefore that only polysome associated mRNA and tRNA are altered.

The nature of the molecular alteration is unknown. The increased size of the mRNA's from interferon treated cells could, in principle mean that totally different information is contained in the mRNA's from interferon treated cells. This appears extremely unlikely; (a) such an effect would undoubtedly produce a different cell from untreated cells, and would likely be toxic, and (b) one would not expect to have a point by point parallelism between the two curves if different information was what we see here. It appears more reasonable to think that an additional piece is added to each of the RNA's from the interferon treated cells. Based on comparison between 4S and 5S RNA's it can be calculated that the increased size could be accounted for by 4-8 additional nucleotides although we do not know if indeed the additional piece consists of nucleotides. Such a piece would probably not contain coding information, but might play a role in recognition control.

That these molecular alterations are induced by the interferon in the preparations rather than impurities is indicated by several control experiments mentioned, i.e. several different interferons bring about the effect, the species specificity of the effect, the parallelism in dose and time effects, pH 2 stability, and a few other things.

Ever since it was demonstrated that translation of viral mRNA is inhibited in interferon treated cells with little or no effect on translation of cell mRNA, the question has existed as to how the interferon treated cell distinguishes between its mRNA's and that of the virus, since both are so similar in essential structural characteristics. The present data indicate that in interferon treated cells, endogenous messenger is modified, and perhaps tRNA as well. The so-called "antiviral protein" of the interferon system might then be the enzyme(s) that is responsible for the modification of RNA. It is tempting to think that interferon treated cell rejects all but the modified type mRNA, whether it be of virus origin, or from a heterologous normal cell. Implicit in this suggestion is the need not only for a difference in recognition sites on the message, but also for a modification in the recognition or initiation mechanisms, perhaps involving tRNA. If the above suggestion should be correct, one would expect inadequate binding of viral RNA, and impaired initiation of its translation.

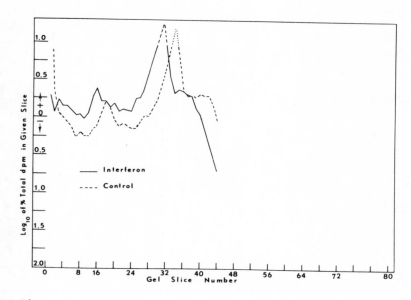

Fig. 1.   Effect of treatment of mouse L cells with 50 u/ml of mouse tissue culture interferon on electrophoretic patterns of m ribonucleoprotein in 7% polyacrylamide gels. See text for details.

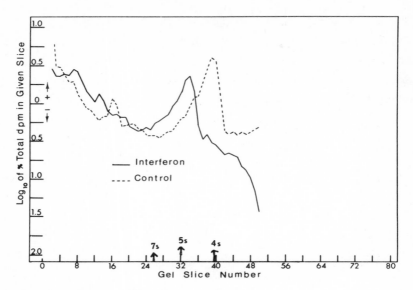

Fig. 2.   Same as Fig. 1.

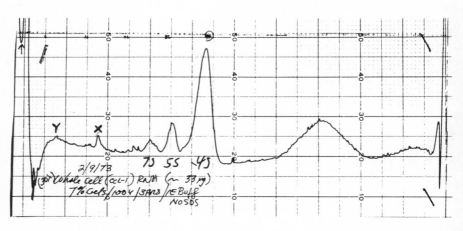

Fig. 3.   Optical density profile at 260 nm of whole L cell
RNA on 7 % polyacrylamide gels.

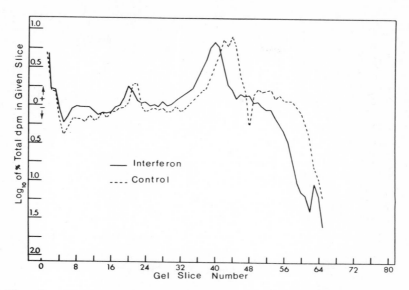

Fig. 4. Effect of treatment of mouse L cells with 100 u/ml of mouse tissue culture interferon on gel electrophoretic patterns of ribonucleic acid.

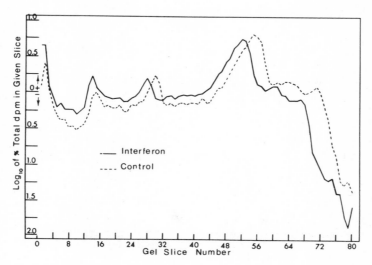

Fig. 5. Effect of treatment of mouse L cells with 100 u/ml of mouse tissue culture interferon on gel electrophoretic patterns of mRNA in the presence of 0.2% sodium dodecyl sulfate.

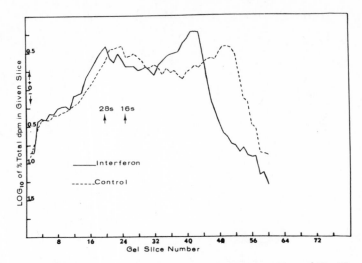

Fig. 6. Effect of treatment of mouse L cells with 60 u/ml of mouse tissue culture interferon on electrophoretic patterns of m ribonucleoprotein in 2% polyacrylamide gels. See text.

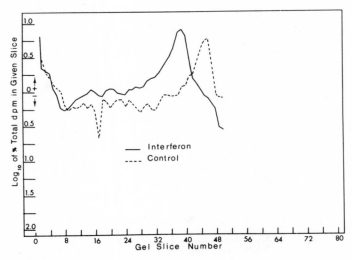

Fig. 7. Effect of treatment of L mouse embryo cells with 50 u/ml of mouse tissue culture interferon on electrophoretic patterns of m ribonucleoprotein in 7% polyacrylamide gels.

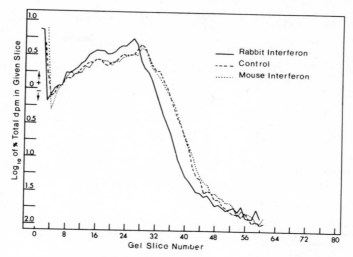

Fig. 8. Effect of   treatment of primary rabbit kidney cells with 100 units/ml of rabbit tissue culture interferon, or 1000 units/ml of mouse tissue culture interferon, on electrophoretic patterns in 7 % polyacrylamide gels of m ribonucleoprotein.

DISCUSSION

<u>Pitha</u>: I've probably missed it but I was wondering, all the gels you show, were they run separately or did you ever run them together with double labelling?

<u>Levy</u>: We tried double labelling experiments in our first attempts, but the rates of labelling of different messenger RNAs with a tritiated uridine and a C 14 uridine are different. If we just ran two control preparations, one labelled with tritiated uridine and the other with C 14 uridine, we could not get sufficient identity between them. So, we ran two gels in each case that I presented here. The gels were prepared at the same time, run at the same time but separate gels.

Pitha: The other thing I have probably missed is: for how long did you label?

Levy: I think that all the experiments here were 3 hour labelling. There were some experiments where we had longer labelling and some where we had shorter labelling. They gave us no differences in the results.

Pitha: The last question I wanted to ask you: you have a very small difference in the movement. Wouldn't you see also the difference if you would have the same molecular size, but one of the molecules would be much more heavier? Let's say one of the RNA would have much more methylated bases than the other. Wouldn't you also see difference in the movement?

Levy: I think that what we are seeing here is the distribution of many different messenger RNAs which are being separated from each other by the gel.

Pitha: All the interferon RNAs seem to move slowly, don't they?

Levy: All the molecular species that go on to the 7 % or the 2 % gel move more slowly than do the control ones.

Pitha: Does it mean that all should be either larger as you suggested, or I wonder if they wouldn't move also slowly if they would be heavier?

Levy: Well, what's heavier as contrasted with larger.

Pitha: You wouldn't add nucleotides, but you would modify: for example, you would add more methylated groups on them.

Levy: Oh yes, we have not established that there are additional nucleotides. I said that if the slower movement was due

to nucleotides then that could be accounted for by 4 to 8 nucleotides. It could be a big piece of carbohydrate or something else
in there. It's not protein. We pretty well removed protein because many of these things were double-labelled with amino acids
as well, and after the phenol treatment all the labelled amino
acids were gone.

Friedman: I think your data require a lot of analysis and
looking at it before one can really agree or disagree with it.
One thing in your theory that is interesting, however, is that
you might predict that addition of exogenous messenger to a cell-
free system from cells which had been treated with interferon,
would unless the messenger has your added piece, not result in
translation, even if it is a normal cellular messenger. Everybody whom I know of who has worked with the cell-free system and
has used exogenous messenger such as globin messenger has found
much to their dismay that the messenger has not been translated
as well as it should have been in interferon-treated cells. So,
it's possible that your theory is reasonable and even though you
take the responsibility, but not the blame for it, maybe it's
all right.

Levy: Well, what should happen of course is that if you
took a translation system prepared from interferon-treated cells
and added interferon messenger RNA, or messenger RNA from interferon-treated cells, this should be translated well; and conversely, messenger RNA from interferon-treated cells when added
to a translation system from normal cells should not be translated very well. This is something I would like to have you do, Bob.

Revel: Have you ever seen the change in the transfer RNA
moiety without the change in what you assume is messenger RNA?
Have you looked in the kinetics of appearance of these changes?
It would be surprising that the two changes would be identical.

One possibility for the messenger, for example, would be that
you have a few more A nucleotides at the end since it is known
that during aging of messenger RNA by translation the poly A is
degraded. If you have a slowing down of translation you have
more poly A. This would not apply to tRNA, so you might expect
the two phenomena to appear separately. Did you observe that?

Levy: We haven't done kinetic studies on the rate at which
these two effects develop. We have, of course, thought of the
differences in poly A possibility and we have done a number of
experiments to see whether or not there is a difference in poly
A content. These differences are so small really that we are
pushing the methodology maximally but I don't think that we can
say that we have seen any differences in poly A content. That
was the first thing that struck us, but we haven't looked at the
kinetics of the development of the two different types of RNA.

Rozee: A few years back we did tRNA methylase studies
with interferon-treated cells and in our first five experiments
we showed really very significant increases in tRNA methylases.
In the next five we couldn't show anything at all, so we abandon-
ed the attempt. But not being a biochemist, we didn't know what
was wrong with the system. The system stopped, but perhaps we
were right the first time and wrong the second.

Levy: I think five experiments are enough.

Colby: I have a comment and then a question. Most of the
gel patterns that I've seen of L cell RNA indicate that histone
message which is there in a very small percentage is approximately 9 or 10 S. But the gross majority of cell message is between
say 18 and 30 S and it wouldn't really be expected to go in your
gels. Most of the patterns of changes that you're seeing I think
are probably in the small molecular weight species. The notion

needs to be, I think, more heavily directed towards a theory
that incorporates a change in the small molecular weight RNA
rather than in the messenger per se. The question is, what do
these gels look like just in terms of counts per minute before
the computer gets a hold of the data?

Levy: There are loads of counts in them, up to 10,000 dpm
per slice.

Colby: In terms of the differences. It was very difficult
for me to try, with my imagination, to duplicate what the computer was doing to the data.

Levy: Well, the computer took the counts. We have a counter which has an absolute activity analyser on it so that it
presents disintegration per minute rather than counts per minute and each of these slices contained anywhere from 400 dpm to
maybe 5,000 to 8,000 dpm. And they were counted to a high level
of statistical accuracy. The computer just determined the percentage distribution of the total that was present in each of
the slices and then plotted it on a logarithmic basis. The reason for doing that was that the quantitative recovery of polysomes from two cell cultures are never identical, and this was
a matter of normalizing; that's the reason for doing it that
way. This procedure enables us to compare two gels more closely.
We have, of course, plotted the actual data and you can see, if
you look at it, the comparable shifts in the peaks. To answer
your earlier question: the reason I did that 2% gel, of course,
was just to look at those other larger species of RNA. I was a-
fraid I would be running into the possible contamination with
ribosomal RNA, that's why most of the studies were done with 7%.
As it is, we could have used 2% gels because we had very little
ribosomal RNA contamination. The difference shows up in all the
species of messenger RNA, big and little.

INTERFERON AND ADENOVIRUS-SIMIAN VIRUS 40 HYBRID VIRUSES

The synthesis of Hybrid Adenovirus 2-Simian Virus 40 RNA
Molecules in Cells Infected with a Nondefective Adenovirus 2-Simian Virus 40 Hybrid Virus

Michael N. Oxman, Myron J. Levin and Andrew M. Lewis, Jr.

Virus Research Unit, Division of Infectious Diseases,
Children's Hospital Medical Center and the Departments
of Pediatrics and Microbiology and Molecular Genetics,
Harvard Medical School, Boston, Massachusetts 02115
Laboratory of Viral Diseases, National Institute of
Allergy and Infectious Diseases, National Institutes
of Health, Bethesda, Maryland 20014

Introduction

Adenovirus (Ad)-SV40 hybrid viruses contain SV40 DNA covalently linked to Ad DNA, and induce the synthesis of both SV40
and Ad-specific RNA and antigens in infected cells (1-12). Because SV40 and Ad differ markedly in their sensitivity to interferon, SV40 being approximately 100 times more sensitive than Ad
(13,14), we have been able to use interferon to probe the effect
of this covalent linkage on the control of both SV40 and Ad gene
expression. Such studies, undertaken with several Ad-SV40 hybrid
viruses, revealed a marked reduction in the interferon sensitivity of SV40 T antigen formation when the synthesis of this early
SV40 antigen was induced by Ad-SV40 hybrid viruses. In fact,
SV40 T antigen synthesis induced by these hybrid viruses was as
resistant to interferon as Ad T antigen synthesis (14). In contrast, the characteristically high sensitivity of SV40 T antigen
synthesis induced by SV40 itself was not altered in cells simulta-

neously infected with SV40 and nonhybrid (wild-type) adenoviruses (14). Thus the decreased interferon sensitivity of hybrid
virus-induced SV40 T antigen synthesis could not be explained by
the production of a diffusible Ad-induced substance or by an Ad-
induced alteration in cellular metabolism. Instead, it appeared
to be a consequence of the covalent linkage of SV40 and Ad DNA
in the genomes of these hybrid viruses.

While interferon has been reported to inhibit translation
in a number of viral-cell systems (15-19), recent observations
indicate that in SV40 infection interferon acts blocking transcription. That is, in interferon treated cells, the synthesis
of early SV40 RNA is inhibited to the same extent as the synthesis of SV40 T antigen (20). It also appears that the relative
resistance of Ad T antigen synthesis to interferon is paralleled by a comparable resistance of Ad RNA synthesis (M.J. Levin et
al., unpublished observations). Furthermore, whereas SV40 RNA
synthesis is sensitive to interferon in cells infected with SV40,
it is relatively resistant to interferon in hybrid virus infected cells, as is the synthesis of SV40 T antigen (M.J. Levin et
al., unpublished observations; 20). These observations suggest
that it is the interferon resistance of transcription of SV40
genetic information in the hybrid virus genomes which is responsible for the interferon resistance of hybrid virus-induced SV40
T antigen synthesis. Such an alteration in the interferon sensitivity of SV40 transcription might reflect the initiation of
transcription of SV40 genetic information in an adjacent region
of Ad DNA, rather than at the usual (interferon sensitive) site
in SV40 DNA. If so, this should result in the synthesis of polycistronic RNA molecules which contain both Ad and SV40 nucleotide
sequences.

To further explore this possibility, we have extended our

studies of interferon sensitivity to the nondefective Ad2-SV40 hybrid virus, $Ad2^+ND_4$ (10,11), and have examined the virus-specific RNA synthesized in $Ad2^+ND_4$ infected cells by means of sequential hybridization with Ad2 DNA, elution, and rehybridization with SV40 DNA. As was the case for the previously studied hybrid viruses, the induction of SV40 T antigen by $Ad2^+ND_4$ is as resistant to interferon as the induction of Ad T antigen. Furthermore, a significant proportion of SV40 RNA synthesized in $Ad2^+ND_4$ infected cells is covalently linked to Ad RNA. These findings, which support the hypothesis that transcription of SV40 genetic information in Ad-SV40 hybrid viruses is initiated in an adjoining region of Ad DNA, may explain the relative resistance to interferon of hybrid virus-induced SV40 T antigen synthesis.

Materials and methods

Tissue culture. The Vero line (21) of African green monkey kidney (AGMK) cells was grown in Eagle's minimal essential medium containing penicillin (250 units/ml), streptomycin (250 μg/ml) and 2 mM glutamine (EMEM) plus 10 % fetal bovine serum (EMEM-10) and maintained in EMEM plus 2 % fetal bovine serum (EMEM-2). The BSC-1 (22) and CV-1 (23,24) AGMK cell lines, as well as commercially obtained primary AGMK cells, were grown in Dulbecco's modified Eagle's medium containing the same concentrations of penicillin, streptomycin and glutamine (DUL) plus 10 % fetal bovine serum (DUL-10) and maintained in DUL plus 2% fetal bovine serum (DUL-2). Roller and stationary cultures were refed biweekly until confluent monolayers were formed. All cell lines were repeatedly shown to be free of mycoplasma by anaerobic culture on Hayflick's medium (25).

Viruses. SV40 (strain 777) (26) was produced in BSC-1 and

CV-1 cells by low multiplicity (approximately 10^{-5} plaque forming units [PFU] /cell) infection using an inoculum of virus from
a single seed pool ($10^{9.3}$ PFU/ml) as previously described (9).

$Ad2^+ND_4$ (10) was grown in primary AGMK cells infected with
a multiplicity of 1-5 PFU/cell. The virus pools employed in
these experiments represent the second passage after plaque purification. The derivation and biological properties of $Ad2^+DN_4$
have previously been described (10).

Nonhybrid Ad2 (strain adenoid 6) was grown in suspension
cultures of human (KB) cells and purified as previously described (11).

The Indiana strain of vesicular stomatitis virus (VSV) was
propagated in BSC-1 cells.

Interferon. Sendai virus-induced human leukocyte inter -
feron (27,28) partially purified by selective precipitation was
the generous gift of Dr. K. Cantell (State Serum Institute,
Helsinki). By assay in human cells, this preparation contained
2×10^6 "international" units per mg of protein (assayed in parallel with the British Standard of human interferon, code 69/19;
Division of Biological Standards, National Institute for Medical
Research, Mill Hill, London, UK). In Vero (monkey) cells the antiviral activity of the human interferon proved to be approxi -
mately 1/25th of that in human cells. Since all of our experiments were performed in Vero cells, a unit of interferon is defined here as the amount required to produce a 50 % reduction in
VSV plaque formation in the Vero cells employed. This corresponds
to approximately 25 "international" units.

To determine the effect of interferon on SV40 and Ad T antigen formation, confluent monolayers of Vero cells in 35 mm

Falcon plastic petri dishes containing glass coverslips were exposed for 18-20 hr at 37°C to 2 ml of various concentrations of interferon diluted in EMEM-2. The monolayers, each of which contained approximately 10^6 cells, were then thrice washed with 2 ml EMEM-2 and infected with 1 ml of EMEM-2 containing either SV40 alone (4.5×10^8 PFU), nonhybrid Ad2 alone (3.7×10^7 PFU), SV40 (4.5×10^8 PFU) plus nonhybrid Ad2 (3.7×10^7 PFU), or $Ad2^+ND_4$ (1.6×10^7 PFU). After two hr an additional 1 ml of EMEM-2 was added and incubation continued at 37°C. Coverslips were fixed 25 hr after infection and stored at -70°C for subsequent fluores - cent antibody (FA) staining. Two or three replicate cultures were employed for each point.

T Antigen Assays. SV40 and Ad2 T antigens were assayed by an indirect FA procedure, using serum pools from hamsters bearing virus-free transplants of virus-induced tumors, and using fluorescein-conjugated goat antihamster globulin. Coverslips were bisected so that one-half could be stained for SV40 T antigen and the other half stained for Ad2 T antigen. Procedures for fixing, staining, and quantitation have been described elsewhere (29).

Preparation of virus and extraction of viral DNA. Both Ad2 and SV40 were purified from cells and medium by a previously described (9) modification of the technique of Burnett et al. (30). After cushioning onto CsCl (density = 1.45 gm/ml), the viruses were further purified by two cycles of equilibrium density gradient centrifugation in CsCl (density = 1.34 gm/ml).

DNA was extracted from purified virions by digestion with 1 mg/ml of self-digested pronase (B grade, nuclease free, Calbiochem) in the presence of 3 mg/ml sodium dodecyl sulfate (SDS), followed by phenol extraction and dialysis against 0.1 x SSC (SSC = 0.15 M sodium chloride + 0.015 M sodium citrate, pH 6.9)

(31). Form I SV40 DNA, free of detectable host cell (monkey) nucleotide. sequences, was prepared by subjecting purified SV40 viral DNA to additional cycles of CsCl equilibrium density centrifugation in the presence of ethidium bromide as previously described (32). Escherichia coli DNA was extracted by the method of Marmur (33). The concentrations of DNA solutions were determined by a modified diphenylamine reaction (34) using calf thymus DNA as a standard.

Preparation of radiolabelled RNA. Radiolabelled RNA from $Ad2^+ND_4$ infected and Ad2 infected Vero cells was prepared from confluent, 32 oz bottle cultures infected with 20-50 PFU/cell of these viruses. Four hours after infection, sufficient uridine-5-^3H (25-30 Ci/mM) was added to yield a final concentration of 100 μCi/ml. The cells were harvested by scraping 24 hr after infection, and washed cell pellets were stored at -70°C for subsequent RNA extraction.

Radiolabelled early SV40 RNA (SV40-specific RNA transcribed from the DNA of input virions in the absence of SV40 DNA replication) and late SV40 RNA (SV40-specific RNA transcribed after SV40 DNA replication has commenced) were prepared in roller bottle cultures of Vero cells as previously described (9). For the preparation of early SV40 RNA, 20 μg/ml of cytosine arabinoside (CA) was present throughout infection to prevent SV40 DNA replication. RNA was extracted by a hot phenol-SDS procedure (35) and stored at -70°C in 2 x SSC plus 0.05% SDS.

RNA-DNA hybridization. Radiolabelled RNA was hybridized with Ad2 or SV40 DNA immobilized on nitrocellulose membrane filters (Millipore Corporation; 0.45 μ, HAWP) (35,36). The hybridization reaction was either carried out in a solution consisting of equal parts of formamide and 10 x SSC for 18 hr at 37°C, or in 2 x SSC + 0.05% SDS for 18 hr at 60°C. Filters were then re-

moved and extensively washed with 2 x SSC, first at 37°C and then
at 60°C. Filters not destined for elution were then treated with
pancreatic ribonuclease (20 μg/ml) and ribonuclease T_1 (10 units/
ml) for one hr at room temperature, washed again with 2 x SSC at
60°C, and counted in a Packard Tri-Carb liquid scintillation
spetrometer. Control filters, containing an equivalent amount of
E. coli DNA, were included in each hybridization reaction.

   Elution and rehybridization of virus-specific RNA. After
washing with 2 x SSC at 60°C, filters from the hybridization reaction were eluted, first with formamide: 0.01 x SSC = 9:1 at 37
°C and at 45°C, and then with 0.01 x SSC at 100°C. The eluted RNA
was then rehybridized with fresh DNA filters. All rehybridized
filters were RNAase treated before counting. These procedures
are described in detail elsewhere (32). The SV40-specific CPM
were determined by subtracting the CPM bound to the E. coli DNA
filters from the CPM bound to the SV40 DNA filters. The SV40-
specific RNA recovered following elution and rehybridization
with SV40 DNA (Tables 1 and 2) represent the sum of the SV40 -
specific CPM recovered from the formamide eluent and from the
0.01 x SSC eluents.

Results

   Interferon sensitivity of SV40 and Ad2 T antigen formation
in Vero cells infected with SV40, with Ad2, and with mixtures of
SV40 and Ad2. In cultures infected with SV40 alone, in the absence of interferon, more than 99% of the cells contained SV40
T antigen. However, in replicate cultures, even the lowest dose
of interferon employed (1 unit/ml) produced a significant reduction in the proportion of T antigen positive cells, and a dose
of 7 units/ml resulted in 95% inhibition of SV40 T antigen formation (Fig. 1-A). This reduction in the proportion of T antigen

positive cells was roughly paralleled by a reduction in the intensity of FA staining in those few cells which were positive.

Simultaneous infection with nonhybrid Ad2 did not change the proportion of SV40 T antigen positive cells, nor did it affect the intensity or morphology of SV40 T antigen staining. Of more importance, the interferon sensitivity of SV40-induced SV 40 T antigen formation was not altered in cells simultaneously infected with Ad2 (Fig. 1-A).

The synthesis of Ad2 T antigen in Ad2 infected cells was relatively resistant to interferon, and this was not altered by simultaneous infection with SV40 (Fig. 1-B). Pretreatment with 50 units/ml of interferon had no measurable effect, and 200 units/ml produced less than a 50% inhibition of Ad2 T antigen formation.

Interferon sensitivity of SV40 and Ad2 T antigen formation in Vero cells infected with Ad2$^+$ND$_4$. In cultures infected with Ad2$^+$ND$_4$, in the absence of interferon, approximately 90% of the cells contained SV40 T antigen. However, in contrast to wild-type SV40 infection, doses of interferon as high as 50 units/ml did not reduce the proportion of SV40 T antigen positive cells or alter the intensity or morphology of FA staining (Fig. 1-A). Pretreatment with 200 units/ml did produce a moderate inhibition of SV40 T antigen formation. Thus more than 100 times as much interferon was required to inhibit SV40 T antigen induction by Ad2$^+$ND$_4$ than was required to inhibit SV40 T antigen induction by SV40, indicating that the induction of SV40 T antigen by this hybrid virus is more than 100-fold less sensitive to interferon than is the induction of the same SV40 antigen by wild-type SV40.

In contrast to the marked difference in the interferon sensitivity of SV40 T antigen induction by wild-type SV40 and by

$Ad2^{+}ND_{4}$, there was little difference in the interferon sensitivity of Ad2 T antigen induction by wild-type Ad2 and by $Ad2^{+}ND_{4}$.
Ad2 T antigen formation by $Ad2^{+}ND_{4}$ was relatively resistant to
interferon (Fig. 1-B). In fact, the $Ad2^{+}ND_{4}$-induced synthesis of
both the SV40 and the Ad2 T antigens showed comparable sensitivity to interferon (cf.Fig. 1-A and 1-B).

Detection of RNA molecules containing both SV40 and Ad2
nucleotide sequences. To determine whether the decreased interferon sensitivity of $Ad2^{+}ND_{4}$-induced SV40 T antigen synthesis
might be explained by the initiation of transcription of SV40
genetic information in an adjacent region of Ad2 DNA, we sought
to detect the synthesis of polycistronic RNA molecules containing covalently linked Ad2 and SV40 nucleotide sequences in $Ad2^{+}$
ND_{4} infected cells. The procedure employed to detect such hybrid
RNA molecules is diagrammed in Fig. 2.

Radiolabelled RNA extracted from virus infected cells was
first hybridized with denatured (single-stranded) Ad2 DNA immobilized on nitrocellulose filters. After hybridization the filters were extensively washed, but not RNAase treated. The re -
tained Ad2-specific RNA (together with a small amount of RNA nonspecifically bound to the filters) was then eluted, and the eluted RNA rehybridized with SV40 DNA. The SV40 DNA filters were
then washed and incubated with RNAase to remove any RNA that was
not hybridized with DNA on the filters. The ^{3}H-RNA remaining
after this step consisted exclusively of SV40 RNA sequences.

Only SV40 RNA sequences which are covalently linked to Ad2
RNA will be retained by the first (Ad2 DNA) filter and thus be
carried into the eluent to be detected by the second (SV40 DNA)
filter (see $Ad2^{+}ND_{4}$ ^{3}H-RNA in Fig. 2). Unlinked SV40 RNA sequences will not be retained by the first (Ad2 DNA) filter, and

thus will not be carried forward into the eluent. Ad2 RNA se -
quences, though retained by the first (Ad2 DNA) filter and carried forward into the eluent, will not hybridize with the second
(SV40 DNA) filter. Consequently, mixtures of Ad2 and SV40 RNA
molecules should not contain nucleotide sequences which can hybridize sequentially with both Ad2 and SV40 DNA (see Fig.2).

Table 1 summarizes the results obtained with several preparations of ^{3}H-RNA from cells infected with Ad2, SV40 and Ad2$^+$
ND$_4$. Preparations of ^{3}H-RNA from Ad2 infected cells, and from
cells infected with SV40 in the presence (early SV40 RNA) or absence (late SV40 RNA) of CA, did not hybridize sequentially with
both Ad2 and SV40 DNA. Early SV40 RNA was employed in these control reactions because the SV40-specific RNA induced by Ad2$^+$ND$_4$
consists primarily of early SV40 RNA sequences (12). In contrast,
a significant proportion of the SV40-specific CPM in each of
three preparations of ^{3}H-RNA from Ad2$^+$ND$_4$ infected cells were
retained by the Ad2 DNA filter and could then be eluted and rehybridized to SV40 DNA.

In a final experiment a mixture of early SV40 RNA plus Ad2
RNA was compared with the RNA extracted from Ad2$^+$ND$_4$ infected
cells (Table 2). When the mixture was hybridized with Ad2 or E.
coli DNA and the filters eluted, the eluents contained no SV40
RNA. As expected, an SV40 filter retained a significant amount
of SV40 RNA, which could then be eluted and detected on rehybridization with SV40 DNA; 21.8 % of the SV40-specific CPM initially
present in the mixture were recovered as RNAase-resistant CPM on
the final SV40 DNA filter. When Ad2$^+$ND$_4$ RNA was similarly examined, both Ad2 and SV40 DNA filters retained SV40 RNA, which
could then be eluted and rehybridized with SV40 DNA. When the
first filter contained SV40 DNA,41.2 % of the SV40-specific CPM
initially present were recovered as RNAase-resistant CPM on the

final SV40 DNA filter. The discrepancy between this figure and
the 100% recovery expected on a theoretical basis may be explained by incomplete removal of SV40-specific CPM by the first filter (Table 2), together with losses occurring during the elution
and rehybridization procedures. When the first filter contained
Ad2 DNA, 11.2% of the SV40-specific CPM initially present were
recovered as RNAase-resistant CPM on the final SV40 DNA filter.
A comparison of this recovery to that obtained when both the
first and the final filters contained SV40 DNA indicates that at
least 27% $\left(\frac{11.2}{41.2} \times 100\%\right)$ of the SV40-specific ^{3}H-RNA CPM synthesized in Ad2$^+$ND$_4$ infected cells were covalently linked to Ad2RNA.

This conclusion was further supported by an examination of
the fluids remaining after the initial hybridization (Table 2).
With the mixture of early SV40 RNA and Ad2 RNA, only hybridization with SV40 DNA removed a significant number of SV40-specific
CPM, whereas in the case of Ad2$^+$ND$_4$ RNA, SV40-specific CPM were
removed by hybridization with both Ad2 and SV40 DNA.

Discussion

Ad2$^+$ND$_4$, the nondefective Ad2-SV40 hybrid virus employed
in these experiments, contains 43% of the wild-type SV40 genome
covalently linked to Ad2 DNA (11,37). This SV40 genetic information, which includes all of the early SV40 nucleotide se -
quences (12), is inserted as a single segment of SV40 DNA at a
point approximately 14% in from one end of the Ad2 genome (37).
We have demonstrated that at least some of the RNA sequences
transcribed from the SV40 segment of this hybrid virus are contained in polycistronic RNA molecules which also contain Ad2 nucleotide sequences (Tables 1 and 2). Unless we suppose that separate Ad2 and SV40 RNA molecules are covalently joined at some
time after transcription, the presence of Ad2 and SV40 nucleotide sequences in the same RNA molecules implies that transcrip-

tion is initiated in the DNA of one virus(Ad2 or SV40) and continues without interruption across the point of juncture into
the DNA of the other virus.

Low doses of interferon block the synthesis of both early
SV40 RNA and SV40 T antigen in cells infected with SV40 (14,20,
38,39). Moreover, preliminary results indicate that the relative
resistance of Ad2 T antigen formation to inhibition by interferon
is paralleled by a comparable resistance of Ad RNA synthesis,
and that Ad2-SV40 hybrid virus-induced SV40 and Ad2 RNA synthesis
are both relatively resistant to interferon, as are hybrid virus
induced SV40 and Ad T antigen synthesis (M.J. Levin et al, unpublished observations). These observations suggest that differences in the interferon sensitivity of SV40 and Ad antigen synthesis are the result of differences in the interferon sensitivity of the transcription of the corresponding viral genes. If
this is true, the relative resistance to interferon of $Ad2^+ND_4$-
induced SV40 T antigen synthesis (Fig. 1-A) implies a marked decrease in the interferon sensitivity of the transcription of the
corresponding SV40 genetic information. Since there was no de -
crease in the interferon sensitivity of SV40 T antigen synthesis
in cells doubly infected with both SV40 and wild-type Ad2, this
change cannot be explained by the simultaneous presence and activity of the Ad2 and SV40 genomes in the same cells. Rather, it
would appear to be related to the covalent linkage of SV40 and
Ad2 DNA in the $Ad2^+ND_4$ genome. Moreover, the similarity between
the interferon dose response curves of $Ad2^+ND_4$-induced SV40 and
Ad2 T antigen synthesis (cf. Fig. 1-A and 1-B) suggests that, at
least with respect to the interferon system, the expression of
SV40 genetic information in $Ad2^+ND_4$ (and thus presumably the
transcription of the corresponding region of SV40 DNA) is indistinguishable from Ad2 gene expression (and thus presumably indistinguishable from the transcription of Ad2 DNA).

The synthesis of hybrid RNA molecules in $Ad2^+ND_4$ infected cells and the reduced interferon sensitivity of $Ad2^+ND_4$-induced SV40 T antigen formation can both be explained by hypothesizing that transcription of the SV40 genetic information in $Ad2^+ND_4$ is initiated in an adjacent region of Ad2 DNA. The initiation of SV40 transcription in Ad2 DNA would explain the synthesis of RNA molecules containing both Ad2 and SV40 RNA sequences, and the interferon resistance of Ad2 transcription would account for the unexpected resistance of SV40 transcription (and thus of SV40 T antigen formation) in $Ad2^+ND_4$ infected cells. Since according to this model transcription of hybrid RNA molecules is initiated in Ad2 DNA, the 5'-OH ends of the hybrid RNA molecules found in $Ad2^+ND_4$ infected cells should contain Ad2, rather than SV40, nucleotide sequences. Experiments to test the validity of this prediction are presently underway in our laboratory.

A comparable alteration in the interferon sensitivity of SV40 T antigen synthesis has also been observed in SV40 transformed 3T3 cells (40), in which the SV40 genome is thought to be covalently linked to cellular DNA (41). The synthesis of SV40 T antigen by these cells is refractory to interferon (40), and high concentrations of interferon do not inhibit their synthesis of SV40-specific RNA (M.N. Oxman et al., manuscript in preparation).The failure of interferon to inhibit their synthesis of SV40 T antigen suggests that in SV40 transformed cells the expression of this viral genetic information is under the control of the cell genome. The reported presence of both cell- and virus-specific sequences in the same molecules of nuclear RNA from SV40 transformed 3T3 cells (42) is consistent with the hypothesis that the transcription of the integrated SV40 DNA is initiated in a region of adjacent cell DNA (40,43). Thus, Ad2-SV40 hybrid viruses and SV40-transformed cells represent two situations in which a marked change in the interferon sensitivity of SV40 gene

expression is associated with the covalent linkage of SV40 and
a heterologous DNA and, perhaps, with the initiation of the transcription of SV40 genetic information in that heterologous DNA.

The results of heteroduplex mapping (37,44,45) and hybrid-
ization-competition (12) studies of Ad2$^+$ND$_4$ and the other closely related nondefective Ad2-SV40 hybrid viruses (10) have re -
vealed the relative position of the three identifiable early SV
40 genetic function in the Ad2$^+$ND$_4$ genome. In addition, Morrow
et al. (44) have shown that the SV40 DNA segment in Ad2$^+$ND$_4$ is
colinear with wild-type SV40 DNA, and Khoury et al. (46) have
presented data which indicate that during SV40 infection the direction of transcription of the early region of the SV40 genome
is from the T antigen locus toward the U antigen locus. The studies of Patch et al. (47; C.T. Patch et al., submitted for publication), Khoury et al. (48) and Sambrook et al. (49) indicate
that the segment of SV40 DNA in Ad2$^+$ND$_4$ contains some late se -
quences at each end, and suggest that the early template begins
at approximately 0.55 on the circular map of the SV40 genome
(Fig. 3). Together, these observations indicate that the region
of the SV40 DNA molecule in which the transcription of the early SV40 genes is initiated is present in the SV40 segment of
Ad2$^+$ND$_4$. Likewise, recovery (by cocultivation with permissive
monkey cells) of SV40 virions which are fully sensitive to interferon from the SV40 transformed mouse cells described above
(in which SV40 T antigen synthesis is refractory to interferon)
implies that a normal initiation site for early SV40 transcription is present in these cells as well. Why then should the
function of this site be superseded by that of an initiation
site in covalently linked Ad2 (or cellular) DNA? The answer to
this question may lie in the conformational change which occurs
when SV40 DNA is integrated into the linear Ad2 or host cell
genomes.

The segment of the superhelical form I SV40 DNA molecules
in the region of the putative site of initiation of early SV40
RNA transcription (0.45 to 0.55 on the circular map of SV40; Fig.
3) has certain unique properties. It is the most readily denatured portion of the molecule (50), it is the only portion of the
molecule to bind the T4 gene 32 protein (51), and is one of only two regions (the only one in the presence of high salt) to be
cleaved by the single strand-specific (S_1) endonuclease of As -
pergillus oryzae (52). Furthermore, these properties are markedly influenced by the configuration of the SV40 DNA molecule. For
example, the S_1 nuclease will cleave SV40 DNA in this region only so long as the molecule is supercoiled; it fails to act on
closed circular but non-superhelical molecules, or on linear duplex molecules of SV40 DNA (52). In view of these observations,
we should consider two possible consequences of the loss of superhelical structure that occurs when the SV40 DNA molecule is
integrated into linear host cell (or Ad) DNA:

(i) If the initiation site for early RNA transcription requires the superhelical configuration for its integrity, the
loss of superhelical configuration would necessitate initiation
elsewhere - presumably in adjacent host cell (or Ad) DNA. This
could account for both the synthesis of hybrid RNA molecules and
the altered sensitivity of SV40 gene expression to interferon.

(ii) The loss of superhelical configuration of the initiation site in transformed cells (or in Ad-SV40 hybrid viruses)
might alter its capacity to bind the interferon-induced "antiviral protein", just as its interaction with the S_1 nuclease is
altered when supercoiling is lost. This might also explain the
loss of interferon sensitivity of SV40 T antigen and SV40 RNA
synthesis in SV40 transformed cells and Ad-SV40 hybrid viruses.
Though highly speculative, these models are amenable to laboratory investigation.

Summary

The effect of interferon on SV40 and Ad2 T antigen synthesis has been examined in cells infected with SV40, with Ad2, and with a nondefective Ad2-SV40 hybrid virus, $Ad2^+ND_4$. The induction of SV40 T antigen by SV40 was highly sensitive to interferon, whereas the induction of Ad2 T antigen by Ad2 was resistant. This difference in interferon sensitivity was not altered in cells simultaneously infected with both viruses. However, the induction of SV40 T antigen by $Ad2^+ND_4$, which contains covalently linked SV40 and Ad2 DNA, was as resistant to interferon as the induction of Ad2 T antigen. When RNA extracted from $Ad2^+ND_4$ infected cells was examined by means of sequential hybridization with Ad2 DNA, elution, and rehybridization with SV40 DNA, 27% of the SV40-specific RNA was found to be linked to Ad2 RNA. No such linkage was detected in control mixtures of Ad2 and SV40 RNA. The presence of Ad2 and SV40 nucleotide sequences in the same RNA molecule implies that, in $Ad2^+ND_4$ infection, transcription is initiated in the DNA of one virus(Ad2 or SV40) and continues without interruption across the point of juncture into the DNA of the other virus. Furthermore, the interferon resistance of $Ad2^+ND_4$-induced SV40 T antigen synthesis suggests that transcription of the genetic information for SV40 T antigen is initiated in a region of Ad2 DNA.

Acknowledgements

This investigation was supported by Public Health Service grants CA-12557 from the National Cancer Institute and AI-01992 from the National Institute of Allergy and Infectious Diseases.

Michael N. Oxman is the recipient of a Faculty Research Award (PRA-89) from the American Cancer Society.

Myron J. Levin is a Cancer Research Scholar of the American Cancer Society, Massachusetts Division.

References

1. Huebner, R.J.,Chanock, R.M., Rubin, B.A., and Casey, M.J. (1964). Proc. Nat. Acad. Sci. USA 52, 1333.

2. Rowe, W.P. and Baum, S.G. (1964). Proc. Nat. Acad. Sci. 52, 1340.

3. Rapp, F., Melnick, J.L., Butel, J.S. and Kitahara, T. (1964). Proc. Nat. Acad. Sci. USA 52 , 1348.

4. Rapp, F., Tevethia, S.S. and Melnick, J.L. (1966). J. Nat. Cancer Inst. 36, 703.

5. Rowe, W.P. and Pugh, W.E. (1966). Proc. Nat. Acad. Sci. USA 55, 1126.

6. Baum, S., Reich, P.R., Hybner, C., Rowe, W.P. and Weissman, S,M. (1966). Proc. Nat. Acad. Sci. USA 56, 1509.

7. Lewis, A.M.,Jr. and Rowe, W.P. (1971). J.Virol.7, 189.

8. Levin, M.J., Crumpacker, C.S., Lewis, A.M.,Jr., Oxman, M.N., Henry, P.H. and Rowe, W.P. (1971).J. Virol. 7 , 343.

9. Oxman, M.N., Levine, A.S., Crumpacker, C.S., Levin, M. J., Henry, P.H. and Lewis, A.M., Jr. (1971). J. Virol. 8, 215.

10. Lewis, A.M., Jr., Levine, A.S., Crumpacker, C.S., Levin, M.J., Samaha, R.J. and Henry, P.H. (1973). J. Virol. 11, 655.

11. Henry, P.H., Schnipper, L.E., Samaha, R.J., Crumpacker,

C.S., Lewis, A.M., Jr. and Levine, A.S. (1973). J. Virol. 11, 665.

12. Levine, A.S., Levin, M.J., Oxman, M.N. and Lewis, A.M. Jr. (1973). J. Virol. 11, 672.

13. Gallagher, J.G. and Khoobyarian, N. (1969). Proc. Soc. Exp. Biol. Med. 130, 137.

14. Oxman, M.N., Rowe, W.P. and Black, P.H. (1967). Proc. Nat. Acad. Sci. USA 57, 941.

15. Friedman, R.M. and Sonnabend, J.A. (1970). Arch. Intern. Med. 126, 51.

16. Joklik, W.K. and Merigan, T.C. (1966). Proc. Nat. Acad. Sci. USA 56, 558.

17. Metz, D.H. and Esteban, M. (1972). Nature 238, 385.

18. Friedman, R.M., Metz, D.H., Esteban, M., Tovell, D.R., Ball, L.A. and Kerr, I.M. (1972). J. Virol. 10, 1184.

19. Falcoff, E., Falcoff, R., Lebleu, B. and Revel, M. (1973). J. Virol. 12, 421.

20. Oxman, M.N. and Levin, M.J. (1971). Proc. Nat. Acad. Sci. USA 68, 299.

21. Yasumura, P. and Kawakita, Y. (1963). Nippon Rinsho 21, 1201.

22. Hopps, H., Bernheim, B.C., Nisalak, A., Tjio, J.H. and Smadel, J.E. (1963). J. Immunol. 91, 416.

23. Jensen, F.C., Girardi, A.J., Gilden, R.V. and Koprowski, H. (1964). Proc. Nat. Acad. Sci. USA 52, 53.

24. Robb, J.A., and Martin, R.G. (1970). Virology 41, 751.

25. Hayflick, L. (1965). Tex. Rep. Biol. Med. 23, 285.

26. Black, P.H. and Rowe, W.P. (1964). J.Nat.Cancer Inst. 32, 253.

27. Strander, H. and Cantell, K. (1966). Ann. Med. Exp. Biol. Fenn. 44, 265.

28. Strander, H. and Cantell, K. (1967). Ann. Med. Exp. Biol. Fenn. 45, 20.

29. Pope, J.H. and Rowe, W.P. (1964). J.Exp.Med.120,121.

30. Burnett, J.P., Summers, A.O., Harrington, A.S. and Dwyer, A.C. (1968). Appl.Microbiol. 16, 1245.

31. Kelly, T.J., Jr. and Rose, J.A. (1971). Proc. Nat. Acad. Sci. USA 68, 1037.

32. Oxman, M.N., Levin, M.J. and Lewis, A.M., Jr. (1974). J. Virol. 13, 322.

33. Marmur, J. (1961). J. Mol. Biol. 3, 208.

34. Burton, K. (1956). Biochem. J. 62, 315.

35. Levin, M.J., Oxman, M.N., Diamandopoulos, G.Th., Levine, A.S., Henry, P.H. and Enders, J.F. (1969). Proc. Nat. Acad. Sci. USA 62, 589.

36. Gillespie, D. and Spigelman, S. (1965). J.Mol.Biol.12, 829.

37. Kelly, T.J., Jr. and Lewis, A.M., Jr. (1973). J.Virol. 12, 643.

38. Oxman, M.N. and Black, P.H. (1966). Proc. Nat. Acad. Sci. USA 55, 1133.

39. Oxman, M.N. and Takemoto, K.K. (1970). L'Interferon. Colloq. de L'I.N.S.E.R.M., Nº 6, p. 429-442.

40. Oxman, M.N., Baron, S., Black, P.H., Takemoto, K.K., Habel, K. and Rowe, W.P. (1967). Virology 32, 122.

41. Sambrook, J., Westphal, H., Srinivasan, P.R. and Dulbecco, R. (1968). Proc.Nat.Acad.Sci. USA 60, 1288.

42. Wall, R. and Darnell, J.E. (1971). Nature N. Biol.232, 73.

43. Oxman, M.N. (1967).Archiv. ges. Virusforsch. 22, 171.

44. Morrow, J., Berg, P., Kelly, T.J., Jr. and Lewis, A.M., Jr. (1973). J. Virol. 12, 653.

45. Morrow, J.F. and Berg, P. (1972). Proc. Nat. Acad. Sci. USA 69, 3365.

46. Khoury, G., Martin, M.A., Lee, T.N.H., Danna, K.J. and Nathans, D. (1973). J. Mol. Biol. 78, 377.

47. Patch, C.T., Lewis, A.M., Jr. and Levine, A.S.(1972).
Proc. Nat. Acad. Sci. USA 69, 3375.

48. Khoury, G., Lewis, A.M., Jr., Oxman, M.N. and Levine,
A.S. (1973). Nature N. Biol. 246, 202.

49. Sambrook, J., Sugden, B., Keller, W. and Sharp, P.A.
(1973). Proc. Nat. Acad. Sci. USA 70, 3711.

50. Mulder, C. and Delius, H. (1972). Proc. Nat. Acad. Sci.
USA 69, 3215.

51. Morrow, J.F. and Berg, P. (1973). J. Virol. 12, 1631.

52. Beard, P., Morrow, J.F. and Berg, P. (1973). J. Virol.
12, 1303.

TABLE 1

Detection of hybrid RNA molecules containing both SV40 and Ad2 nucleotide sequences

RNA	Virus-specific ^{3}H-RNA CPM initially present[a]		Recovery of SV40-specific RNA following hybridization with Ad2 DNA, elution and rehybridization with SV40 DNA	
	SV40	Ad2	CPM	% Recovery[b]
Early SV40	750	0	0	0
Early SV40	11,724	0	27	0.23
Late SV40	5,100	0	0	0
Ad2	0	170,000	26	<0.02
Ad2$^+$ND$_4$	446	N.D.	42	9.4
Ad2$^+$ND$_4$	900	4,500	54	6.0
Ad2$^+$ND$_4$	24,940	80,360	1,720	6.9

[a]Each number represents the average of duplicate or triplicate determinations. The virus-specific CPM is the net of the CPM bound to 1 μg SV40 or Ad2 DNA filters less the CPM bound to 1 μg E. coli DNA (control) filters. In all cases the CPM bound to the E. coli filters was less than 1/8 the CPM bound to the viral DNA filters.

[b](Recovered SV40-specific CPM/input SV40-specific CPM) x 100 %. The net SV40-specific CPM was determined with 1 μg SV40 and E. coli DNA filters.

TABLE 2

Detection of hybrid RNA molecules containing both SV40 and Ad2 nucleotide sequences

RNA	Virus-specific ³H-RNA CPM initially present[b]		First filter (2 µg DNA)	% removal of SV40-specific RNA[c]	Recovery of SV40-specific RNA following hybridization with first filter, elution and re-hybridization with SV40 DNA[d]	
	SV40	Ad2			CPM	% Recovery
Early SV40[a] + Ad2	8,440	429,000	Ad2	0	1	<0.02
			SV40	88	1,834	21.8
			E. coli	0	2	<0.03
Ad2⁺ND₄	15,450	114,000	Ad2	53	1,736	11.2
			SV40	68	6,364	41.2
			E. coli	0	6	<0.04

[a] Early SV40 RNA and Ad2 RNA were separately extracted and mixed in 2xSSC+0.05% SDS.

[b] Each number represents the average of duplicate or triplicate determinations. The virus-specific CPM is the net of CPM bound to 2 µg SV40 or Ad2 DNA filters less the CPM bound to 2 µg E. coli DNA (control) filters. In all cases the CPM bound to the E. coli filters was less than 1/10 the CPM bound to the viral DNA filters.

c(initial SV40-specific CPM) - (remaining SV40-specific CPM) x 100 %. The remaining SV40-specific
(initial SV40-specific CPM)
CPM was determined by adding a fresh 1 μg SV40 DNA filter to the hybridization fluid remaining
from the initial hybridization.

d(Recovered SV40-specific CPM/input SV40-specific CPM) x 100 %. The net SV40-specific CPM was determined with 1 μg SV40 and E. coli DNA filters.

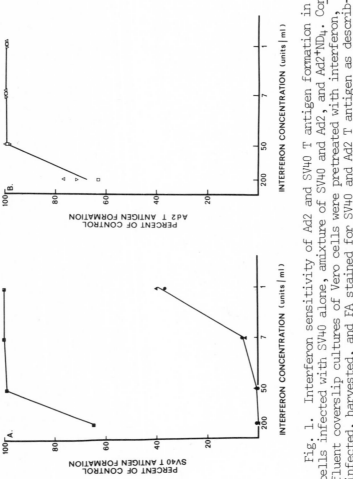

Fig. 1.   Interferon sensitivity of Ad2 and SV40 T antigen formation in cells infected with SV40 alone, amixture of SV40 and Ad2, and Ad2⁺ND₄. Confluent coverslip cultures of Vero cells were pretreated with interferon, infected, harvested, and FA stained for SV40 and Ad2 T antigen as described in Materials and methods. A. SV40 T antigen: ● = SV40 infection; ▲ = SV40 plus Ad2 infection; ■ = Ad2⁺ND₄ infection. B. Ad2 T antigen: ▽ = Ad2 infection; △ = SV40 plus Ad2 infection; □ = Ad2⁺ND₄ infection.

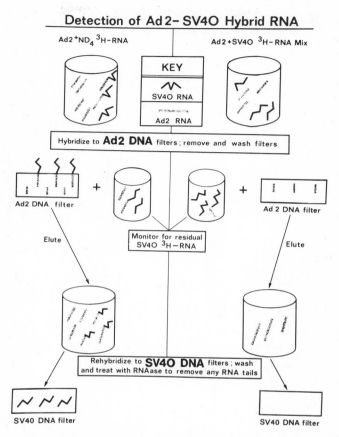

Fig. 2. Procedure for the detection of Ad2-SV40 hybrid RNA molecules.

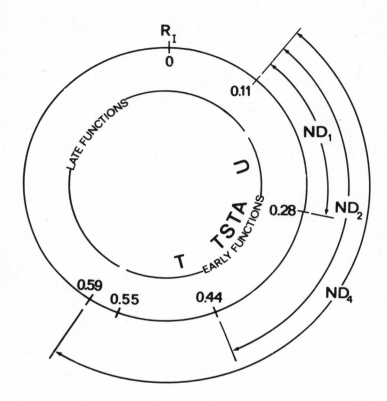

Fig. 3. Physical map of the SV40 genome indicating the SV40
DNA segments contained in Ad2$^+$ND$_1$ (ND$_1$), Ad2$^+$ND$_2$ (ND$_2$) and Ad2$^+$
ND$_4$ (ND$_4$). The approximate location of the regions associated
with T, TSTA and U antigen synthesis are indicated.

DISCUSSION

Chany: Your explanations concerning the insensitivity of the T antigens induced by SV40 or by adenovirus are not clear to me. It has been known for many years that as soon as SV40 or adenovirus penetrate into the cell, within a few hours, the cellular sensitivity to interferon decreases when assayed with VSV. Don't you think there can be a cellular factor involved?

Oxman: In our experiments, the cells were pretreated with interferon overnight, so that the antiviral state is fully developed prior to infection. Moreover, the interferon sensitivity of SV40 T antigen synthesis was not reduced in the cells which were doubly infected with SV40 and wild-type (nonhybrid) adenoviruses.

Levy: The earliest times that you and Dave Mecs looked recently were 25 hours after infection. Is that the earliest time you can measure early messenger RNA effects?

Oxman: No, but if you pick a very much earlier time you have considerably less early SV40 RNA. These experiments require that SV40 infection be limited to early events. That is, that transcription occurs only from input viral templates. Under these circumstances there is never much SV40 RNA synthesized.

Colby: Mike, do you have some preliminary experiments of the type that you would be reluctant to talk about in the formal presentation, but perhaps you might mention in the discussion concerning the sequential hybridization to the two types of DNA which you labelled with gama-labelled triphosphate?

Oxman: I am not being coy. We simply haven't done those experiments.

OXMAN, LEVIN & LEWIS, Jr.

Costa: In the course of your second hybridization step with SV40 DNA, have you tried to get nuclease cleavage of the nonhybridized adeno RNA fragments in order to get a so-called pure SV40 RNA segment in your hybrid?

Oxman: If we use RNAase after the first hybridization, we will of course hydrolyze the free SV40 portion of any hybrid RNA molecules which are bound to the adenovirus DNA filter by adenovirus end. However, in the second hybridization (with the SV40 DNA filter) we do use RNAase to insure that all of the RNA bound at this point consists of SV40 nucleotide sequences.

Tan: Does SV40 virus induce chromosome aberrations, one of which might alter the genetics of interferon response?

Oxman:. SV40, as well as just about every other oncogenic and nononcogenic virus known, is capable of inducing chromosomal damage. It is not clear to me how this relates to SV40-induced transformation because if you look very early after transformation the SV40 transformed cells do not appear to have significant chromosomal abnormalities. Moreover, I have not observed consistent differences in the interferon sensitivity of normal and transformed mouse 3T3 cells.

Chany: I just want to confirm what Dr. Oxman has just said. Dr. Cassingena in Paris has studied very extensively morphological chromosomal aberrations due to SV40. They appear very late, and I don't think that they can explain anything in short term experiments.

VII - MISCELLANEOUS

INTERFERON AND INFECTIOUS, VIRUS-INDUCED, DOUBLE-STRANDED RNA*

R. Perez-Bercoff, G. Carrara, F. Ameglio, A. Degener
and G. Rita

Institute of Virology - University of Rome
Viale di Porta Tiburtina, 28 - 00185
Roma, Italy

During the past few years the biological properties of virus-induced, double-stranded RNAs have been studied with increasing interest.

Among the properties of this molecule, we shall mention only three; the replicative form (RF) of picornaviruses is:

a) infectious,

b) blocks protein synthesis, and

c) in adequate conditions can induce interferon (IF) production.

The first two properties are pertinent to our subject.

It was already known that the replicative form of picornaviruses is infectious, but the mechanism of this remains still
obscure.

Using different blocking agents we have been recently able
to demonstrate:

1) that a cellular function is involved in the very early
steps of the replication cycle initiated by mengovirus RF; and

---

* This work was supported by grant N° 115/0107 72.00294/44 of
the Consiglio Nazionale delle Ricerche, Rome (Italy)

2) that cellular transcription must be conserved for RF to replicate.

Obviously, this is not the case for mengovirus single-stranded RNA and this implies that double-stranded and single-stranded mengovirus RNAs initiate their replication cycle by different ways.

The problem of the mechanism responsible of replication of RF was further complicated by the fact that this molecule blocks protein synthesis in several systems (1,3).

As far as in vitro experiments are concerned, it has been described that addition of poliovirus RF in a protein-synthezising, cell-free system results in an almost immediate blockade of labeled amino acid incorporation and in active dissociation of the initiation complex.

Similar results were further reported to occur in vivo: addition of inactivated, non-infective RF in a cell culture resulted in a complete cessation of protein synthesis within fifteen minutes (4).

Since interferon severely impairs viral infectivity without drastic alterations of cellular synthesis, it seemed to be appropriate tool for studying the differences between the mechanism responsible of replication of mengovirus single and double-stranded RNAs.

First of all we tried to determine wether the replication cycle initiated by mengovirus RF was sensitive or not to interferon.

Confluent monolayers of L cells were treated overnight with different doses of IF (from 0 to 100 units per ml). Then, fluids were discarded, cell sheets were carefully washed, pre-treated with DEAE-dextran and infected with either mengovirus or

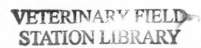

mengovirus RF. After one hour adsorption at 37°C, inocula were
eliminated, cells were washed four times with ice-cold PBS, prewarmed medium was added and incubation at 37°C continued for
eight hours (that is, the lenght of a single replication cycle).
Cultures were then frozen at -80°C, virus release was helped by
freezing and thawing, and the virus yields were titrated by plaque assay.

Results are shown in Table 1. It can be seen that treatment with IF decrease the yield of mengovirus-infected cultures
by more than 90%, and that the infectious cycle initiated by
mengovirus RF is as sensitive to IF as that initiated by mengovirus.

To get further information we analyzed the evolution of
protein synthesis in RF-infected cells and the influence of IF-
treatment.

In order to do this, IF-treated L cells and untreated controls were incubated at 37°C for 30 minutes with DEAE-dextran
and afterwards each culture was labeled with 0.1 μC of ^{14}C-al-
gal hydrolisate. After 15 minutes cells were infected (or mock
infected) with mengovirus RF. Incubation at 37°C continued for
3 hours and at different times incorporation of labeled amino
acids into the protein fraction was determined. Fig. 1 shows the
results of a representative experiment. It can be seen:

1) that IF-treatment does not alter amino acid incorporation;

2) addition of infective mengovirus RF does not result in
a blockade of protein synthesis, but in an almost immediate enhancement of amino acid incorporation. This is a very early e-
vent: as soon as 10 minutes after infection there is an increase
in the incorporation rate.

3) this enhancement of amino acid incorporation might be
related to replication of RF, since suppression of infectivity

by IF-treatment results in the disappearance of RF-induced enhancement during the first 2 hours.

4) infection with RF in IF-treated cells results in a delayed establishment of the blockade of protein synthesis.

We tentatively interpret this as a degradative process within the cell, which results in the transformation of the incoming RF into an <u>inactive</u>, <u>non-infective</u> molecule. But other interpretations are not excluded.

At this point some conclusions may be drawn:

1) Despite the marked differences existing in the early steps of the replication cycle initiated by mengovirus and mengovirus RF, interferon is equally active on both. That means: IF exerts its action at the level of a common step.

2) It has been suggested that the appearance of RF in picornavirus-infected cells is responsible of virus-induced blockade of cellular synthesis. As far as <u>infective</u>, <u>active</u> RF is concerned, this seems not to be the case.

3) On the contrary, <u>infective</u> RF promotes a very early marked <u>increase</u> in amino acid incorporation and we are currently investigating the nature of active polysomes in order to ascertain wether or not <u>all</u> these syntheses are virus-directed.

REFERENCES

1. Ehrenfeld, E., and Hunt, T. (1971). Proc. Nat. Acad. Sci. USA <u>68</u>, 1075.

2. Robertson, H., and Mathews, M. B. (1973). Proc. Nat. Acad. Sci. USA <u>70</u>, 225.

3. Chao, J., Chao, L., and Speyer, J. (1971). Biochem. Biophys. Res. Comm. <u>45</u>, 1096.

4. Cordell-Stewart, B., and Taylor, M.W. (1973). J. Virology <u>11</u>, 232.

T A B L E I

Interferon activity on the replication of mengovirus and infectious,
double-stranded mengovirus RNA

IF treatment U/ml	Mengovirus		d-s mengovirus RNA	
	Virus yield (PFU/ml)	% of control	Virus yield (PFU/ml)	% of control
0	9.0×10^4	100	7.0×10^3	100
1.0	2.7×10^4	30	1.0×10^3	14.2
3.2	1.1×10^4	12.2	1.0×10^2	1.4
10	5.2×10^2	0.5	--	--
32	--	--	--	--

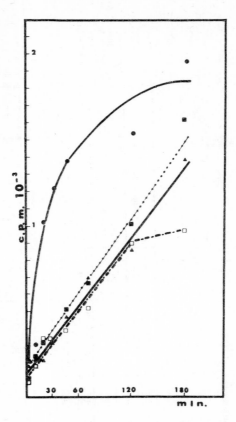

Fig. 1. Effect of mengovirus-induced RF and mouse IF ; la-
beled-amino acid incorporation in L-cells: ▲——▲ control cells;
●——● d-s RNA infected cells; ■••••■ mouse IF treated cells;
□–·–·–□ mouse IF pre-treated and then d-s RNA infected cells.

DISCUSSION

Levy: We recently did some work studying the effect of
double-stranded poly I:C on protein synthesis in cells and tissue culture and we also found an increased incorporation of amino-acids into proteins; but if we examined the specific activity of the acid soluble precursor pool, we found that this was
also increased. In other words, at least with poly I:C the increased incorporation of amino-acids into proteins was probably
at least largely a reflection of increased radioactive amino-acids in the pool. Did you look at the effect of the double-stranded RNA on the radioactivity in the acid soluble fractions in
those cells? Because if you had more radioactivity in the precursor fraction, this would reflect itself in more radioactivity
in the protein without really being increased protein synthesis.

Rita: We have to point out two things. The first one is:
we have digested our TCA-precipitable fraction in alcaline conditions and results were not modified. This excluded the spuri-
ous apport of radioactivity of charged t-RNA. Secondly, we did
not determine the size of the soluble precursor pool of amino -
acids in RF infected cells, but the increased incorporation of
labeled amino-acids into proteins in RF-infected cells cannot be
explained as reflecting a modification of the pool, because such
an increase in protein synthesis needs full infectivity of RF,
and not its mere presence on the cell. Figure 2 shows that neither IF-treatment nor IF-treatment followed by RF infection modified the rate of amino-acid incorporation.

SERUM INTERFERON LEVELS AND VIRAL RESISTANCE FOLLOWING REPEATED ADMINISTRATION OF DS-RNA

D. N. Planterose

Beecham Research Laboratories, Brokham Park
Betchworth, Surrey, England

We have been engaged on a programme of work in evaluating the biological activity of pure double-stranded RNA (BRL 5907) isolated from a virus infected fungus. A battery of biological tests was employed including antiviral activity in a number of species, immunological tests, assay of serum interferon, anti-tumour activity and certain aspects of toxicology.

During the course of this work the broad biological activity of double-stranded RNA (ds-RNA) became apparent, and in this presentation I have drawn together the data, mainly repeat dose studies, that suggests ds-RNA may be mediating its antiviral action by mechanisms other than the induction of serum interferon. The facts emerging from these repeat dose studies must be taken into account in drawing up hypotheses on the regulation of induction of interferon and on the antiviral state in the animal.

We have already presented data showing that antiviral activity is retained during the hyporeactive state of interferon induction (1). Briefly, groups of mice were given 0.5 mg/kg of ds-RNA intraperitoneally once daily and bled at 3, 5 and 24 hr. after each dose. Serum interferon was assayed using primary mouse cell monolayers which were challenged with encephalomyocarditis virus. Equivalent groups of mice were challenged daily with

100 and 1 000 LD_{50} of encephalomyocarditis virus (intraperitoneally) 5 hr. after each dose of inducer. The well-known hyporeactive state of serum interferon induction was obtained, no stimulation of interferon being found with the third or subsequent
dose of inducer (Fig. 1). However, equal or better protection
against virus challenge was shown by second or subsequent doses
of ds-RNA. Thus mice were equally protected by either a single
dose of inducer (giving a high serum interferon level) or by the
last of a series of doses of inducer (giving no detectable interferon).

We have observed that aerosol dosing of mice gives the
best protection against influenza (2), so we have done similar
experiments to that just described with repeated aerosol dosing
of ds-RNA (1 mg/ml) and an influenza virus challenge (Ao/PR 8).
Repeated daily dosing was started 10 days before virus challenge,
and this was compared with the optimum dosage schedule (dosing
at 30 and 6 hr. before and 18 hr. after infection). It can be
seen from Fig. 2 that the antiviral effect was not diminished by
repeated dosing before infection.

With the availability of relatively large amounts of ds -
RNA the optimum dosage schedule has been worked out for farm pigs
challenged by the introduction into the compound of pigs infected with foot and mouth disease. Daily dosing (-2 to +7) of 0.1
mg/kg of ds-RNA subcutaneously was better than dosing every 2
days or every 3 days (Fig. 3) (3). This would hardly be observed
if there was a hyporeactive state of protection generated by the
first dose.

During our investigations on the biology of ds-RNA, it was
observed that our ds-RNA was immunogenic in some species (4). We,
therefore, investigated the possibility that the presence of antibody to ds-RNA would affect the ability of ds-RNA to induce
interferon and the antiviral state (5). The results are shown in

Table I. The control mice were given Freunds complete adjuvant
plus saline and when they were subsequently given ds-RNA (0.5
mg/kg intraperitoneally) high levels of serum interferon (as -
sayed on L-cells) were produced and good protection observed a-
gainst encephalomyocarditis virus challenge (intraperitoneal).
In mice immunised with ds-RNA in adjuvant, high levels of antibody were observed 28 days later. When these mice were given ds-
RNA only low levels of interferon were observed, but protection
was as good as in the mice exhibiting high levels of interferon.

Because of certain limitations of ds-RNA itself, such as
lack of duration of activity, its toxicity, etc., we have studied a number of complexes between ds-RNA and polybases (6). Depending upon the polybase and the complexing conditions, complexes are formed which are either soluble or insoluble in physiological saline. If ds-RNA is totally neutralised with polybrene an
insoluble complex (BRL 10733) is produced. It gives a more prolonged antiviral state than free ds-RNA. However, virtually no
serum interferon is produced (Fig. 4).

In Summary, protection is observed whenever there is a significant level of serum interferon, but in the circumstances
mentioned here protection by an inducer is also observed where
only low levels of serum interferon are obtained. There are several possible mechanisms to account for the observed facts:
1. IF rapidly taken up therefore not seen in serum
2. IF secretion by cells is reduced
3. Maintenance antiviral state possible with small IF concentration
4. IF not important.

Most of these results are consistent with the possibility
that interferon once produced primes the animal to take up interferon more rapidly, so giving only low levels of serum interferon

on repeated doses of inducer. Alternatively, the amount of interferon secreted by cells may be greatly reduced, or perhaps maintainance of the antiviral state may be possible with only small
amounts of interferon. These possibilities are susceptible to
experimentation. On the other hand, the fact that ds-RNA may induce the antiviral state by mechanisms other than interferon
must be considered seriously in view of the wide biological activity of our ds-RNA; such as antitumour activity (7), adjuvancy
(8), and macrophage activation (9). Furthermore no-one has suggested that the toxicological manifestations of polynucleotide
inducers are related to interferon, although perhaps the induction process itself leads to toxicity. A similar wide biological
activity of Poly (I).Poly (C) has been described (10, 11). There
are, however, little data on repeated dosing with Poly (I). Poly
(C) and subsequent virus challenge, as has been described here
for the natural ds-RNA.

It is concluded that the hyporeactive state of interferon
induction generated by repeated doses of inducer does not prevent
the maintenance of a continuous antiviral state. These facts
must be included in any unifying hypothesis on the regulation of
induction of interferon and of the antiviral state in the animal.

REFERENCES

1. Sharpe, Birch, and Planterose (1971). J. gen. Virology
   12, 331.
2. Boyd, and Planterose, in preparation.
3. Sellers, Herniman, Leiper, and Planterose (1973). Vete-
   rinary Record 93, 90.
4. Naysmith, and Cunnington, in preparation.
5. Naysmith, Planterose, and Sharpe, submitted for publication.

6. Harnden, Brown, Sharpe, and Vere-Hodge (1973). American Chemical Soc. Meeting.

7. Parr, Wheeler, and Alexander (1973). Brit. J. Cancer 27, 370.

8. Cunnington, Naysmith, Feaver, to be published.

9. Evans, and Alexander (1971). Nature New Biology 232, 76.

10. Merigan (1970). Nature 228, 219.

11. Merigan (1970). Symposium on Interferon and Host Response to Virus Infection, Archives of Internal Medicine 126.

TABLE I

Pre-treatment	Antibody level	Interferon at * 2 6 24 hrs			Virus susceptibility* ds-RNA Saline	
Adjuvant + saline	0.5	7o	850	18	1/10	9/10
Adjuvant + ds-RNA	47	<4	105	<4	1/10	7/10

* following 0.5 mg/kg ds-RNA

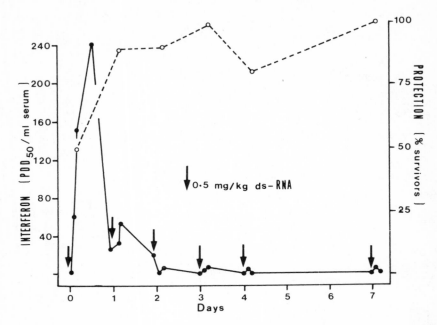

Fig. 1. Antiviral activity during the hyporeactive state of interferon induction. ●———● interferon induction; O----O antiviral activity.

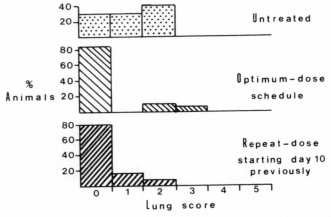

Fig. 2. Treatment of FLU (AoPR8) by aerosol ds-RNA (1 mg/ml).

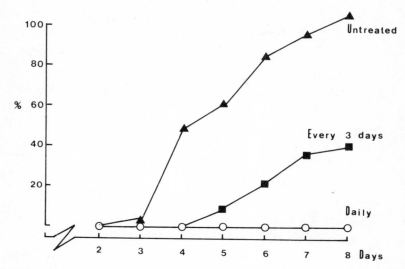

Fig. 3. Percent sites developing lesions in pigs infected
with FMDV. Treatment with 0.1 mg/kg ds-RNA (s.c.).

	Antiviral activity (ED_{50}) mg/kg	Duration	Serum interferon*		
ds-RNA	0.3	+			400
					200
polybrene complex	0.7	+++			

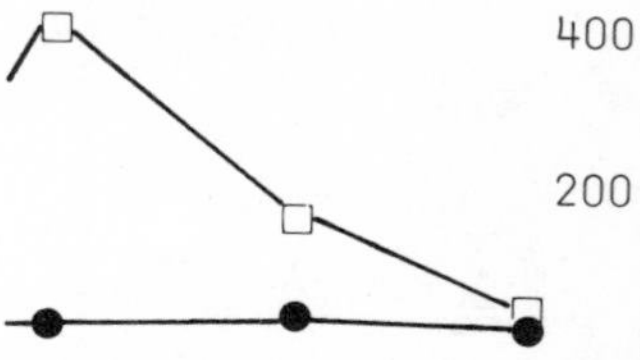

* following 0.5 mg/kg ds-RNA

Fig. 4. Effect of polybrene on the antiviral state and serum interferon production by ds-RNA

DISCUSSION

Baron: There was a recent report that hyporesponsiveness in the animal might occur in some organs and not in others. I think the report indicated that brain was spared of hyporesponsiveness. Have you examined the interferon levels in several organs?

Planterose: No, most of our work has been done in observing virus resistance, because we were more interested in virus resistance than knowing the mechanism behind it. We haven't looked at interferon levels in the brain. I did present data on repeated doses of inducer to the respiratory tract and by the subcutaneous route, with an aerosol challenge.

Dianzani: Perhaps you remember that some years ago we observed an increase of resistance, and also interferon production in mice repeatedly injected with what has been later defined "judicious doses" of poly I:C. Actually these were the highest doses of poly I:C we could use at that period as poly I:C was not fully available. Later it was shown that using higher doses of poly I:C one could have a very strong reduction of interferon production, and the development of hyporeactivity as well, after repeated doses of inducer. Could you tell me if your dosage of poly I:C is high or low? And did you observe any difference between using lower or higher doses of poly I:C?

Planterose: We used 0.5 mg per kilogram in the mouse. I think that's probably not a terribly high dose of double-stranded RNA. Specifically we haven't looked at the hypoactive state generated by different doses of inducer, but there are data in the literature on this.

Ankel: The polymer that you used, what kind of compound is that?

Planterose: The poly base?

Ankel: You fixed the double-stranded RNA to this polymer. How do you do it?

Planterose: The polybase we used was polybrene, a quaternary nitrogen compound with various CH_2 spacers separating the quaternary groups. Enough polybase was added to completely neutralize the double-stranded RNA.

Levy: Is polybrene a rather toxic material to cells?

Planterose: It is. But the amount used in the complex is low.

Pitha: I only wanted to say that polybrene is a polycation usually used as DEAE dextran. We use it in the XC test (for example) to the increase and adsorption of MLV virus.

PURIFICATION OF MOUSE INTERFERON BY
ANTIBODY AFFINITY CHROMATOGRAPHY[1]

K. Paucker, K. Berg[2], C. A. Ogburn

Department of Microbiology
The Medical College of Pennsylvania
Philadelphia, Pa. 19129, U.S.A.

At this meeting a number of papers have been presented in which certain non-antiviral properties of interferon preparations were discussed. When dealing with such controversial aspects of interferon expression, it becomes especially important to ascertain that one is in fact describing a bona fide effect of interferon and not of one of the many contaminants present in most interferon materials under study. The availability of a highly purified product is, therefore, essential to permit proper interpretation of any experimentation dealing with the more fundamental aspects of interferon action.

Unfortunately, efforts to purify interferons have not enjoyed the same attention or successes reported for some other areas of interferon research, and a pure product has thus far eluded those few laboratories which have dared to venture into this field. However, the record shows that the purity of interferon preparations available for study has steadily improved in

[1] This work was supported in part by Contract NO1 AI 02126 from the Infectious Disease Branch, National Institute of Allergy and Infectious Diseases.

[2] Fellow in Medical Microbiology, Aarhus University, Denmark.

recent years and that a number of laboratories have availed
themselves of such highly purified products in their investigations (1-4).

Two general approaches have been used in attempts to purify interferons. The first of these is physicochemical and relies
on the segregation of interferon proteins from other cellular or
noncellular contaminants by virtue of their distinctive differences in molecular configuration and composition. However, the
cell makes a myriad of metabolic products some of which resem-
ble interferon proteins in closest detail. It is not surprising,
therefore, that the most highly purified interferons prepared
by physicochemical methods contain, as far as one can tell, components devoid of interferon activity (5-7). Whether these represent possible developmental forms of interferon, inactivated
interferon proteins, or entirely unrelated factors is a question
which the techniques employed have not been able to resolve. As
a rule, recoveries of the purified product accounted at most for
a few percent of the biological input activity (8), and the heterogeneous nature of interferon proteins (9) often made it necessary to select arbitrarily given components for further purification steps. Workable quantities to study this material could
not be obtained with but rare exceptions (7).

The second approach is immunological and relies on the
existence of specific antigenic groupings on the interferon molecule which are distinct from those of all other cellular proteins. The basis for this assumption rests on the well documented findings that interferon activity can be specifically neutralized by sera from animals immunized with interferon (10,11)
but neither by antibodies to normal cellular and noncellular
constituents (11) nor by those directed against interferons from
other hosts (12) unless serological crossrelationships have been
established (13).

Selecting the immunological approach for the purification of interferons, two avenues present themselves. In the one instance, the aim would be to bind anti-interferon globulins to a solid matrix, then to specifically adsorb interferon to the attached antibody and, finally, to elute interferon under well defined conditions. The capacity of the immunosorbent would thus be restored and it could be used over and over again. Experience has shown, however, that unless care is taken to eliminate antibodies to other impurities, the purification that can be achived in this way is limited (14).

Alternatively, one might envision the use of antibodies to impurities rather than to interferon, in which case the contaminants would be bound and interferon collected in the void volume. This technique has been used to advantage in the purification of the C3 component of human complement (15) but gave less than optimal results in the interferon system for reasons which time or space do not permit to detail further. We favored, therefore, the first approach, namely the use of anti-interferon globulin, for the purification of interferon.

A number of rabbits were immunized at monthly intervals with crude concentrated interferon preparations emulsified in Freund's complete adjuvant. Each immunizing dose contained in the vicinity of 1×10^7 interferon units and was administered intramuscularly, subcutaneously and into the hind foot pads. As shown in Table 1, interferon-neutralizing antibodies became first detectable after three months and increased steadily thereafter, until a plateau was reached some 11 months later. However, the neutralizing antibody response varied considerably among animals and some failed to reach detectable titers even after a protracted course of injections. On the other hand, antibodies to various contaminants rose earlier and more uniformly, attaining maximum levels within two to three months.

Sera with high neutralizing antibody content were subjected to extensive absorptions with contaminant antigens bound to bentonite (16). In this manner, antibodies to all identified impurities were reduced by more than 99.9% without diminution of interferon neutralizing activity.

In a subsequent step, ammonium sulfate precipitated globulin fractions of anti-interferon serum, control serum (from rabbits which did not develop neutralizing antibodies), and of normal rabbit serum were bound to CNBr-activated Sepharose 4B according to established procedures (17, 18). Passage of crude, concentrated L cell interferon through the anti-interferon globulin-Sepharose column permitted free flow-through of all impurities against which antibodies had been eliminated by prior absorption of the antiserum. Interferon was bound and then eluted in a steep pH gradient (19). Recovery of biological activity was quantitative and purification during the chromatography step alone about 50-fold. Interferons produced by ultraviolet (uv) irradiated Newcastle disease virus and by poly I:poly C were purified to a similar degree, yielding preparations with specific activities in the vicinity of 1×10^8 NIH reference units per milligram protein (19). On the other hand, interferon was totally excluded from Sepharose-bound control and normal rabbit globulins.

Interferon purified in the manner described was then concentrated 10-fold by pressure dialysis to yield approximately 500 µg of protein per milliliter. This material was tested by immunodiffusion against nonabsorved anti-interferon and control sera (without measurable neutralizing antibodies). Both antisera gave three identical precipitin bands with the purified material, suggesting that it contained antigenic components other than interferon, which were either of normal or induced cell derivation. This was confirmed by passive hemagglutination test (20) as shown in Table 2, in which sheep red cells coated with highly purified interferon, obtained by affinity chromatography, were tested for agglutination by anti-interferon and control sera as well as by antiserum from a rabbit injected with normal L cell extract. It can be seen that both anti-interferon and control sera agglutinated the antigen-coated red cells to a similar degree. Serum prepared against normal L cell extract, obviously devoid of neutralizing antibodies, also agglutinated the coated erythrocytes but to a far lesser extent. These data were interpreted to mean that the highly absorbed anti-interferon globulin used for affinity chromatography contained antibodies to normal host components which we had failed to recognize and consequently eliminate by immunoabsorption. Normal L cell extracts used for this purpose were apparently a poor source of these antigens, since immunization of rabbits with this material yielded but low antibody titers.

This observation prompted the following experiment in which "spent" media that had been in contact with induced and noninduced L cell cultures for varying periods of time were analyzed by hemagglutination inhibition (HAI) test (19) for the accumulation of L cell proteins during incubation. For this purpose a limiting dilution of a reference antiserum containing from 4 to 8 agglutinating units was first permitted to react with equal volumes of serial dilutions of the test material before addition of red cells coated with L cell proteins. The results presented in Table 3 show that in both types of cultures cellular proteins were gradually released into the culture medium. The accumulation of L cell product was possibly greater in the induced set of cultures which also liberated considerable amounts of interferon. The significance of this marginal difference is not clear and might reflect a generally increased rate of protein synthesis in induced as compared to unstimulated cells.

Additional absorptions of anti-interferon globulins were, therefore, indicated but this necessitated also an enrichment procedure whereby normally released L cell proteins could be obtained in amounts suitable for immunoabsorption. The method schematically depicted in Fig. 1 was selected for this purpose. Approximately 30 liters of "spent" L cell tissue culture medium were passaged in instalments through a 100 ml bed volume column of Sepharose-bound control serum which contained high titers of antibodies to liberated L cell proteins. At intervals, reflecting the saturation capacity of this affinity column, L cell and other contaminant proteins were eluted, and the regenerated column was reused on numerous occasions to adsorb additional quantities of L cell proteins. Pooled eluates, after dialysis against distilled water were lyophilized and bound in turn to CNBr-activated Sepharose 4B. Small quantities of preabsorbed anti-interferon serum, a few milliliter at a time, were then passed repeatedly through the "antigen cocktail" column, which was regenerated at intervals, to exhaust the anti-interferon serum of antibodies against the residual contaminants. This method was highly successful in reducing HAI titers to liberated L cell proteins by greater than 99.9%. The reabsorbed anti-interferon globulin excluded from the second column was then bound to CNBr-activated Sepharose to see whether improved purification of interferon could be obtained.

Figure 2 contrasts chromatographies carried out with partially absorbed anti-interferon globulin bound to Sepharose (right side) and the readsorbed immune globulin (left side). Void volumes and peak fractions were assayed by HAI test for presence of L cell antigens and the elution profiles of interferon and proteins were determined in each instance. In the case of the less completely absorbed antiserum (19) both interferon and a major portion of L cell proteins normally released in-

to the growth medium were bound to and eluted from the affinity
column. A small amount of the L cell contaminants (about 20% of
input), was collected in the void volume and represented excess
of those antigens over and above the capacity of the column. On
the other hand, chromatography of interferon on anti-interferon
globulin which had been subjected to the reabsorption procedure
described resulted in the collection of nearly 90% of the residual impurities in the exclusion volume whereas interferon was
eluted in the usual way and quantitatively recovered. Disappoint-
ingly, the reduction in elutable proteins was improved only a-
bout two-fold, not enough to result in a meaningful amelioration
of specific activity in the purified product. This could indicate that the low concentration range of interferon proteins and
impurities, and possibly a reduced biological stability of the
interferon under these conditions, all may have concurred in
affecting the reliability of assays employed. However, in spite
of the negligeable enhancement in specific activity, examination
of a concentrated preparation of this type in Ouchterlony tests
(180 µg protein per milliliter) with the antisera previously
mentioned disclosed that two of the immune bands recognized earlier had been eliminated. The remaining band, showing an identi-
ty reaction with anti-interferon and both control sera listed
in Table 2 was barely detectable and estimated to account at most
for 10% of the total protein content of this material. Interest-
ingly enough, the major portion of proteins in this preparation,
in spite of the more than adequate level of concentration available, failed to show visible precipitation with hyperimmune anti-interferon globulin.

These observations raise two important points with regard
to interferon purification. One, the absence of immune precipitation suggests that interferon may belong to those classes of
compounds which, due to small size or distribution pattern of

antigenic determinants, fail to show visible lattice formation.
The same restriction would, of course, also apply to any other
possible contaminant which has so far gone undetected. Second,
the expression of interferon purity solely in terms of units per
milligram of protein may be misleading and inadequately describe
the extent of purification achieved, unless the presence or absence of residual impurities is verified by sensitive serological
procedures. As the biological activity of interferon appears to
be more readily destroyed than its antigenic composition, structural studies of interferon proteins specified as described may
be closer at hand than currently anticipated. The present investigation stresses the fact that reliance on antigenic differences
between interferon and host proteins represents a new valuable
dimension in efforts to purify interferons and is worthy of further exploration. Preliminary studies with human interferons
have confirmed the general validity of this concept.

References

1. Friedman, R.M., Metz, D.H., Esteban, R.M., Tovell, D.
    R., Ball, L.A., and Kerr, I.M. (1972). J. Virol. 10,
    1184.

2. Gresser, I., Bandu, M., Tovey, M., Bodo, G., Paucker,
    K., and Stewart II, W.E. (1973). Proc. Soc. Exp. Biol.
    Med. 142, 7.

3. Stewart II, W.E., De Clercq, E., De Somer, P., Berg,
    K., Ogburn, C.A., and Paucker, K. (1973). Nature New
    Biol. 246, 141.

4. Chester, T.J., Paucker, K., and Merigan, T.C. (1973).
    Nature 246, 92.

5. Stancek, D., Golgher, R.R., and Paucker, K. (1970). J. Gen. Physiol. 56, 134s.

6. Yamazaki, S., and Wagner, R.R. (1970). J. Virology 5, 270.

7. Kawade, Y., Jap. J. Microbiol. 17, 129, 1973.

8. Ng, M.H., and Vilcek, J. (1972). In Advances in Protein Chemistry, Ed. by C.B. Anfinsen, J.T. Edsall and F.M. Richard, Vol. 26, p. 173, Academic Press, New York.

9. Fantes, K.H. (1973). In Interferons and Interferon Inducers, Ed. by N.B. Finter, 2nd edition, Vol. 2, 171, North Holland Publishing Company, Amsterdam.

10. Nagano, Y., and Kojima, Y. (1960). C.R. Séances Soc. Biol. Filiales 154, 2172.

11. Paucker, K., and Cantell, K. (1962). Virology 18, 145.

12. Paucker, K. (1965). J. Immunol. 94, 371.

13. Levy-Koenig, R.E., Golgher, R.R., and Paucker, K.(1970). J. Immunol. 104, 791.

14. Sipe, J.D., DeMaeyer-Guignard, J., Fauconnier, B., and DeMaeyer, E. (1973). Proc. Natl. Acad. Sci. 70, 1037.

15. Molenaar, J.L., Müller, M., and Pondman, K.W. (1973). J. Immunol. 110, 1570.

16. Cheng, W.C., and Talmadge, D.W. (1969). J. Immunol. 103, 1385.

17. Cuatrecasas, P., and Anfinsen, C.B. (1971). In Methods in Enzymology, Ed. by W.B. Jacoby, Vol. 22, p. 345, Academic Press, New York.

18. Pharmacia Publication Maj 1972-1, Appelbergs tryckeri, Sweden.

19. Ogburn, C.A., Berg, K., and Paucker, K. (1973). J. Immunol. 111, 1206.

20. Boyden, S.V. (1951). J. Exptl. Med. 93, 107.

TABLE 1

Development of antibodies in a rabbit
immunized with crude NDVuv-induced L cell interferon

Immunizations		Antibody titer per ml against[b]				
Month	No. of injections[a]	IF	L	NDV	AF	CS
0	0	8	8	8	8	8
1	2	8	2,000	64,000	4,000	64,000
4	3	200	16,000	128,000	4,000	64,000
6	4	2,000	8,000	128,000	4,000	64,000
9	6	16,000	16,000	256,000	4,000	128,000
11	7	32,000	8,000	256,000	4,000	128,000

a 1x10^7 reference units per dose in Freund's adjuvant(complete).

b Determined 2 weeks after the most recent injection. Abbreviations denote: Interferon (IF), normal L cell extract (L), Newcastle disease virus (NDV), allantoic fluid (AF) and calf serum (CS). Titers measured by neutralization (IF) or passive hemagglutination (others).

TABLE 2

Hemagglutination test with selected antisera
and red cells coated with L cell interferon
prepared by affinity chromatography

| Antiserum against | Antibody titer per ml[c] measured by | |
	Interferon Neutralization	Red cell Agglutination
Interferon[a]	8,000	64,000
Interferon (control)[b]	8	128,000
Normal L cell extract	<8	512

[a]Absorbed to remove antibodies to all identified impurities.
[b]Rabbit immunized with interferon which failed to develop
neutralizing antibodies.
[c]Reciprocal of endpoint dilution.

TABLE 3

Accumulation of normal L cell product in media of
NDVuv-induced and noninduced cultures

| Hours of incubation | Activities in units per milliliter[a] | | | |
| | Induced cells | | Noninduced cells | |
	Interferon	L protein	Interferon	L protein
0	<10	<2	<10	<2
2	<10	4	<10	2
4	20	8	<10	4
6	400	16	<10	4
22	>32000	64	<10	32

[a]Determined by CPE inhibition of VSV for interferon, and by passive hemagglutination inhibition (HAI) test for liberated L
cell proteins.

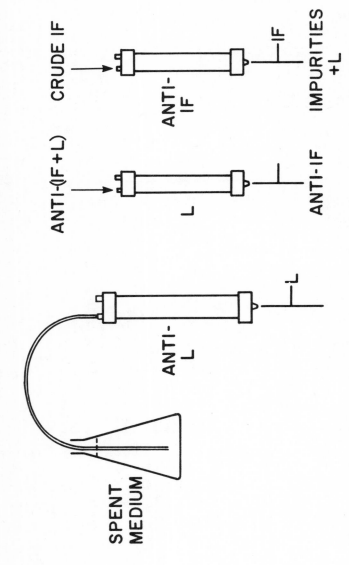

Fig. 1. Schematic representation of affinity chromatography steps used to remove antibodies to liberate L cell proteins from anti-interferon serum. Vertical and horizontal bars at outflow of columns indicate excluded and eluted products, respectively. For explanation see text.

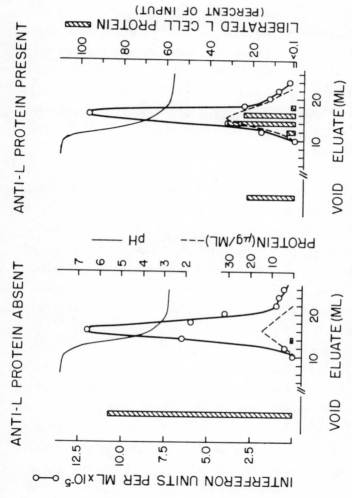

Fig. 2. Affinity chromatography of NDVuv-induced L cell interferon on Sepharose-bound anti-interferon globulin before and after removal of antibodies to liberated normal L cell proteins. Technical details were described elsewhere (19).

DISCUSSION

Pereira: This paper illustrates in a beautiful way the
difficulties involved in getting a really pure protein of any
kind, especially when your starting material is not plentiful.
It is a little bit like: which comes first, the chicken or the
egg? You have to have one element pure if you are going to use
immunological methods for purification and I can foresee hopefully the point when you will have enough of your really pure
interferon to make a column with which to prepare pure interferon antibody and then carry on from there until the thing snow-
balls and soon we'll have lots of very pure interferon. I con-
gratulate you on these beautiful results.

Chany: You were very pessimistic about the use of anti -
bodies against impurities and I think it is perfectly right. But
I wonder if this could not be used as a complementary step for
purification? I have tried this type of approach some years ago
with Dr. Avrameas when activated Sepharose was not available.
We used polymers of antibodies and found that both interferon
and impurities were adsorbed. Did you ever try this approach as
a complementary step?

Paucker: Yes, we tried. We have worked with double column
procedures but unfortunately, I think, that as you purify your
interferon, any additional steps such as re-dialysis or concentration, reduce the recovery. I have not emphasized that recovery in this procedure is quantitative. In other words, you get
slightly more out than you put in, and this, of course, is the
main virtue of the technique. We prefer to have a single step
procedure. The reason for not using antibodies to impurities is
really that, first of all, they are so plentiful that you would

have to have a gigantic column in order to really bind all of
the contaminants present. Furthermore, you cannot reuse or regen-
erate effectively a column made with antibodies against impurities because not all antigen-antibody systems dissociate under
the same elution conditions. The restoration of such a column
is thus limited, whereas an anti-interferon column which is
clean or fairly clean can be used indefinitely. We have used
ours more than fifty times until it was wiped out by contamination due to break down of the central airconditioning system,
but its use is really unlimited and its capacity fully retained.
It is for this reason that we like our approach better.

Pereira: That is why I was saying that one has grounds to
be hopeful. The beauty of it is the fact that you can reuse
these columns so many times.

Tovey: Is your highly purified material obtained from
your affinity columns, stable in terms of biological activity?

Paucker: It is stable; well, I think that it will be stable if you have enough of it. The work of Dr. Kawade, who unfortunately could not be here, pointed out that if you have enough
interferon protein, in your preparation it would be stable. So
far we have not reached this condition, but we have also not
been able to completely inactivate this material. Without the
addition of bovine plasma albumin, we lose approximately from
80% to 90% of the activity but the remainder, for some reason or
other, is perfectly stable. So, for our biological studies we
still have to add bovine plasma albumin until such time as the
capacity of our column is increased to the point where we don't
need this anymore. Unfortunately, we have not yet been able to
devise a test for the detection of interferon-specific protein

without testing for its biological activity. We are working on
that but it just is not quite ready yet.

Ankel: I think rabbit interferon shows several bands upon
electrofocusing due to different amounts of sialic acid. I was
just wondering, does mouse interferon behave in the same fashion
if you treat it with neuraminidase?

Paucker: We have treated mouse interferon (this is unrelated to the present study), but we have treated purified mouse
interferon preparations with neuraminidase and then subjected
them to polyacrilamide gel electrophoresis. The effect was very
similar to that described for rabbit interferon by Schone, I believe, some years ago, in that there was a homogenizing effect
and out of a broad distribution of activities we now obtained
one single peak.

Ankel: May I ask another question? In most glycoproteins
sialic acid is bound to galactose. In the case of rabbit interferon it was possible to label the terminal galactose with tri-
tium. Have you tried that?

Paucker: No, we haven't tried it, but preliminary amino
acid analyses of mouse interferons purified by immune affinity
chromatography suggest that earlier results from this laboratory describing the incorporation of other labelled precursors into less extensively purified interferons may have to be re-eval-
uated. Therefore we prefer to wait with new studies of this type until the purity of our material has been better established.

Stewart: One of the objectives of purifying interferon
is to show that the activities we are observing are in one unit

one effector. I have taken interferons from various sources to
determine the ratio of antiviral and non-antiviral activities,
with increasing specific activities. We have interferons from
various sources with various specific activities and plotting
the antiviral activity against the particular non-antiviral activity, with a range of specific activity of approximately 10^2
up to now approximately 10^8 the ratio remains constant through
this purification regardless of the source of the interferon. I
have what I call a trace challenge and full challenge and with
the poly I:C toxicity it takes more interferon to enhance the
susceptibility of the cells to 2 micrograms than to 10; here a-
gain the ratios stay parallel. I've also determined the ratios
of priming activities to the antiviral activity of these preparations, again with specific activities of approximately 10^2 to
10^8 with intermediates, and the ratios again stay constant with
both full priming dose and trace priming. Full priming is the
amount that gives the maximum yields of interferon with the induction (the inducer here is poly I:C which doesn't induce in
mouse L cells normally) and the trace priming is just the unit
of interferon that, in terms of antiviral activity, gives just
detectable interferon in the system.

Tan: Referring to an earlier quetion of Dr. Ankel, Drs.
Hans Wieldili and Lengyel have shown that highly purified preparations are homogeneous on isoelectric focusing after treatment with neuraminidase.

Friedman: With your purified preparations, have you found
any evidence for Carter-like polymeric forms of interferon?

Paucker: We have not tested for that but this type of
work is now in progress. So, I cannot comment on it yet.

AFFINITY OF MURINE INTERFERON FOR CONCANAVALIN A

F. Besançon and M. F. Bourgeade

Institut National de la Santé et
de la Recherche Médicale
Unité 43 de Recherche sur les Virus
Hôpital St. Vincent de Paul
74, avenue Denfert-Rochereau
75014 Paris, France

The hypothesis of the presence of polysaccharide components in the interferon molecule is supported i) by its sensitivity to periodate and ii) by the modification of its molecular weight and electrical charge following treatment by neuraminidase (1).

In addition, the affinity of many glycoproteins for lectins (such as Concanavalin A) is well documented (2). In all of the here presented experiments, Concanavalin A, covalently fixed to Sepharose 4B beads, was used to test the affinity of murine interferon for this lectin.

Murine interferon was prepared using LM cells induced by the Hertfordshire strain of Newcastle disease virus (NDV), irradiated with UV (5000 erg/mm^2). Interferon was separated from the virus and assayed, using routine techniques.

In order to saturate residual free binding groups which might persist on activated Sepharose-Con A beads, they (10^7 beads) were first treated with ethanolamine 1M pH 8 overnight at 4°C and washed with the following buffer: NaCl 1 M, CH_3 COONa 10^{-1} M pH 6, $MgCl_2$ 10^{-3} M, $CaCl_2$ 10^{-3} M, Mn SO_4 10^{-3} M. The beads were then centrifuged at 1000 rpm and 4 ml of murine interferon

(50000 ref. units/ml) were added. The mixture was incubated for 2 1/2 h at 20°C.

In parallel sets of experiments, the Sepharose-Con A was incubated with the following sugars: D-glucose (0.2 M), D-galactose (0.2 M), or α methyl-D-mannoside (0.2 M). Each of these sugars were present during the binding period of interferon to Sepharose-Con A. After coupling, the preparation was washed 6 times with 30 ml of buffer to eliminate unbound interferon. L cells were incubated for 24 h at 37°C with 1 bead/50 cells of each of the different sets. The cells were then challenged with vesicular stomatitis virus (VSV) at the m.o.i. = 0.1 pfu/cell for 16 h. The viral yield was assayed by routine plaque tech - niques.

The results are presented in Table 1. The Sepharose-Con A treated with murine interferon alone, or with interferon and galactose or glucose, was able to induce the antiviral state to the same extent. However, this activity disappeared when the beads were treated simultaneously with α methyl-D-mannoside and interferon. This sugar has a very strong affinity for Concanavalin A (3). Thus, these results suggest a competition between interferon and α methyl-D-mannoside for sugar receptor sites on Concanavalin A.

In spite of the fact that α methyl-D-mannoside prevents the fixation of interferon on Concanavalin A, the addition of this sugar to the interferon-Con A complex, after coupling, did not displace (in our experimental conditions) the interferon already complexed. However, the Sepharose-Con A-interferon beads, in contact with sensitive cells, release detectable amounts of interferon in the tissue culture medium (Table 2) and were able to protect cells located at distance from the beads.

Discussion

The binding of murine interferon to Concanavalin A is inhibited by α methyl-D-mannoside. However, when D-galactose and D-glucose are used, no such activity can be observed. The affinity of interferon for Concanavalin A and its inhibition by α methyl-D-mannoside are in favor of the glycoproteinic structure of this molecule. Our results agree with a recent report by Dorner, Scriba and Weil, who demonstrated the affinity of rabbit interferon for another lectin: phytohemagglutinin (4). This agglutinin has a strong affinity for galactose. In their experiments, interferon could also not be displaced by this sugar. Nevertheless, the addition of glycopeptides from human erythrocytes released almost all of the interferon molecules bound. We can postulate, therefore, that in our experiments, the binding of Concanavalin A with the cell membrane might induce changes in the interferon-Con A complex, resulting in the release of interferon.

The role of these polysaccharide components on the biological activity of interferons has not yet been elucidated.

References

1. Schonne, E., Billiau, A., and De Somer, P. (1970). Symp. Ser. Immunobiol. Stand, 14, 61.

2. Allan, D., Auger, J., and Crumpton, M.J. (1972). Nature New Biol. 236, 23.

3. Goldstein, I.J., Hollerman, C.E., and Smith, E.E. (1965). Biochem. 4, 876.

4. Dorner, F., Scriba, M., and Weil, R. (1973). Proc. Nat. Acad. Sci. 70, 1981.

TABLE 1

	Control	D-mannoside	D-glucose	D-galactose
Control Sepharose-Con A	3×10^6	2.1×10^6	7×10^6	5.6×10^6
Interferon-treated Sepharose-Con A	8×10^3	2.6×10^6	6.8×10^4	2×10^4

Effect of different sugars on the fixation of interferon on Sepharose-Con A beads: virus yield of VSV-infected cells after treatment by beads (pfu/ml).

TABLE 2

	Exp. 1	Exp. 2	Exp. 3
(1) Supernatant of cells treated with Sepharose-Con A	7×10^5	3×10^6	4×10^5
(2) Supernatant of cells treated with interferon Sepharose-Con A	4.7×10^3	10^4	1.2×10^4

Virus yield (pfu/ml) of L cells infected by VSV after a 16 h incubation period in the presence of:
1) the supernatant of L cells treated with control Sepharose-Con A;
2) the supernatant of L cells treated with interferon-bound Sepharose-Con A.

DISCUSSION

Kerr: Are there any questions for any of the speakers before we finish?

There is one thing I would like to do because I don't think there will be any other opportunity to do it. I'm sure you would like to join me in thanking Charles Chany for all the work he has put into this. Certainly as one of the Chairmen who was supposed to help in organizing, I found my load extremely light, which really meant that someone else was doing all the work, and I know who that someone else was. So will you join me in thanking him now?

Chany: I want to thank you all first for having accepted to come, and secondly for having contributed in such a very interesting manner to the success of the meeting. I also wish to express my gratitude to the Gulbenkian Foundation and to Dr. Artur Geraldes, whose efficient organization made this meeting such a great success.